Second Edition

Appleton & Lange's Review of RESPIRATORY CARE

Second Edition

Appleton & Lange's Review of RESPIRATORY CARE

Crystal L. Dunlevy, EdD, RRT
Assistant Professor
Director of Clinical Education
Respiratory Therapy Program
The Ohio State University
Columbus, Ohio

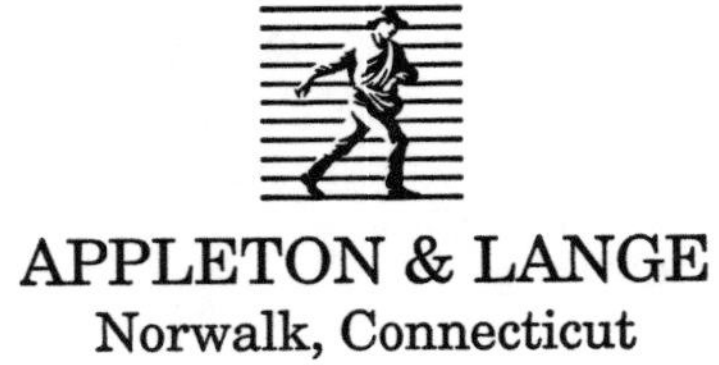

APPLETON & LANGE
Norwalk, Connecticut

Notice: The author and the publisher of this volume have taken care to make certain that the doses of drugs and schedules of treatment are correct and compatible with the standards generally accepted at the time of publication. Nevertheless, as new information becomes available, changes in treatment and in the use of drugs become necessary. The reader is advised to carefully consult the instruction and information material included in the package insert of each drug or therapeutic agent before administration. This advice is especially important when using new or infrequently used drugs. The publisher disclaims any liability, loss, injury, or damage incurred as a consequence, directly or indirectly, or the use and application of any of the contents of the volume.

95 96 97 98 99 / 10 9 8 7 6 5 4 3 2 1

Prentice Hall International (UK) Limited, *London*
Prentice Hall of Australia Pty. Limited, *Sydney*
Prentice Hall Canada, Inc., *Toronto*
Prentice Hall Hispanoamericana, S.A., *Mexico*
Prentice Hall of India Private Limited, *New Delhi*
Prentice Hall of Japan, Inc., *Tokyo*
Simon & Schuster Asia Pte. Ltd., *Singapore*
Editora Prentice Hall do Brasil Ltda., *Rio de Janeiro*
Prentice Hall, *Englewood Cliffs, New Jersey*

Library of Congress Cataloging-in-Publication Data

Dunlevy, Crystal L.
Appleton & Lange's review of respiratory care. — 2nd ed. / Crystal L. Dunlevy.
p. cm.
Rev. ed. of: Respiratory care : national board review / C.A. Brainard, with the assistance of Michael J. Wirth and contributions by Arnie L. Kosmatka. Bowie, MD : Brady, c1985.
Includes bibliographical references.
ISBN 0-8385-8414-4
1. Respiratory therapy—Problems, exercises, etc. 2. Respiratory therapy—Examination, questions, etc. I. Brainard, C. A., 1947- Respiratory care. II. Title. III. Title: Review of respiratory care.
[DNLM: 1. Respiratory therapy—examination questions. Review of respiratory care.]
RC735.I5B73 1995
615.8′36′076—dc20
DNLM/DLC
for Library of Congress 94-23439
CIP

ISBN 0-8385-4149-4

Acquisitions Editor: J. Alex Schwartz
Production Editor: Jennifer Sinsavich

PRINTED IN THE UNITED STATES OF AMERICA

to Bill and Cole and Blair

and to all of my students,
past and present,
who inspire, entertain, and enlighten me

Contents

Preface

The revision of this review text after ten years proved to be a major undertaking. The respiratory care profession has changed greatly in the past ten years, and with it the credentialling examinations offered by the National Board for Respiratory Care (NBRC) have changed. Respiratory therapists enjoy expanded roles in home care and rehabilitation. They are expected to be familiar with a much broader variety of ventilator modes and management techniques, and to exhibit greater sophistication in the areas of hemodynamic monitoring and patient assessment. All of these changes are reflected in the most recent NBRC job analysis, examination matrices (released in 1993), and in this text.

The format of the text remains unchanged from the first edition—there is a review of pertinent calculations, situational sets, review of hemodynamics, review of examination content (all with pretests), and practice posttest examinations. All pretest questions are referenced to respiratory care texts likely to be available to the exam candidate and are accompanied by explanations. Posttest examination answers are categorized by NBRC examination content area. Each section is identified as applicable either to the entry level exam candidate, advanced practitioner exam candidate, or both. Because students already have a reference library in their academic texts, minimal text appears in this book. Candidates preparing for the NBRC examinations will find this text useful because it includes a review of *both* the CRTT and RRT examinations.

The intent of this review book is to help the graduate pass the NBRC examination(s) by providing NBRC-type practice questions that will jog the memory, stimulate the search for more information, and provide the direction to do so.

Acknowledgments

Thanks to my editor, J. Alex Schwartz, for his guidance, always provided constructively and with a sense of humor, throughout this endeavor. Thanks to my best friends (who also happen to be my family) Bill, Cole, and Blair, who offered love, support, and coffee while I completed this manuscript. Thanks to my colleagues, Herb and Tim, for expanding my reference library; and to Kathy and Kay, who cheered me on and listened to much whining. Thanks to my students, who make my job fun, and who I feel fortunate to consider my friends.

Introduction

A. How to Use This Book

An alarmingly large number of candidates for the National Board for Respiratory Care® (NBRC®) examinations fail to pass by a frustrating few percentage points. These individuals probably had the necessary background to pass, but something just didn't "click" on examination day. This situation is best avoided with the proverbial ounce of prevention. This book is no panacea, but it can provide the following two useful functions: (1) to jog your memory and (2) to teach you how to take the NBRC Examination.

When was the last time you used the Fick equation? How long has it been since you calculated V_D/V_T or FEF_{25-75}? All of us could use a good jog in the memory department from time to time. Turn to the Mathematics Review and Pretest and look up some of your least favorite equations. If that doesn't jog your memory, try the case histories in the Hemodynamics Review and Pretest. If that doesn't work, you need more help than this text can give you!

When taking a test, some people answer the question at hand and then, like efficient little test-taking machines, move confidently to the next question and so on, until they have finished the test. Others find themselves getting bogged down right from the start. Awash in a sea of confusion, they waste their time trying to figure out what the question is asking, rather than trying to determine the correct answer. They cannot get beyond the technical details to see how the problem at hand relates to actual patient care. How does one learn not to get hung up on the mechanics of the NBRC Examination? Well, usually a little extra practice is all that it takes to fine-tune those test-taking instincts. With over 1100 NBRC type questions, this book should provide ample opportunity for that.

Text Structure

This text is divided into a Pretest and Review Section and a Posttest and Mastery Section. Section I contains four pretest and review units. Unit I is a complete review of the mathematics of respiratory care. From tank factors to sophisticated hemodynamic calculations, 34 separate mathematics pretest modules are presented along with a brief discussion of clinical significance. Unit II contains 22 situational sets of the type found on the Entry Level Examination. Unit III is a review of hemodynamics for the advanced practitioner candidate. An increasing number of questions on this examination require an understanding of such concepts as the pulmonary wedge pressure and pulmonary vascular resistance. Unit IV contains 50 separate pretests, one for each NBRC Entry Level and Advanced Practitioner Examination category. For the really serious candidate, this unit represents the heart of the book. The questions are designed to assess each of the specific competencies listed in the NBRC Composite Examination Matrix.

Section II contains one full-length Entry Level Examination (Unit I) and one full-length Advanced Practitioner Examination (Unit II). These posttests are constructed according to specifications outlined in the NBRC Composite Examination Matrix. Posttests, especially when taking under examination-like conditions, are a reliable way of assessing a candidate's mastery and overall preparedness for the NBRC Examination.

Important

Before you begin to review the pretest sections, please examine the remainder of this introductory section carefully. It contains valuable information regarding examination content, type of question, and number of questions in each category. Some of the information can also be found in your NBRC Candidate Handbook (which you should also read carefully). Much of it, such as the description of each individual examination category, can only be found there and will allow you to use this text much more efficiently.

B. Examination Content

Approximately every five years, the NBRC performs a job analysis in order to create a national "job description" for the Respiratory Care Practitioner. This job analysis is conducted for both entry level and advanced level practitioners. The most recent job analysis was conducted in 1992, and the NBRC examination matrix was revised in order to reflect that data. The revised content outlines were approved by the Board of Trustees and were implemented for the July 1994 Entry Level CRTT Examination and the December 1994 Written Registry Examination.

The goal of NBRC examinations is to determine whether the candidate possesses cognitive skills necessary to practice respiratory therapy at the entry level (CRTT) or the advanced level (RRT). Candidates are tested on their ability to recall, apply, and analyze information. The content outlines contain hundreds of competencies for which the candidate is responsible.

To use your time most efficiently, you must first know which topics are going to be assessed on a given examination. For instance, if a candidate spent a considerable amount of time studying chest physical assessment while preparing for the Advanced Practitioner Examination, valuable time would be wasted because this is assessed *primarily* on the Entry Level Examination. *This is not to say that the advanced practitioner candidate should not have a thorough understanding of the principles of chest physical assessment or any of the topics emphasized in the Entry Level Examination.* For example, the advanced practitioner's decision to recommend chest tube placement for a patient with a tension pneumothorax could not possibly be made without the ability to assess chest physical data. In examining the Entry Level and Advanced Practitioner Examination category descriptions on the next few pages, you will note that many topics are assessed on one examination only. This should not prove confusing if you remember the following statement:

> The entry level candidate need concern himself or herself only with the topics described in the Entry Level Examination category section. Advanced practitioner candidates should concern themselves with Advanced Practitioner examination category topics in particular but must also be able to demonstrate a general understanding of basic concepts.

The latter should not prove difficult because these individuals are already Certified Respiratory Therapy Technicians.

It is extremely important that you determine what is on the examination before you begin studying. To do this, please read the next pages carefully, since they present a detailed account of the content of each examination. Should you have further questions regarding an examination category, please refer to the pretest module for that particular content area as presented in Unit IV of Section I.

C. Entry Level Examination Matrix

The following is the Entry Level Examination matrix. It lists the number of items assessed on each performance level. These represent the hierarchy of cognitive (intellectual) skills in order of complexity.

TABLE I. ENTRY LEVEL EXAMINATION CONTENT OUTLINE MATRIX

Content Area	Complexity Level			
	Recall	*Application*	*Analysis*	*Number of Items*
I. Clinical Information				35
A. Examine patient records; suggest additional procedures	2	4	0	6
B. Collect and assess clinical information	3	7	2	12
C. Perform and evaluate therapeutic procedures	3	7	2	12
D. Evaluate the respiratory care plan	1	1	3	5
II. Equipment				35
A. Select appropriate equipment and assure cleanliness	5	7	0	12
B. Assemble, check, and troubleshoot	9	14	0	23
III. Therapy				70
A. Perform patient education; communicate verbally and in writing; maintain sterility	2	5	1	8
B. Maintain patent airway	3	5	0	8
C. Ensure ventilation	2	6	2	10
D. Ensure oxygenation	3	5	0	8
E. Evaluate patient response	2	6	2	10
F. Recommend alternative therapy based on patient's response	4	4	13	21
G. Perform emergency cardiopulmonary resuscitation	1	3	1	5
Totals	40	74	26	140

1. *Recall.* These questions test the ability to recall or recognize specific information. For example, a question may ask that the candidate recognize the average length of the adult trachea.
2. *Application.* These questions ask that the candidate be able to relate knowledge or facts to a new or changing situation. For example, if the candidate is informed that a 70-kg patient has a minute alveolar ventilation of 2.5 L/min, it could safely be assumed that the patient is hypoventilating.
3. *Analysis.* This is the most complex of the performance levels, built on the foundation of the first two. These questions ask that complex information be analyzed in order to arrive at a solution. For example, the candidate may be asked to evaluate a patient's aerosol therapy and make recommendations to modify that therapy based on the patient's response.

D. Entry Level Examination Categories

The preceding examination matrix lists 13 content areas. The following is a brief description of each of these. These descriptions are designed to provide an overview to help map out a study plan. For a more detailed explanation, please refer to the Table of Contents and look up the specific examination category in Unit IV of Section I.

I. Clinical Information
   A. Examine patient records; suggest diagnostic procedures. Questions in this category assess the candidate's ability to interpret existing data from progress notes, patient history and physical, respiratory therapy orders, pulmonary function tests, blood gases, chest x-rays, and respiratory and cardiovascular monitoring. The candidate must also be able to recommend procedures and/or tests that will provide additional data about the patient's cardiopulmonary status.
   B. Collect and assess clinical information. Questions in this category assess the candidate's ability to assess a patient's overall cardiopulmonary status through inspection, palpation, auscultation, and interview. Candidates are also tested on their ability to recognize proper endotracheal or tracheostomy tube placement on a chest x-ray.
   C. Perform and evaluate procedures. This category of questions requires the candidate to interpret the results of procedures performed at the bedside, such as pulse oximetry, tidal volume, minute volume, I:E, maximum inspiratory pressure (MIP), peak flow, timed forced expiratory volumes, tracheal tube cuff pressure, lung mechanics, alveolar ventilation, blood gas analysis, and maximum expiratory pressure. Candidates are also expected to be able to interpret co-oximetry results, and spirometry pre and post bronchodilator.
   D. Evaluate the respiratory care plan. These questions assess the candidate's ability to determine whether or not the prescribed respiratory care plan is appropriate, recommend modifications (if appropriate), and be involved with the development of the respiratory care plan.

II. Equipment
   In the clinical setting, the respiratory therapy practitioner must select, assemble, check proper function, and troubleshoot for various types of respiratory therapy equipment.
   A. Select appropriate equipment and assure cleanliness.
      1. Medical gas storage, delivery, metering, and analyzing devices
         a. Medical gas cylinders
         b. Regulators and reducing valves
         c. Flowmeters
         d. Oxygen and blood gas analyzers
         e. Air compressors
         f. Air/oxygen blenders
         g. Pulse oximeters
      2. Oxygen administration devices
         a. Low-flow delivery systems (cannula, simple mask, face tent, partial rebreather)
         b. High-flow delivery systems (all air entrainment devices, nonrebreathers)
         c. Oxygen hoods and tents
      3. Humidity and aerosol therapy devices
         a. Bubble, passover, cascade, wick, and condensing humidifiers
         b. Pneumatic and electric aerosol generators, and aerosol mist tents
      4. Airway care and resuscitation devices
         a. Bag-valve resuscitators
         b. Mouth-to-valve mask resuscitators
      5. Positive pressure (IPPB, CPAP, PEEP valve) and incentive breathing devices
      6. Continuous mechanical ventilators (pneumatic, electric, and microprocessor ventilators)
      7. Artificial airways (pharyngeal, endotracheal, tracheostomy, and intubation equipment)
      8. Suctioning equipment (catheters, collection traps, hypopharyngeal suctioning devices)
      9. Gauges and manometers
      10. Percussors/vibrators (electric, pneumatic)
      11. Metered dose inhalers and spacing devices

      Also included in this Equipment category are questions assessing the candidate's ability to ensure cleanliness and/or sterilization of all equipment.

B. Assemble, check, and troubleshoot. Questions here evaluate the candidate's ability to put together, check for proper function, and, if necessary, troubleshoot, the equipment listed under section A above.

III. Therapy

A. Perform patient education; communicate verbally and in writing; and maintain sterility. Questions in this category assess the candidate's ability to explain respiratory therapy clinical goals in simple and understandable terms so that the patient may benefit optimally from his or her therapy. Candidates should also be able to demonstrate competence in both verbal and written communication. Candidates must understand and be able to perform infection control procedures.

B. Maintain patent airway. Questions in this category assess the candidate's ability to:
1. Appropriately use humidity and aerosol therapy
2. Insert pharyngeal airways (both oral and nasal)
3. Maintain proper cuff inflation and position
4. Instruct patients on proper cough techniques
5. Use chest physical therapy
6. Perform suctioning techniques
7. Administer aerosolized medication

C. Ensure ventilation. Questions in this category assess the candidate's ability to:
1. Use intermittent positive pressure breathing (IPPB) therapy
2. Use deep breathing and incentive spirometry therapy
3. Administer medication
4. Place a patient on a ventilator, selecting appropriate settings

D. Ensure oxygenation. Questions in this category assess the candidate's ability to:
1. Administer oxygen therapy
2. Administer positive end-expiratory pressure (PEEP) and continuous positive airway pressure (CPAP) therapy to prevent hypoxia
3. Prevent hypoxemia that may be caused by performing certain procedures (suctioning)

E. Evaluate patient response. Questions in this category are designed to test the candidate's ability to:
1. Note hazardous and adverse reactions to all forms of therapy
2. Monitor effectively all parameters necessary to evaluate a patient's cardiopulmonary status on a *basic* level (vital signs, pulse oximetry, chest auscultation, subjective response to therapy, etc.)

F. Recommend alternative therapy based on the patient's response. Questions in this category are designed to assess the candidate's ability to:
1. Terminate therapy based on patient's adverse response
2. Modify effectively all respiratory therapy modalities based on the patient's response

G. Perform emergency cardiopulmonary resuscitation. Questions in this category are designed to assess the candidate's ability to initiate, modify, or conduct basic cardiopulmonary resuscitation (CPR) techniques in an emergency setting.

E. Advanced Practitioner Examination Matrix

The following is the Advanced Practitioner Examination matrix. It lists the number of items assessed on each performance level. These represent the hierarchy of cognitive (intellectual) skills in order of complexity.

1. *Recall.* These questions test the ability to recall or recognize specific information. For example, a question may ask that the candidate recognize normal values for the physiologic shunt fraction ($\dot{Q}_S/\dot{Q}_T$) for various types of patients.
2. *Application.* These questions ask that the candidate be able to relate knowledge or facts to a new or changing situation. For example, the candidate may be informed that a patient whose oxygen consumption is normal, has a $C(a\text{-}\bar{v})O_2$ of 7.5 vol%. Given this information, the candidate should recognize that the cardiac output is reduced.
3. *Analysis.* This is the most complex of the performance levels, built on the foundation of the first two. These questions ask that complex information be analyzed in order to arrive at a solution. For example, the candidate may be asked to evaluate a patient's cardiopulmonary status and make recommendations regarding that patient's respiratory care plan.

F. Advanced Practitioner Examination Categories

The preceding examination matrix lists 10 content areas. The following is a brief description of each of these. These descriptions are designed to provide a general overview to help you map out a study plan. For a more detailed explanation, please refer to the Table of Contents and look up the specific examination categories in Unit IV.

I. Clinical Information

A. Examine patient records; suggest additional procedures. Questions in this category assess the candidate's ability to review and interpret existing clinical data, collect and/or

TABLE II. ADVANCED PRACTITIONER EXAMINATION CONTENT OUTLINE MATRIX

Content Area	Complexity Level			
	Recall	***Application***	***Analysis***	***Number of Items***
I. Clinical Information				***20***
A. Examine patient records; suggest additional procedures	2	2	2	6
B. Collect and assess clinical information	1	2	4	7
C. Perform and evaluate diagnostic procedures, and facilitate development of the respiratory care plan	1	2	4	7
II. Equipment				***20***
A. Choose appropriate equipment and assure cleanliness	2	3	0	5
B. Assemble, check, troubleshoot, and perform quality control	3	3	9	15
III. Therapy				***60***
A. Assess, observe, and record patient response	2	3	8	13
B. Maintain a patent airway, assuring ventilation and tissue oxygenation	1	3	1	5
C. Recommend alternative therapy based on patient response	6	6	18	30
D. Perform respiratory therapy procedures in emergency situations	2	4	1	7
E. Provide assistance to physicians and administer pulmonary rehabilitation/home care	1	3	1	5
Totals	21	31	48	100

recommend the collection of additional data, and recommend modifications to the patient's therapy based on that data. Many of the questions in this section are of the analysis type. This category tests the candidate's knowledge about the following:

1. Laboratory results, including electrolytes, CBC, hemoglobin and hematocrit, fluid balance (intake and output)
2. Results of cardiovascular monitoring, including cardiac output, pulmonary capillary wedge pressure, pulmonary artery pressures, central venous pressures, ECG mixed venous oxygen levels, $C(a\text{-}\bar{v})O_2$
3. Results of respiratory monitoring, including dead space to tidal volume ratio (V_D/V_T), shunt studies ($\dot{Q}_S/\dot{Q}_T$), capnography, inspiratory and expiratory flow, volume, and pressure waveforms, and transcutaneous O_2/CO_2
4. Culture, sensitivity, and/or Gram's stain results from sputum, blood, or other body fluids (pleural fluid, urine, etc.)
5. Results of upper airway x-rays
6. Perinatal/neonatal data, including maternal and perinatal history, APGAR scores, gestational age, L/S ratio and/or other studies to determine lung maturity
7. Results of sleep studies and ventilation/perfusion scans
8. Pulmonary stress testing results

Candidates are also tested on their ability to recommend the following procedures to obtain additional data:

1. Laboratory tests, including electrolytes, CBC, sputum culture and sensitivity, and blood gases
2. Chest and upper airway x-rays
3. Pulmonary function tests, including maximum voluntary ventilation (MVV), flow-volume loops, pre and post bronchodilator spirometry, diffusing capacity, nitrogen washout distribution, FRC, total lung capacity (TLC)
4. Insertion of arterial, umbilical, and/or central venous pressure monitoring lines

B. Collect and assess clinical information. Questions in this category are designed to assess the candidate's ability to determine a patient's cardiopulmonary status using physical examination techniques—inspection, palpation, auscultation, as well as through patient interviews. Candidates are also tested on their ability to examine and interpret chest and lateral neck x-rays. Last, candidates are expected to be able to perform and understand the following bedside techniques:

1. Transcutaneous O_2/CO_2 monitoring, pulse oximetry
2. V_D/V_T
3. Cardiac output, pulmonary capillary wedge pressure, pulmonary artery pressures, central venous pressures
4. Shunt studies
5. Capnography
6. Sampling of mixed venous blood
7. Lung compliance, ventilatory parameters (tidal volume, minute volume, etc.), I:E

8. Calculation of $P(A\text{-}a)O_2$
9. ECG
10. Apnea monitoring, sleep studies

C. Perform and evaluate diagnostic procedures, and facilitate development of the respiratory care plan. Questions in this category are designed to assess the candidate's ability to perform and evaluate hemodynamic data, sleep studies, and the results of pulmonary laboratory tests on an *advanced* level. Candidates are expected to utilize this information to make judgments about the patient's physiologic status and to contribute to the development of an appropriate respiratory care plan.

II. Equipment

In the clinical setting, the advanced respiratory therapy practitioner must select, assemble, check proper function, and troubleshoot for a variety of respiratory therapy apparatus.

A. Choose appropriate equipment and assure cleanliness (monitor sterilization procedures) of the following:
1. Ventilators (including pneumatic, electric, fluidic, high frequency, BiPAP, transport, and home care types)
2. Artificial airways
3. Resuscitation apparatus (demand-valve)
4. Patient breathing circuits
5. Gauges and manometers
6. Fiberoptic bronchoscopes
7. Analyzing, gas delivery, and measuring devices (transcutaneous O_2, CO_2, co-oximeter, canograph, oxygen concentrators, liquid oxygen portable systems)
8. Positive expiratory pressure (PEP) masks
9. Helium/oxygen therapy
10. Flow-sensing devices, respirometers
11. Electrocardiography equipment (12-lead ECG)
12. Hemodynamic monitoring apparatus (arterial and pulmonary artery catheters)

B. Assemble, check, troubleshoot, and perform quality control.
1. Put together and check equipment for proper function, all of the equipment listed in section II.A. above, in addition to the following:
   a. Oxygen delivery devices (including transtracheal oxygen systems)
   b. Vacuum systems for pleural drainage
2. Correct any equipment-related problems associated with all types of respiratory therapy equipment (refer to section II.A. above and section II.A. under Entry Level Examination matrix)
3. Perform quality control on the following:
   a. Pulmonary laboratory equipment
   b. Ventilator calibration (flow, pressure, and volume)
   c. Blood gas analyzers, co-oximeters
   d. Noninvasive monitors (pulse oximetry, transcutaneous O_2/CO_2, etc.)
   e. Gas measuring devices

III. Therapy

A. Assess, observe, and record patient response. Questions in this category are designed to assess the candidate's ability to:
1. Evaluate a patient, noting response to therapy based on the following (candidates should be able to perform, recommend, and/or interpret results of each item):
   a. Subjective response
   b. Chest x-ray
   c. Mean airway pressure
   d. Transcutaneous monitoring of O_2/CO_2
   e. Co-oximetry, arterial, mixed venous, and capillary blood gases
   f. Central venous pressure, pulmonary artery pressure, pulmonary capillary wedge pressure, cardiac output
   g. Fluid balance
   h. Electrolytes, CBC, and other blood chemistries
   i. Lung compliance and airway resistance
   j. Hemodynamic calculations (shunt studies, cardiac index, pulmonary vascular resistance, systemic vascular resistance, stroke volume)
   k. V_D/V_T, $P(A\text{-}a)O_2$, and $C(a\text{-}\bar{v})O_2$
2. Record and appropriately communicate the following information:
   a. Vital signs
   b. Physical examination findings
   c. Cough/sputum production
   d. Subjective response of the patient to therapy
   e. Smoking cessation counseling

B. Maintain a patent airway, assuring ventilation and tissue oxygenation. This section contains questions that evaluate the candidate's ability to:
1. Maintain a patent airway, making sure that the patient is optimally ventilated and oxygenated:
   a. Perform endotracheal intubation and extubation
   b. Select appropriate endotracheal tubes
   c. Perform tracheostomy tube changes
2. Perform therapy that is designed to provide sufficient spontaneous or mechanical ventilation:
   a. Teach the technique of inspiratory muscle training (IMT)
   b. Adjust ventilator settings, whether they are specified or not
   c. Supply other modes of ventilation (inverse ratio ventilation, airway pres-

sure release ventilation, pressure control ventilation, negative pressure ventilation)
   d. Provide nasal/mask ventilation

C. Recommend alternative therapy based on patient response. Questions in this category are designed to assess the candidate's ability to:
   1. Terminate therapy modalities based on patient response (each respiratory therapy procedure is included here, including medication adjustments, incentive breathing devices, aerosol and humidity therapy, medical gas therapy, bronchial hygiene therapy, airway maintenance, mechanical ventilation, IPPB therapy)

D. Perform respiratory therapy procedures in emergency situations. These questions assess the candidate's ability to perform the following:
   1. ECG
   2. Monitor pupillary size and reactivity
   3. Intubate
   4. Participate in transport (land or air)
   5. Assess endotracheal tube placement via CO_2 detector
   6. Suggest pharmacologic administration and instill medication into the endotracheal tube
   7. Assess the patient's need for bicarbonate

E. Provide assistance to physicians and administer pulmonary rehabilitation/home care. Questions in this category are designed to assess the candidate's ability to assist the physician in performing or providing the following:
   1. Bronchoscopy
   2. Transtracheal aspiration
   3. Thoracentesis
   4. Tracheostomy
   5. Stress testing
   6. Placement of transtracheal catheters
   7. Sleep studies
   8. Cardioversion
   9. Intubation
   10. Pulmonary rehabilitation and/or home care services including:
      a. Define therapeutic goals
      b. Begin and monitor a graded exercise program
      c. Provide and maintain respiratory therapy equipment used in the home
      d. Monitor infection control and safety
      e. Provide patient education to patients and their families
      f. Assess patient progress
      g. Maintain apnea monitors
      h. Modify respiratory therapy techniques for home use

G. NBRC Type Questions

There are three specific types of questions used on NBRC written examinations. Unfortunately, many candidates may only be familiar with the first one or two of these types.

I. Simple Multiple Choice

Question:
Which of the following most accurately represents the $Pa{O_2}$ for a healthy 60-year-old patient?

A. 50 mm Hg
B. 60 mm Hg
C. 70 mm Hg
D. 80 mm Hg

Answer: D
This type of question requires the selection of the *one best response* from four plausible choices. To make guessing difficult, most NBRC questions are written so that all four of the choices are *possible.* In addition, two or even three of the choices may be *very nearly correct.* However, *for each question there is only one correct answer.* There are other methods of increasing the difficulty of these questions. One is to bait the candidate with fashionable therapeutic modes. For example, the candidate may be asked to select between a volume or pressure-cycled ventilator for use in providing continuous ventilatory support. Clinically, the candidate may never have even *seen* a pressure-cycled ventilator used for this purpose. However, if the settings presented for the volume ventilators are obviously wrong, no other choice would be reasonable and thus correct.

II. Multiple True–False Type Questions

Question:
Three days post total hip replacement surgery, a 50-kg, 73-year-old woman experiences pleuritic pain, tachypnea, and tachycardia. Bedside examination reveals grossly distended neck veins and a cough productive of a small amount of blood-streaked sputum. The following laboratory and bedside data are made available at this time:

$FI{O_2}$	0.21
$Pa{O_2}$	58 mm Hg
$Pa{CO_2}$	42 mm Hg
pH	7.37
HCO^-_3	24 mEq/L
Base excess	+0.6 mEq/L
Minute ventilation	26 L/min
V_D/V_T	0.78

Which of the following statements is (are) true regarding this patient's status?

I. The patient's hypoxemia is due to hypoventilation.
II. A blood gas laboratory error is present.

III. Ventilatory support is indicated.
IV. Pulmonary embolus is a likely cause of distress.

A. II and III
B. I only
C. II and IV
D. III and IV

Answer: D

Many candidates find these questions difficult. This may be due either to the large amount of information they contain or to a lack of familiarity with this type of question. Whatever the reason, these questions generally become simpler once a systematic approach is employed, as follows:

A. Evaluate the information presented in the question's opening statement.
B. Go down the list of presented choices and make a mark beside the statements that are true.
C. Select the corresponding combinations of choices.
D. If still in doubt, make an educated guess. Remember, *there is no penalty for guessing on NBRC written exams.*
E. Practice taking as many of these questions as possible. This book contains hundreds of them. More will be found in the candidate handbook. Study them all very carefully until you are comfortable with their format.

III. Situational Sets

Situational sets are mini case histories. They consist of a scenario followed by three to five questions. Like a clinical simulation, they place the candidate in charge of a patient management problem. An example of a situational set appears below.

Directions:

Each group of questions below concerns a certain situation. In each case, first study the description of the situation. Then, choose the one best answer to each question following it. A 64-year-old man with a history of chronic obstructive pulmonary disease (COPD) is brought to the emergency department after several days of increasing distress that did not respond to his home respiratory care program. Arterial blood gas data on room air and 2 L nasal oxygen are as follows:

	Room Air	2 L O_2
Pa_{O_2}	36 mm Hg	65 mm Hg
Pa_{CO_2}	68 mm Hg	65 mm Hg
pH	7.28	7.35
HCO_3^-	35 mEq/L	37 mEq/L

1. Based on the above information, the respiratory therapy practitioner should now recommend which of the following?

A. Increase oxygen to 3 L/min
B. Leave oxygen flow unchanged
C. Decrease oxygen to 1 L/min
D. Place patient on a 35% air entrainment mask

Answer: B

2. Which of the following is (are) most likely to be responsible for this patient's arterial hypoxemia?

I. Low V/Q
II. Physiologic shunting
III. Hypoventilation

A. I only
B. I and III
C. II only
D. II and III

Answer: B

3. This patient has a long history of bronchiectasis. Which of the following would be the most valuable adjunct in helping maintain bronchial hygiene?

A. Aerosol therapy
B. Continuous ventilatory support
C. Breathing retraining
D. Postural drainage techniques
E. Bronchodilator therapy

Answer: D

4. Seven days later, the patient is beginning to improve. Acid-base and blood gas data obtained at this time are as follows:

FI_{O_2}	0.21
Pa_{O_2}	63 mm Hg
Pa_{CO_2}	69 mm Hg
pH	7.60
HCO^-_3	37 mEq/L
Base excess	+16 mEq/L

Based on the above data, which of the following is the most correct interpretation of this patient's acid-base status?

A. Acute respiratory alkalosis and metabolic alkalosis exist.
B. An overcompensated respiratory acidosis exists.
C. A laboratory error exists.
D. Fully compensated metabolic alkalosis exists.

Answer: C

With the exception of the branching-logic clinical simulation, these situational sets are the most complex devised by the NBRC. Many candidates find them even more difficult than the multiple true–false type. Performance on these questions can be improved by using the following approach:

A. *Read the questions very carefully.* Read and reread the scenarios until you grasp the intent of the situation. Often, the set will follow a particular patient throughout his or her hospitalization. In this case, information presented in each preceding question must be considered before selecting an answer.

B. *Practice taking situational set type questions.* Like branching-logic clinical simulations, these questions can be very confusing. Fortunately this problem is usually alleviated with a little practice. This book contains many such sets. The candidate handbook will contain more. Study them all very carefully.

H. References

Every attempt has been made to reference each question in this book to the latest edition of sources that are part of a candidate's library. In the next few pages there is a list of 21 references used in developing these test items. Please note in particular that most of the questions herein have been referenced to texts that would most likely form the core of the candidate's library, as recommended by the NBRC.

Throughout the text the questions are referenced using the following representative format:

(3:321–3; 8: Chap 1)

Each set of parentheses gives the reference number on the left of the colon and the pages or chapters on the right.

References

1. Burton GG, Hodgkin JE, Ward JJ: *Respiratory Care: A Guide to Clinical Practice,* 3rd ed. Philadelphia, JB Lippincott Co., 1991.
2. McPherson SP: *Respiratory Therapy Equipment,* 4th ed. St. Louis, CV Mosby, 1990.
3. Scanlan CL, Spearman CB, Sheldon RL: *Egan's Fundamentals of Respiratory Care,* 5th ed. St. Louis, CV Mosby, 1990.
4. Shapiro BA, Kacmerek RM, Cane RD, et al: *Clinical Application of Respiratory Care,* 4th ed. St. Louis, Mosby–Year Book, 1991.
5. Darovic GO: *Hemodynamic Monitoring.* Philadelphia, WB Saunders, 1987.
6. Ruppel G: *Manual of Pulmonary Function Testing,* 6th ed. St. Louis, Mosby–Year Book, 1994.
7. Rau JL Jr.: *Respiratory Care Pharmacology,* 4th ed. St. Louis, Mosby–Year Book, 1994.
8. Des Jardins T: *Clinical Manifestations of Respiratory Disease,* 2nd ed. Chicago, Year Book Medical Publishers, 1990.
9. Farzan S: *A Concise Handbook of Respiratory Diseases,* 3rd ed. Norwalk, CT, Appleton & Lange, 1992.
10. Aehlert B: *ACLS Quick Review Study Guide.* St. Louis, Mosby–Year Book, 1994.
11. May DF: *Rehabilitation and Continuity of Care in Pulmonary Disease.* St. Louis, Mosby–Year Book, 1991.
12. Haas F, Axen K, eds: *Pulmonary Therapy and Rehabilitation,* 2nd ed. Baltimore, Williams and Wilkins, 1991.
13. Barnes TA: *Core Textbook of Respiratory Care Practice,* 2nd ed. St. Louis, Mosby–Year Book, 1994.
14. Koff PB, Eitzman D, Neu J: *Neonatal and Pediatric Respiratory Care,* 2nd ed. St. Louis, Mosby–Year Book, 1993.
15. Pilbeam SP: *Mechanical Ventilation,* 2nd ed. St. Louis, Mosby–Year Book, 1992.
16. Pierson DJ, Kacmerek RM: *Foundations of Respiratory Care.* New York, Churchill Livingstone, 1992.
17. Kacmerek RM, Mack CW, Dimas S: *The Essentials of Respiratory Care,* 3rd ed. St. Louis, Mosby–Year Book, 1990.
18. White GC: *Basic Clinical Lab Competencies for Respiratory Care,* 2nd ed. Albany, NY, Delmar Publishers, 1993.
19. Shapiro BA, Peruzzi WT, Templin R: *Clinical Application of Blood Gases,* 5th ed. St. Louis, Mosby–Year Book, 1994.
20. Hodgkin JE, Connors GL, Bell CW: *Pulmonary Rehabilitation: Guidelines to Success,* 2nd ed. Philadelphia, JB Lippincott, 1993.
21. National Board for Respiratory Care Composite Examination Matrix, National Board for Respiratory Care, 1993.

Second Edition

Appleton & Lange's Review of

RESPIRATORY CARE

I

EXAMINATION PRETEST AND REVIEW

UNIT I

Mathematics Review and Pretest

There is a bewildering array of formulas and equations for which the respiratory therapy practitioner is responsible. A glance at the NBRC Composite Examination Matrix (see reference 21) confirms this. From tank factors to sophisticated hemodynamic measurements, the practitioner may, at times, feel overwhelmed by an avalanche of laboratory and clinical data. This need not be the case. With a sound knowledge of the metric system and the ability to organize and solve basic algebraic equations, the calculations used in respiratory care can be done correctly and with confidence.

Important

According to the NBRC Composite Examination Matrix, the Entry Level Examination candidate should be familiar with all but the following calculations contained in this mathematics review section.

1. $\dot{Q}_S/\dot{Q}_T$ determinations
2. $C(a-\bar{v})O_2$ calculations
3. Fick equation
4. a/A ratio and respiratory index calculations
5. Pulmonary vascular resistance calculations
6. Spirometry calculations
7. Residual volume determinations

The candidate for the Advanced Practitioner Examination should be familiar with all of the material presented in this unit, in addition to the above calculations.

PART 1

Medical Gas Therapy Calculations

Contents

A. Conversion Factor Pretest

Questions in this category are designed to assess the practitioner's ability to use medical gas therapy conversion factors. For example, being able to convert cubic feet of gaseous oxygen to liters of gaseous oxygen would be beneficial in helping the therapist determine actual cylinder contents. The following pretest was developed to help the candidate become proficient in this area. References are provided for each question, and candidates will find correct answers, including explanations, at the end of Unit I.

1. How many liters of oxygen are contained in 1 cubic foot of gaseous oxygen?

   A. 14.7
   B. 7.52
   C. 13.4
   D. 28.3
   E. 24.9

   (3:591)

2. How many liters of gaseous oxygen are contained in a full E cylinder?

   A. 622
   B. 687
   C. 590
   D. 486
   E. 930

   (2:22–3; 3:590)

3. How many liters of gaseous oxygen are contained in a full H cylinder?

   A. 9600
   B. 5300
   C. 7400
   D. 6900
   E. 4700

   (2:22–3; 3:590)

4. How many cubic feet of gaseous oxygen are contained in 1 cubic foot of liquid oxygen?

   A. 920
   B. 283
   C. 314
   D. 860
   E. 750

   (2:31; 3:593)

5. A full D cylinder of oxygen contains 356 liters of oxygen. What is the tank factor for a D tank of oxygen?

   A. 0.28
   B. 0.16
   C. 0.67
   D. 1.42
   E. 1.86

   (3:591)

B. Cylinder Duration Pretest

Questions in this category are designed to assess the practitioner's ability to determine the amount of time that a particular medical gas cylinder will run before going dry under the clinical conditions stated in the question. In answering these questions, the candidate must be able to recall that the tank factors for E-, G-, and H-size oxygen cylinders are 0.28, 2.41, and 3.14, respectively. These factors must then be inserted into the following equation:

$$\text{Cylinder duration (min)} = \frac{\text{Actual cylinder gauge pressure (psig)} \times \text{Tank factor}}{\text{Actual delivered liter flow (L/min)}}$$

The above equation gives cylinder duration in minutes. This means that the value must be divided by 60 in order to convert it to hours of cylinder duration. The following pretest was developed to help the candidate become proficient in this area.

1. The respiratory care practitioner is asked to set up a full E cylinder of oxygen to deliver 3 L/min to a patient with chronic obstructive pulmonary disease. How long will it take for the cylinder to run empty at the above liter flow?

   A. 3 hr and 46 min
   B. 3 hr and 25 min
   C. 2 hr and 43 min
   D. 4 hr and 10 min
   E. 3 hr and 12 min

   (2:31; 3:592)

2. A G cylinder of oxygen contains 1600 psig and is running at a rate of 5 L/min. At this flow rate, how long will it take for the cylinder to run completely dry?

   A. 11 hr and 49 min
   B. 11 hr and 30 min
   C. 12 hr and 5 min
   D. 12 hr and 51 min
   E. 12 hr and 15 min

   (2:31; 3:592)

3. At a flow rate of 4 L/min, how long will it take for a full H cylinder to run completely dry?

   A. 19 hr and 55 min
   B. 29 hr and 15 min
   C. 47 hr and 20 min
   D. 30 hr and 10 min
   E. 28 hr and 47 min

   (2:31; 3:592)

4. An H cylinder of oxygen has 700 psig and is delivering a flow of 7 L/min. Approximately how long will it take before it runs completely dry?

   A. 6 hr and 45 min
   B. 5 hr and 30 min
   C. 6 hr and 15 min
   D. 5 hr and 45 min
   E. 5 hr and 15 min

   (2:31; 3:592)

C. General FIO_2 Formula Pretest

Even when an oxygen analyzer is not available, the respiratory therapy practitioner can determine a patient's fractional inspired oxygen concentration (FIO_2). This may be crucial in an emergency situation. The appropriate formula is as follows:

$$FIO_2 = \frac{[(0.21)\ (\text{Liters Air})\ ] + [(1.00)\ (\text{Liters Oxygen})]}{\text{Total system liter flow}}$$

The following pretest was developed to help the candidate become proficient in this area.

1. The respiratory care practitioner is blending 6 L/min of oxygen and 9 L/min of air into an oxygen hood. Approximately what concentration of oxygen will be administered under these circumstances?

   A. 25%
   B. 30%
   C. 35%
   D. 45%
   E. 50%

   (2:73; 3:614)

2. The respiratory care practitioner is blending 5 L/min oxygen with 15 L/min air. What concentration of oxygen will be administered under these circumstances?

   A. 30%
   B. 55%
   C. 45%
   D. 40%
   E. 50%

   (2:73; 3:614)

D. PIO_2 Formula Pretest

Because it is part of the alveolar air equation, the PIO_2 formula has important laboratory and clinical applications. The formula is as follows:

$$PIO_2 = (FIO_2)\ (P_B - PH_2O)$$

The following pretest was developed to help the candidate become proficient in this area.

1. Calculate a patient's PIO_2 given the following clinical conditions:
   - PB 760 mm Hg
   - FIO_2 0.21
   - PH_2O 47 mm Hg

   A. 160 mm Hg
   B. 150 mm Hg
   C. 140 mm Hg
   D. 185 mm Hg
   E. 137 mm Hg

   (1:183)

2. Calculate a patients PIO_2 given the following clinical data:

   FIO_2 0.40
   P_B 727 mm Hg
   PH_2O 47 mm Hg

   A. 250 mm Hg
   B. 240 mm Hg
   C. 270 mm Hg
   D. 243 mm Hg
   E. 120 mm Hg

   (1:183)

3. Calculate the PIO_2 given the following clinical conditions:

   FIO_2 0.70
   P_B 420 mm Hg
   PH_2O 47 mm Hg

   A. 480 mm Hg
   B. 235 mm Hg
   C. 260 mm Hg
   D. 295 mm Hg
   E. 280 mm Hg

   (1:183)

E. Alveolar Air Equation Pretest

Because the alveolar oxygen tension must be known in order to calculate the $P(A\text{-}a)_{O2}$ and the intrapulmonary shunt fraction (when using the modified clinical shunt equation), the alveolar air equation is used very frequently by the respiratory care practitioner. Unfortunately, there are multiple versions of this equation. Thus, confusion sometimes exists concerning which equation is most appropriate. *Although this is certainly not the case in all laboratory and clinical situations on NBRC examinations, any one of the alveolar air equations is sufficiently accurate for the candidate to determine the correct answer.* I recommend that the candidate learn one of the simpler versions when preparing for these examinations. The suggested alveolar air equations appear below:

$$PAO_2 = [FIO(P_B - PH_2O)] - (PaCO_2/R)$$

or

$$PAO_2 = [FIO_2 (P_B - PH_2O)] - [(PaCO_2) \times (1.25)]$$

These equations are suggested because they are accurate and relatively easy to remember. In the clinical setting, when the patient is receiving an FIO_2 greater than 0.60, the correction for R can be eliminated.

The following pretest was developed to help the candidate to become proficient in this area.

1. Calculate the PAO_2 given the following clinical information:

   P_B 760 mm Hg
   FIO_2 0.21
   $PaCO_2$ 40 mm Hg

   A. 100 mm Hg
   B. 120 mm Hg
   C. 108 mm Hg
   D. 95 mm Hg
   E. 90 mm Hg

   (1:183–4)

2. Calculate the PAO_2 given the following conditions:

   P_B 640 mm Hg
   FIO_2 1.0
   $PaCO_2$ 30 mm Hg

   A. 520 mm Hg
   B. 540 mm Hg
   C. 560 mm Hg
   D. 490 mm Hg
   E. 590 mm Hg

   (1:183–4)

3. Given the following clinical data, which of the following choices most accurately represents a patient's PAO_2?

   P_B 730 mm Hg
   FIO_2 0.40
   $PaCO_2$ 55 mm Hg

   A. 205 mm Hg
   B. 225 mm Hg
   C. 240 mm Hg
   D. 180 mm Hg
   E. 195 mm Hg

   (1:183–4)

F. Air Entrainment Formula Pretest

The air entrainment formula allows the respiratory care practitioner to determine how many liters of room air are entrained by a particular air entrainment valve per liter of source gas. It is assumed that this source gas is 100% oxygen. The formula is as follows:

$$\frac{100 - FIO_2}{FIO_2 - 21^*} = \frac{\text{Liters of air entrained}}{\text{Liters of oxygen}}$$

This air:oxygen ratio should always be computed so that the number for liters of oxygen = 1. For example, if FIO_2 = 70%, air:oxygen ratio is 0.6:1.

To solve the above equation, the practitioner must know the FIO_2 of the air entrainment valve being used. The most common practical application of this equation is the determination of total flow rate as delivered by a given air entrainment system. The formula for this is as follows:

Total system flow rate
= total number of liters of gas (liters of entrained air + liters of oxygen) × liter flow of the source gas

From this system it can be seen that in the case of a 3:1 ratio (such as exists with a 40% air entrainment system), a source gas flow of 10 L/min will yield a total flow of 40 L/min.

3 L of air + 1 L of oxygen = 4 L of gas

4 L × 10 L/min of source gas = 40 L/min total flow

The following pretest was developed to help the candidate become proficient in this area.

1. The respiratory therapy practitioner is using an air entrainment valve that is designed to deliver an FIO_2 of 0.4. To do this it must entrain how many parts room air for each part source gas?

   A. 3
   B. 4
   C. 5
   D. 10
   E. 20

   (2:73; 3:619–20)

2. An air entrainment valve is designed to deliver an FIO_2 of 0.6. To do this it must entrain how many parts room air for each part driving gas?

   A. 1.4
   B. 1.3
   C. 1.5
   D. 1.7
   E. 1.0

   (2:73; 3:619–20)

3. According to the air entrainment formula, how many parts room air must be entrained for each part driving gas to obtain an FIO_2 of 0.24?

   A. 10
   B. 15
   C. 20
   D. 25
   E. 30

   (2:73; 3:619–20)

4. An all-purpose pneumatic nebulizer is being driven by 8 L/min and the air entrainment valve is on the 40% setting. What is the total delivered flow rate?

   A. 37 L/min
   B. 40 L/min
   C. 32 L/min
   D. 27 L/min
   E. 45 L/min

   (2:73; 3:619–20)

5. An all-purpose pneumatic nebulizer is being driven by 12 L/min and the air entrainment valve is set on 65%. What is the approximate total liter flow being delivered to the patient?

   A. 24 L/min
   B. 22 L/min
   C. 18 L/min
   D. 14 L/min
   E. 29 L/min

   (2:73; 3:619–20)

6. A properly functioning 24% air entrainment mask is being driven by 4 L/min. What is the approximate total flow rate being delivered to the patient?

   A. 104 L/min
   B. 80 L/min
   C. 100 L/min
   D. 96 L/min
   E. 26 L/min

   (2:73; 3:619–20)

G. Flowmeter Accuracy Calculations Pretest

Questions in this category are designed to assess the candidate's ability to determine the actual flow rate being administered by properly calibrated flowmeters that are delivering unusual gas mixtures. The following self-study

* 20 is often used in place of 21 to make estimation easier, but for oxygen concentrations equal to or below 30%, 21 must be used.

questions were developed to help the candidate become proficient in this area.

1. A properly calibrated backpressure-compensated oxygen flowmeter is being used to administer a mixture of 80% helium and 20% oxygen. The meter presently reads 10 L/min. Which of the following choices most accurately represents the flow rate in liters per minute that is actually being administered?

   A. 0
   B. 10
   C. 12
   D. 15
   E. 18

   (3:628–9)

2. A properly calibrated backpressure-compensated oxygen flowmeter is being used to administer a mixture of 70% helium and 30% oxygen. The meter presently reads 10 L/min. Which of the following choices most accurately represents the flow rate in liters per minute that is actually being administered?

   A. 10
   B. 14
   C. 16
   D. 20
   E. 22

   (3:628–9)

H. Unusual Atmosphere Calculation Pretest

Questions in this category are designed to assess the candidate's ability to apply his/her knowledge of medical gas therapy and respiratory physiology to patient care situations that involve unusual atmospheric conditions. The most common example of this occurs during the administration of hyperbaric medicine. The following pretest was developed to help the candidate become proficient in this area.

1. Which of the following choices most accurately represents the barometric pressure exerted on a diver who is submerged to a depth of 100 feet?

   A. One atmosphere
   B. Two atmospheres
   C. Three atmospheres
   D. Four atmospheres
   E. Five atmospheres

   (1:342)

2. Given a sample of gas under the following conditions, what is the partial pressure of oxygen (P sample 0_2) of the gas?

   P_B 2.0 atmospheres
   FIO_2 0.21
   PH_2O 47 mm Hg

   A. 340 mm Hg
   B. 310 mm Hg
   C. 280 mm Hg
   D. 420 mm Hg
   E. 330 mm Hg

   (1:183)

3. A patient is in a hyperbaric chamber breathing 100% 0_2 at 1.5 atmospheres. If his $PaCO_2$ is 40 mm Hg and his respiratory exchange ratio is 0.8, which of the following most closely approximates this patient's PAO_2?

   A. 1420 mm Hg
   B. 1660 mm Hg
   C. 1050 mm Hg
   D. 1010 mm Hg
   E. 1130 mm Hg

   (1:183–4)

PART 2

Humidity and Aerosol Therapy Calculations

Contents

A. Terminology Pretest

Questions in this category are designed to assess the practitioner's understanding of medical and scientific terms and symbols that are fundamental to the study of aerosol and humidity therapy. The following pretest was developed to help the candidate become proficient in this area.

1. Which of the following sets of conditions are represented by the term *STPD?*

   I. 273° Kelvin; one atmosphere; $PH_2O = 0$ mm Hg
   II. 0° Centigrade; 713 mm Hg; $PH_2O = 0$ mm Hg
   III. 459° Kelvin; 760 mm Hg; $PH_2O = 44$ mm Hg
   IV. O° Centigrade; 760 mm Hg; $PH_2O = 0$ mm Hg
   V. 273° Kelvin; 1034 g/cm^2; $PH_2O = 0$ mm Hg

   A. I, II, III, IV, and V
   B. II, III, IV, and V
   C. I, IV, and V
   D. I, II, III, and V
   E. I, II, and IV

   (2:6; 3:44)

2. Which of the following sets of conditions best represents the term *ATPD?*

   A. Ambient temperature; ambient pressure; $PH_2O = 47$ mm Hg
   B. Ambient temperature; ambient pressure; $PH_2O = 0$ mm Hg
   C. Ambient temperature; PB = 713 mm Hg; $PH_2O = 0$ mm Hg
   D. Body temperature; ambient pressure; $PH_2O = 0$ mm Hg
   E. Body temperature; ambient pressure; $PH_2O = 47$ mm Hg

   (3:44)

3. Which of the following sets of conditions are represented by the term *ATPS?*

   A. Ambient temperature; ambient pressure; $PH_2O = 47$ mm Hg
   B. Ambient temperature; ambient pressure; $PH_2O = 0$ mm Hg
   C. Ambient temperature; ambient pressure; 100% relative humidity
   D. Ambient temperature; ambient pressure; $PH_2O = 44$ mm Hg
   E. Ambient temperature; $P_B = 760$ mm Hg; $PH_2O = 0$ mm Hg

   (3:44)

4. Which of the following sets of conditions are represented by the term *BTPD?*

   A. 310° Kelvin; ambient pressure; $PH_2O = 47$ mm Hg
   B. 273° Centigrade; ambient pressure; $PH_2O = 0$ mm Hg
   C. 37° Centigrade; ambient pressure; $PH_2O = 0$ mm Hg
   D. Ambient temperature; ambient pressure; $PH_2O = 0$ mm Hg
   E. 21° Centigrade; ambient pressure; $PH_2O = 0$ mm Hg

   (3:44)

5. Which of the following sets of conditions are represented by the term *BTPS?*

A. 37° Centigrade; ambient pressure; $PH_2O = 47$ mm Hg
B. 273° Kelvin; 760 mm Hg; $PH_2O = 47$ mm Hg
C. 273° Kelvin; ambient pressure; 100% body humidity
D. 37° Centigrade; ambient pressure; $PH_2O = 0$ mm Hg

(3:44)

6. What is the water vapor tension of a sample of alveolar gas at BTPS?

A. 44 mm Hg
B. 47 mm Hg
C. 37 mm Hg
D. 101 mm Hg
E. 52 mm Hg

(2:80; 4:58)

7. Under the following conditions, what is the water vapor tension of a normothermic patient's alveolar gas?

PB	390 mm Hg
FIO_2	0.90
$PaCO_2$	65 mm Hg

A. 47 mm Hg
B. 44 mm Hg
C. 37 mm Hg
D. 100 mm Hg
E. 12 mm Hg

(2:80; 4:58)

8. Which of the following accurately describe alveolar gas?

I. $PH_2O = 44$ mm Hg
II. Absolute humidity = 44 mg/L
III. Relative humidity = 100%
IV. Percent body humidity = 100%
V. Water vapor density = 47 mg/L
VI. Exists at BTPS

A. I, II, III, IV, and V
B. II, III, IV, V, and VI
C. I, II, IV, V, and VI
D. II, III, IV, and VI
E. I, II, III, IV, V, and VI

(4:57–58)

B. Absolute Humidity Pretest

Questions in this category are designed to assess the candidate's understanding of the concepts of absolute humidity. Absolute humidity is defined as the quantity of water vapor actually present in a gas sample. In human physiology this content is usually expressed in milligrams per liter (mg/L). The following pretest was developed to help the candidate become proficient in this area.

1. Which of the following values represents the absolute humidity of a liter of gas at BTPS?

A. 44 mg/L
B. 47 mg/L
C. 100 mg/L
D. 37 g/L
E. 310 g/L

(2:81; 4:57)

2. A normothermic 100-kg patient is on a volume ventilator with a VT of 850 mL. The FIO_2 is 45% and the P_B is 660 mm Hg. For this patient the absolute humidity of a liter of alveolar gas is represented most accurately by which of the following choices?

A. 24 mg/L
B. 44 mg/L
C. 12 mg/L
D. 38 mg/L
E. 47 mg/L

(2:81; 4:57)

3. What is the absolute humidity of a liter of gas that exists at condition of STPD?

A. 37 mg/L
B. 47 mg/L
C. 44 mg/L
D. 0.0 mg/L
E. 97.5 mg/L

(2:79; 4:57)

C. Percent Relative Humidity Pretest

Questions in this category are designed to assess the candidate's understanding of the concept of relative humidity. Relative humidity is defined as the degree to which a sample of gas is saturated with water expressed as a percent. This definition can be written algebraically as follows:

$$\text{Relative humidity} = \frac{\text{Sample gas absolute humidity in mg/L}}{\text{Sample water vapor capacity in mg/L}} \times 100$$

Relative humidity may also be expressed as:

$$\frac{\text{Content}}{\text{Capacity}} \quad \text{or} \quad \frac{\text{Maximum absolute humidity}}{\text{Absolute humidity}}$$

It is also helpful for the candidate to remember that a liter of alveolar gas is capable of holding 44 mg of water vapor when 100% saturated. The following pretest was developed to help the candidate become proficient in this area.

1. Calculate the relative humidity of a liter of gas under the following conditions:

Absolute humidity	31 mg/L
Temperature	37° C

   Which of the following choices most accurately represents this value?

   A. 30%
   B. 40%
   C. 50%
   D. 70%
   E. 100%

   (2:81; 3:67)

2. Calculate the relative humidity of a liter of sample gas under the following conditions:

Absolute humidity	9 mg/L
Temperature	310° K

   Which of the following choices most accurately represents this value?

   A. 15%
   B. 20%
   C. 28%
   D. 33%
   E. 50%

   (2:81; 3:67)

3. If a gas is capable of holding 28 mg H_2O/L when it is fully saturated, calculate the relative humidity if the absolute humidity is 4 mg/L.

   A. 23%
   B. 10%
   C. 29%
   D. 14%
   E. 17%

   (2:81; 3:67)

D. Percent Body Humidity Pretest

Questions in this category are designed to assess the candidate's understanding of the concept of percent body humidity. The term *percent body humidity* is used to describe gases being delivered during aerosol and humidity therapy. The water vapor content of these gases is expressed as a percentage of the water vapor content of gases at BTPS, such as alveolar gas. This definition can be written algebraically as follows:

$$\text{Percent body humidity} = \frac{\text{Sample gas absolute humidity in mg/L}}{44 \text{ mg/L}} \times 100$$

Forty-four milligrams per liter is the absolute humidity of a gas at BTPS. The following pretest was developed to help the candidate become proficient in this area.

1. Which of the following most accurately represents the percent body humidity of a sample of gas with an absolute humidity of 14 mg/L?

   A. 25%
   B. 32%
   C. 40%
   D. 14%
   E. 30%

   (3:67)

2. Which of the following choices represents the percent body humidity of a sample of gas at body temperature (37°C) with a relative humidity of 50%?

   A. 50%
   B. 45%
   C. 30%
   D. 20%
   E. 44%

   (3:67)

E. Humidity Deficit Pretest

Questions in this category are designed to assess the candidate's understanding of the concept of humidity deficit. The term *humidity deficit* is defined as the absolute humidity of alveolar gas (44 mg/L) minus the absolute humidity of the inspired gases. This can be written algebraically as follows:

$$\text{Humidity deficit in mg/L} = (\text{Absolute humidity of alveolar gas (44 mg/L)}) - (\text{Absolute humidity of inspired gas})$$

The following pretest was developed to help the candidate become proficient in this area.

1. Which of the following most accurately represents the humidity deficit if the patient is breathing gas with an H_2O content of 23 mg/L?

   A. 19 mg/L
   B. 24 mg/L
   C. 17 mg/L
   D. 26 mg/L
   E. 21 mg/L

   (1:360–61; 4:58)

2. Which of the following most accurately represents the humidity deficit of a patient who is breathing medical gas with a percent body humidity of 65%?

   A. 30 mg/L
   B. 19 mg/L
   C. 25 mg/L
   D. 15 mg/L
   E. 6 mg/L

(1:360–1; 4:58)

PART 3

Calculations Used in Continuous Ventilatory Support

Contents

A. The Flow Rate Formula Pretest

Few equations or calculations are as fundamental to the practice of respiratory therapy as the flow rate formula. Continuous ventilatory support cannot be administered intelligently without a thorough understanding of the concepts embodied in this formula:

Flow rate (L/sec)
= Tidal volume (L)/Inspiratory time (sec)

This formula will yield a flow rate in liters per second (L/sec). Should the practitioner desire this value in the more commonly used units of liters per minute, the original value must be multiplied by the factor 60 sec/min. As an example, a flow rate of 1 L/sec when multiplied by this factor yields the value 60 L/min.

The above formula, when manipulated algebraically to solve for the other two variables, yields the following forms:

Tidal volume = (Flow rate) (Inspiratory time)

and

Inspiratory time = Tidal volume/Flow rate

The following pretest was developed to help the candidate become proficient at the above calculations and techniques.

1. The respiratory therapy practitioner is using a volume-cycled constant flow generator in the intensive care unit. If the ventilator routinely delivers 850 cc of gas in 0.65 sec, which of the following most accurately represents the average inspiratory flow rate?

   A. 130 L/min
   B. 60 L/min
   C. 78 L/min
   D. 54 L/min
   E. 66 L/min

   (2:163; 3:862)

2. A volume-cycled ventilator is delivering a tidal volume of 500 cc with an inspiratory time of 1.1 sec. Based on this information, which of the following most accurately represents the ventilator's average inspiratory flow rate?

   A. 20 L/min
   B. 25 L/min
   C. 42 L/min
   D. 27 L/min
   E. 35 L/min

   (2:163; 3:862)

3. A tidal volume of 75 cc is delivered over a 0.6-sec inspiratory time. Which of the following is the average inspiratory flow rate?

   A. 75 mL/sec
   B. 7.5 L/min
   C. 150 mL/sec

D. 750 mL/sec
E. 75 L/min

(2:163; 3:862)

4. The inspiratory time for a volume-cycled ventilator with a flow rate of 500 mL/sec and a tidal volume of 650 cc is represented by which of the following choices?

A. 1.3 sec
B. 1.2 sec
C. 3.2 sec
D. 1.0 sec
E. 1.1 sec

(2:163; 3:862)

5. Given a tidal volume of 950 cc and a flow rate of 35 L/min, the inspiratory time will be approximately:

A. 2.1 sec
B. 1.8 sec
C. 3.1 sec
D. 1.7 sec
E. 1.6 sec

(2:163; 3:862)

6. Given a mean flow rate of 50 L/min and an inspiratory time of 1.2 sec, the approximate tidal volume is represented by which of the following choices?

A. 1.0 L
B. 1.1 L
C. 830 cc
D. 1.2 L
E. 900 cc

(2:163; 3:862)

B. I:E Ratio Pretest

Questions in this category are designed to assess the candidate's ability to calculate the I:E ratio of a patient receiving continuous ventilatory support. Probably the simplest and most versatile formula for determining this is as follows:

$$(I + E) = \frac{\text{Inspiratory flow rate (L/min)}}{\text{Minute ventilation (L/min)}}$$

What this formula states is that the numerical total of the inspiratory and expiratory ratio numbers is equal to the patient's minute ventilation divided into the average inspiratory flow rate. This is noted in the example below:

$$\frac{\text{Flow rate} = 60 \text{ L/min}}{\text{Minute ventilation} = 20 \text{ L/min}} = 3$$

Because the I of I:E must always be 1, the appropriate I:E in the above example is 1:2.

From this equation, it can be seen that to obtain an I:E of 1:2, the patient's average inspiratory flow rate must be three times his mechanical minute volume. By the same token, a flow rate four times the minute volume will yield a 1:3 ratio.

It is often useful to manipulate this formula to solve for other unknowns. These formulas are as follows:

$$\text{Flow rate} = (\text{Minute ventilation})\,(I + E)$$

and

$$\text{Minute ventilation} = \text{Flow rate}/(I + E)$$

The following pretest was developed to help the candidate become proficient in the above calculations and techniques.

1. What is the I:E ratio if the flow rate is 60 L/min and the minute ventilation is 20 L/min?

A. 1:1
B. 1:3
C. 1:2
D. 1:4
E. 2:1

(2:163; 3:864)

2. Which of the following most accurately represents the I:E ratio given a tidal volume of 1100 cc, a respiratory rate of 13/min, and an inspiratory flow rate of 40 L/min?

A. 1:2.6
B. 1:3.2
C. 1:2.3
D. 1:2.1
E. 1:1.8

(2:163; 3:864)

3. What is the I:E ratio if the V_T is 25 mL, the respiratory rate is 42/min, and the flow rate is 75 mL/sec?

A. 1:2.8
B. 1:2.6
C. 1:2.4
D. 1:3.3
E. 1:2.9

(2:163; 3:864)

4. What is the mean inspiratory flow rate necessary to maintain an I:E ratio of 1:2 if the tidal volume is 800 mL and the respiratory rate is 23/min?

A. 50 L/min
B. 55 L/min
C. 32 L/min
D. 60 L/min
E. 80 L/min

(2:163; 3:864)

5. What is the mean inspiratory flow rate necessary to maintain an I:E ratio of 1:3 if the ventilator's tidal volume is 300 cc and the respiratory rate is 33/min?

   A. 15 L/min
   B. 25 L/min
   C. 40 L/min
   D. 55 L/min
   E. 79 L/min

(2:163; 3:864)

6. The neonatologist asks the respiratory therapy practitioner to set up high-frequency ventilation on a 1100-g infant with severe infant respiratory distress syndrome. He wants a respiratory rate of 150/min and an inspiratory time of 0.20 second. What will the I:E ratio be under those circumstances?

   A. 1:1
   B. 1:0.5
   C. 1:1.5
   D. 1:1.2
   E. 1:1.3

(2:163; 3:864)

C. Corrected Tidal Volume and System Compliance Pretest

Questions in this category are designed to assess the candidate's ability to determine the actual or corrected tidal volume being delivered to the patient during the administration of continuous ventilatory support. The formula for corrected tidal volume is as follows:

Patient's corrected tidal volume
= Ventilator exhaled tidal volume − Compressed volume

Thus, the actual tidal volume received by the patient is equal to that volume delivered by the ventilator (preferably measured at the exhalation port) minus the volume compressed in the ventilator external tubing and humidifier system. To determine the compressed volume, the following formula must be used:

Compressed volume (cc)
= Corrected peak pressure (cm H_2O)
× System compliance factor (cc/cm H_2O)

There is a variation to this formula that is used whenever the practitioner is calculating the patient's effective static compliance (ESC). In this case, because pressure is measured during intervals of no gas flow, the patient's plateau pressure is substituted for the peak pressure as follows:

Compressed volume (cc)
= Corrected plateau pressure (cm H_2O)
× System compliance factor (cc/cm H_2O)

It must be emphasized that for these and all other ventilator calculations, peak and plateau pressure measurements must be PEEP corrected if they are to be 100% accurate.

The system compliance noted above is frequently assumed to be 3.0 cc/cm H_2O and 1.0 cc/cm H_2O for adult and neonatal systems, respectively. This value can and, particularly for neonatal circuits, should be calculated. This formula is as follows:

$$\text{System compliance (cc/cm } H_2O) = \frac{\text{Test volume (cc)}}{\text{Plateau pressure (cm } H_2O)}$$

These values are obtained by delivering a small test volume (usually about 200 cc for adult and 50 cc for neonatal circuits) into the ventilator system and then noting the plateau pressure obtained at this time.

The following pretest was developed to help the candidate become proficient in these calculations and techniques.

1. The respiratory therapy practitioner is asked to calculate the system compliance for a Bennett MA-I ventilator. In so doing, he obtains an inspiratory plateau pressure of 61 cm H_2O with a test volume of 200 cc. Based on this information, which of the following choices most accurately represents this ventilator's system compliance factor?

   A. 2.8 cc/cm H_2O
   B. 4.4 cc/cm H_2O
   C. 2.3 cc/cm H_2O
   D. 3.0 cc/cm H_2O
   E. 3.3 cc/cm H_2O

(3:756–9)

2. Which of the following most accurately represents the system compliance factor of a Sechrist ventilator if a plateau pressure of 56 cm H_2O is reached after delivering a flow rate of 3.0 L/min for 1 sec into the ventilator system?

   A. 1.25 cc/cm H_2O
   B. 0.75 cc/cm H_2O
   C. 0.50 cc/cm H_2O
   D. 0.90 cc/cm H_2O
   E. 3.0 cc/cm H_2O

(3:756–9)

3. What is the corrected (delivered) tidal volume if the set V_T is 890 mL, the peak pressure is 52 cm H_2O, and the tubing compliance factor is 2. 1 cc/cm H_2O?

   A. 900 cc
   B. 830 cc

C. 740 cc
D. 780 cc
E. 760 cc

(3:756–9)

4. Which of the following most accurately represents the corrected (delivered) tidal volume given the following conditions?

Set V_T	1100 cc
Peak pressure	73 cm H_2O
Compliance factor	3.8 cc/cm H_2O
PEEP	18 cm H_2O

A. 1030 cc
B. 890 cc
C. 930 cc
D. 845 cc
E. 742 cc

(3:756–9)

5. Which of the following most accurately represents the corrected (delivered) tidal volume if the set V_T is 45 cc, the peak pressure is 58 cm H_2O, and the tubing compliance factor is 0.6 cc/cm H_2O?

A. 5 cc
B. 10 cc
C. 15 cc
D. 30 cc
E. 25 cc

(3:756–9)

D. Effective Compliance and Resistance Pretest

Questions in this category are designed to evaluate the candidate's ability to assess pulmonary mechanics by calculating effective compliance and resistance values. The formulas for effective dynamic and static compliance are as follows:

$$\text{Effective dynamic compliance (EDC)} = \frac{\text{Corrected tidal volume (cc)}}{\text{Corrected peak pressure (cm } H_2O)}$$

and

$$\text{Effective static compliance (ESC)} = \frac{\text{Corrected tidal volume (cc)}}{\text{Corrected plateau pressure}}$$

In order for these calculations to be accurate, all peak and plateau pressure measurements must be corrected for PEEP. Additionally, when calculating ESC, compressed *volume determinations should be performed using plateau, not peak, pressure measurements.* (Please see the previous section, C, for further explanation.)

Using readily available data, the patient's effective airway resistance can be determined. The formula is as follows:

$$\text{Effective airway resistance (cm } H_2O\text{/L/sec)} = \frac{\text{(Proximal airway pressure)} - \text{(Plateau pressure)}}{\text{Inspiratory flow rate (L/sec)}}$$

This formula recognizes that the gradient between proximal and plateau pressures is due to nonelastic or "airway" resistance to gas flow. Widening of this gradient most typically occurs during episodes of bronchospasm or when excessive secretions accumulate in the airways. The following pretest was developed to help the candidate become proficient in these calculations and techniques.

1. Which of the following choices most accurately represents a patient's effective dynamic compliance if the corrected tidal volume is 730 cc, the peak pressure is 38 cm H_2O, and the ventilator plateau pressure is 23 cm H_2O?

A. 19 cc/cm H_2O
B. 45 cc/cm H_2O
C. 12 cc/cm H_2O
D. 74 cc/cm H_2O
E. 32 cc/cm H_2O

(3:183; 4:296)

2. What is the effective static compliance if the corrected tidal volume is 620 mL, the ventilator plateau pressure is 42 cm H_2O, and the peak pressure is 59 cm H_2O?

A. 28 cc/cm H_2O
B. 39 cc/cm H_2O
C. 10 cc/cm H_2O
D. 22 cc/cm H_2O
E. 15 cc/cm H_2O

(3:183; 4:296)

3. What is the effective static compliance if the corrected tidal volume is 880 mL, the ventilator plateau pressure is 53 cm H_2O, the peak pressure is 62 cm H_2O, and the patient is on 14 cm H_2O of PEEP?

A. 47 cc/cm H_2O
B. 17 cc/cm H_2O
C. 23 cc/cm H_2O
D. 12 cc/cm H_2O
E. 29 cc/cm H_2O

(3:183; 4:296)

4. What is the effective static compliance if the plateau pressure is 56 cm H_2O, the system compliance factor is 4.2 cc/cm H_2O, and the uncorrected tidal volume is 1200 cc?

A. 32 cc/cm H_2O
B. 17 cc/cm H_2O
C. 21 cc/cm H_2O
D. 48 cc/cm H_2O
E. 11 cc/cm H_2O

(3:183; 4:296)

5. Which of the following choices most accurately represents a patient's effective static compliance under the following clinical conditions?

Uncorrected tidal volume	920 cc
System compliance factor	2.4 cc/cm H_2O
Plateau pressure	44 cm H_2O
PEEP	16 cm H_2O

A. 20 cc/cm H_2O
B. 25 cc/cm H_2O
C. 30 cc/cm H_2O
D. 42 cc/cm H_2O
E. 35 cc/cm H_2O

(3:183; 4:296)

6. Which of the following choices most accurately represents a patient's effective airway resistance under the following clinical conditions?

Corrected tidal volume	1.0 L
Proximal airway (peak) pressure	45 cm H_2O
Plateau pressure	33 cm H_2O
Mean inspiratory flow rate	60 L/min

A. 4 cm H_2O/L/sec
B. 8 cm H_2O/L/sec
C. 12 cm H_2O/L/sec
D. 14 cm H_2O/L/sec
E. 18 cm H_2O/L/sec

(3:387; 4:25)

7. Which of the following choices most accurately represents a patient's effective airway resistance under the following conditions?

Corrected tidal volume	700 cc
Proximal airway (peak) pressure	58 cm H_2O
Plateau pressure	47 cm H_2O
Mean inspiratory flow rate	35 L/min
PEEP	12 cm H_2O

A. 19 cm H_2O/L/sec
B. 12 cm H_2O/L/sec
C. 24 cm H_2O/L/sec
D. 6 cm H_2O/L/sec
E. 34 cm H_2O/L/sec

(3:387; 4:25)

E. PEEP Compliance Study Pretest

In the absence of cardiac output and other values that are only possible in patients with pulmonary artery catheters in place, serial measurement of effective static compliance at different levels of PEEP is thought to be an effective method for determining the most appropriate level of this modality. The preferred level of PEEP is the one that gives the highest effective static compliance. The following pretest was developed to help the candidate become proficient in this technique.

1. The respiratory therapy practitioner is asked to place a patient on the lowest level of PEEP that yields the highest effective static compliance. After calculating the corrected tidal volume, which was adjusted to remain constant during this study, the following data were collected:

Level of PEEP (cm H_2O)	Plateau Pressure (cm H_2O)
3	34
6	35
9	37
12	41
15	45
18	49

Based on the above data, the preferred level of PEEP is:

A. 6 cm H_2O
B. 9 cm H_2O
C. 12 cm H_2O
D. 15 cm H_2O
E. 18 cm H_2O

(4:296)

2. The respiratory therapy practitioner is monitoring a 45-kg patient in the intensive care unit who is receiving continuous ventilatory support via a Servo 900 C ventilator. The patient's pulmonary wedge pressure (PWP) has risen rapidly over the past hour and is now 34 mm Hg. At this time the following clinical data are collected:

Pa_{O_2}	45 mm Hg
$S\bar{v}_{O_2}$	50%
$C(a-\bar{v})_{O_2}$	6.8 vol%
Peak pressure	48 cm H_2O
Plateau pressure	42 cm H_2O
PEEP	0 cm H_2O

Based on this information, the practitioner is asked to place the patient on the lowest level of PEEP that corresponds to the patient's highest effective static compliance. In so doing, the following data are collected:

Corrected Tidal Volume (cc)	Level of PEEP (cm H_2O)	Plateau Pressure (cm H_2O)
550	0	42
550	3	44
550	6	45
550	9	47
550	12	48
550	15	49
550	18	54
550	21	58

Based on the above information, at which of the following levels of PEEP is the patient's effective static compliance highest?

A. 9 cm H_2O
B. 12 cm H_2O
C. 15 cm H_2O
D. 18 cm H_2O
E. 21 cm H_2O

(4:296)

PART 4

Calculations Used to Assess Cardiopulmonary Status

Contents

A. Alveolar Ventilation Pretest

Because ventilation and oxygenation are the two major functions of the body's pulmonary system, few concepts are more fundamental than those of tidal, alveolar, and deadspace ventilation. Their relationship is expressed in the following formula:

$$V_A = V_T - V_D$$

This equation can also be rearranged so the practitioner can solve for the other two variables, as follows:

$$V_T = V_A + V_D$$

$$V_D = V_T - V_A$$

By multiplying the patient's respiratory rate by the tidal, alveolar, or deadspace ventilation, the values for minute alveolar (V_A), deadspace (V_D), and total minute ventilation ($\dot{V}_E$) can be determined.

The following pretest was developed to help the candidate become proficient in these calculations.

1. What is the alveolar ventilation under the following conditions?

V_T	950 cc
V_D	180 cc

A. 490 cc
B. 770 cc
C. 560 cc
D. 680 cc
E. 720 cc

(3:198; 4:266–7)

2. What is the minute alveolar ventilation (V_A) given the following conditions?

V_T	820 cc
V_D	230 cc
Respiratory rate	17/min

A. 13.5 L/min
B. 12.6 L/min
C. 9.3 L/min
D. 10.0 L/min
E. 14.2 L/min

(3:198)

3. What is the minute deadspace ventilation (V_D) given the following conditions?

V_A	260 mL
V_T	420 mL
Respiratory rate	42/min

A. 1.4L
B. 10.3L
C. 5.9L
D. 7.6L
E. 6.7L

(3:198)

B. V_D/V_T Calculation Pretest

Questions in this category are designed to assess the candidate's ability to calculate and use the deadspace to tidal volume ratio (V_D/V_T). This value is most frequently determined by using the Enghoff modification to the Bohr equation. This formula is as follows:

$$V_D / V_T = \frac{Paco_2 - P\bar{E}co_2}{Paco_2}$$

This value is readily determined at the patient's bedside by simultaneously obtaining samples of arterial blood and mixed expired gas and measuring their carbon dioxide tensions.

An application of the V_D/V_T relationship is its use in determining alveolar and physiologic deadspace ventilation by using the following formulas:

$$V_A = (V_T)\,(1 - V_D/V_T)$$

and

$$V_D = (V_T)\,(V_D/V_T)$$

The following pretest was developed to help the candidate become proficient in these calculations.

1. The respiratory therapy practitioner is asked to calculate the V_D/V_T of a patient whose $Paco_2$ is 53 mm Hg and whose mixed expired carbon dioxide tension ($P\bar{E}co_2$) is 31 mm Hg. Which of the following choices most accurately represents this value?

   A. 0.42
   B. 0.53
   C. 0.67
   D. 0.37
   E. 0.32

   (1:707–8)

2. The respiratory therapy practitioner is asked to determine the V_D/V_T given the following clinical data:

$Paco_2$	40 mm Hg
$P\bar{E}co_2$	28 mm Hg

   A. 0.75
   B. 0.67
   C. 0.30
   D. 0.25
   E. 0.39

   (1:707–8)

3. What is the V_D/V_T given the following conditions?

$Paco_2$	85 mm Hg
$P\bar{E}co_2$	33 mm Hg

   A. 0.46
   B. 0.61
   C. 0.29
   D. 0.73
   E. 0.87

   (1:707–8)

4. Given the following clinical conditions, calculate the minute alveolar ventilation (V_A) for a patient who is receiving 50% oxygen by way of a T tube setup.

V_T	830 cc
Respiratory rate	27/min
V_D/V_T	0.45

   Which of the following is the correct choice?

   A. 10.1 L/min
   B. 14.6 L/min
   C. 12.3 L/min
   D. 14.3 L/min
   E. 9.4 L/min

   (3:197–8)

5. What is the minute alveolar ventilation (V_A) given the following conditions?

V_T	1130 cc
Respiratory rate	29/min
V_D/V_T	0.74

   A. 8.5 L/min
   B. 4.7 L/min
   C. 9.3 L/min
   D. 12.4 L/min
   E. 5.1 L/min

   (3:197–8)

C. Oxygen Content Calculation Pretest

Questions in this category are designed to assess the candidate's ability to calculate the content of oxygen in samples of arterial and/or venous blood. To do this the practitioner must remember that the total amount of oxygen in any given sample of blood is equal to the sum of the quantity of oxygen combined with hemoglobin and the quantity of oxygen dissolved in the plasma. This concept is represented by the following formula:

Content O_2 in blood = (Hemoglobin concentration) (1.34) × (Hemoglobin saturation) + (PO_2 × 0.003)

The following pretest was developed to help the candidate become proficient in this calculation.

1. Which of the following choices most accurately represents the content of oxygen dissolved in the plasma of a patient whose PaO_2 is 570 mm Hg?

   A. 1.7 vol%
   B. 2.4 vol%
   C. 1.9 vol%
   D. 7.1 vol%
   E. 1.5 vol%

(4:116–17)

2. The respiratory therapy practitioner is asked to calculate the oxygen content of the arterial blood (CaO_2) given the following clinical data:

PaO_2	61 mm Hg
SaO_2	89%
Hb concentration	13.9 g/dL
O_2 carrying capacity	1.34 mL O_2/g Hb

   Which of the following most correctly represents this value?

   A. 16.8 vol%
   B. 17.9 vol%
   C. 13.0 vol%
   D. 17.2 vol%
   E. 17.4 vol%

(4:116–17)

3. The respiratory therapy practitioner is asked to calculate the arterial oxygen content of a patient given the following clinical conditions:

SaO_2	85%
Hb concentration	22.4 g/dL
O_2 carrying capacity	1.34 mL O_2/g Hb

   Which of the following most correctly represents this value?

   A. 24.2 vol%
   B. 20.9 vol%
   C. 26.7 vol%
   D. 25.5 vol%
   E. 28.4 vol%

(4:116–17)

4. A severely anemic patient is receiving hyperbaric oxygen therapy. The respiratory therapy practitioner is asked to calculate this patient's arterial oxygen content. Given the following clinical data, which of the following most accurately represents this value?

P_B	2.5 atmospheres
$PaCO_2$	35 mm Hg
$P(A–a)O_2$	240 mm Hg
SaO_2	100%
Hb concentration	3.6 g/dL
O_2 carrying capacity	1.34 mL O_2/g Hb

   A. 8.1 vol%
   B. 4.9 vol%
   C. 5.0 vol%
   D. 9.5 vol%
   E. 8.6 vol%

(4:116–17)

D. $P(A–a)O_2$ Calculation Pretest

Questions in this category are designed to assess the candidate's ability to calculate the $P(A–a)O_2$. This is done by determining the alveolar oxygen tension from any one of the alveolar air equations and subtracting from that value the patient's arterial oxygen tension. This value is used to assess patient oxygenation status. In general, values greater than 40 mm Hg in patients breathing room air are an indication for oxygen administration. Values greater than 350 mm Hg in patients receiving high concentrations of oxygen indicate the presence of refractory hypoxemia and usually require continuous ventilatory support with PEEP. The following pretest was designed to help the candidate become proficient at this calculation.

1. Which of the following most accurately represents the $P(A–a)O_2$ for a patient on whom the following clinical data were obtained?

PaO_2	88 mm Hg
P_B	760 mm Hg
FIO_2	0.40
$PaCO_2$	40 mm Hg
Respiratory exchange ratio (R)	0.8

   A. 147 mm Hg
   B. 175 mm Hg
   C. 216 mm Hg
   D. 125 mm Hg
   E. 235 mm Hg

(1:183; 4:113)

2. Given the following clinical data, which of the following most accurately represents the $P(A–a)O_2$?

PaO_2	148 mm Hg
P_B	710 mm Hg
FIO_2	0.85
$PaCO_2$	73 mm Hg
Respiratory exchange ratio (R)	0.8

   A. 285 mm Hg
   B. 343 mm Hg
   C. 316 mm Hg

D. 473 mm Hg
E. 360 mm Hg

(1:183; 4:113)

3. Given the following clinical data, which of the following most accurately represents this patient's Pa_{O_2}?

$P(A\text{–}a)O_2$	486 mm Hg
FI_{O_2}	0.80
P_B	760 mm Hg
Pa_{CO_2}	40 mm Hg
Respiratory exchange ratio (R)	0.8

A. 80 mm Hg
B. 20 mm Hg
C. 47 mm Hg
D. 65 mm Hg
E. 192 mm Hg

(1:183; 4:113)

E. Right-to-left Shunt ($\dot{Q}_S/\dot{Q}_T$) Equation Pretest (Advanced Level Only)

Questions in this category are designed to assess the candidate's ability to calculate $\dot{Q}_S/\dot{Q}_T$ for patients receiving respiratory care. This calculation, like the alveolar air equation, may present some confusion because multiple equations exist. In the interest of brevity and simplicity, only the two most common forms of these equations will be described here.

1. The Modified Clinical Shunt Equation

This is probably the most familiar form of the shunt equation. This stems not from its clinical applicability but from the fact that it is the easiest to understand. This equation is as follows:

$$\dot{Q}_S / \dot{Q}_T = \frac{(P(A-a)O_2)\ (0.003)}{[C(a-\bar{v})O_2] + [P(A-aO_2)\ (.003)]}$$

For this equation to be accurate, the following limited clinical condition must be met. *The patient's hemoglobin must be 100% saturated with oxygen.* This does not occur until the Pa_{O_2} reaches 150 mm Hg. It must be emphasized that this equation is accurate at *all* FI_{O_2}s as long as the Sa_{O_2} is 100%. The actual clinical usefulness of this equation is limited by the fact that the vast majority of patients are managed at Pa_{O_2}s considerably less than 150 mm Hg.

For those clinical situations when this condition does not exist, the practitioner will want to use the classic shunt equation described below.

2. The Classic Shunt Equation

This equation is accurate on all patients regardless of their FI_{O_2} or Pa_{O_2}. The equation is also more concise as can be noted below:

$$\dot{Q}_S / \dot{Q}_T = \frac{Cc'O_2 - Ca_{O_2}}{Cc'O_2 - C\bar{v}O_2}$$

In this equation the content of oxygen in the end pulmonary capillaries ($Cc'O_2$) can be calculated most easily if the patient is receiving an FI_{O_2} of 0.3 or greater. This oxygen concentration should allow for a PA_{O_2} of greater than 150 mm Hg. The tension of oxygen in end pulmonary capillary blood ($Pc'O_2$) is believed to be equivalent to that of those ventilated alveoli that they perfuse. Thus, an $Sc'O_2$ of 100% can be assumed under these circumstances. When the PA_{O_2} is less than 150 mm Hg, the $Sc'O_2$ must be determined by referring to the oxyhemoglobin dissociation curve. For either equation to be accurate, true mixed venous blood must be available. Although the modified clinical shunt equation is perhaps more frequently used, the classic version can be used on a broader patient population. When used on identical sets of patient data, both yield the same shunt fraction.

The following pretest was developed to help the candidate become proficient in these calculations and techniques.

1. The respiratory therapy practitioner is monitoring a 20-year-old patient in the intensive care unit who is receiving an FI_{O_2} of 1.0. A Pa_{O_2} of 265 mm Hg and a Pa_{CO_2} of 40 mm Hg exist at a P_B of 760 mm Hg. At the same time, a $C(a-\bar{v})O_2$ of 2.3 vol% is noted.

   Based on this information, what is the patient's right-to-left shunt fraction ($\dot{Q}_S/\dot{Q}_T$)?

A. 39%
B. 23%
C. 30%
D. 43%
E. 34%

(1:708; 4:244–5)

2. Which of the following most accurately represents the percent right-to-left shunt ($\dot{Q}_S/\dot{Q}_T$) for a patient on whom the following clinical data were collected?

P_B	760 mm Hg
FI_{O_2}	1.0
Pa_{CO_2}	40 mm Hg
Pa_{O_2}	150 mm Hg
Sa_{O_2}	100%
Hb concentration	15.0 g/dL
O_2 carrying capacity	1.34 mL O_2/g Hb
$C\bar{v}O_2$	16.3 vol%
Respiratory exchange ratio (R)	0.8

A. 32%
B. 30%
C. 20%
D. 17%
E. 19%

(1:708; 4:244–5)

3. Which of the following choices most accurately represents the right-to-left shunt fraction (Q_S/Q_T) for a patient on whom the following data were collected?

SaO_2	100%
$P(A\text{–}a)O_2$	500 mm Hg
$C(a\text{-}\bar{v})O_2$	8.0 vol%

A. 12%
B. 19%
C. 32%
D. 47%
E. 16%

(1:708; 4:244–5)

4. Which of the following most accurately represents the right-to-left shunt fraction (Q_S/Q_T) for a patient on whom the following clinical data were collected?

SaO_2	100%
$P(A\text{–}a)O_2$	500 mm Hg
$C(a\text{-}\bar{v})O_2$	2.5 vol%

A. 39%
B. 23%
C. 30%
D. 43%
E. 34%

(1:708; 4:244–5)

5. Which of the following most accurately represents the right-to-left shunt fraction (Q_S/Q_T) for a critically ill patient on whom the following clinical data were collected?

$Cc'O_2$	20.6 vol%
CaO_2	19.8 vol%
$C\bar{v}O_2$	16.3 vol%

A. 10%
B. 24%
C. 38%
D. 19%
E. 14%

(1:708; 4:244–5)

F. a/A Ratio Pretest (Advanced Level Only)

Questions in this category are designed to assess the practitioner's ability to calculate and use the a/A ratio formula:

$$\text{a/A Ratio} = \frac{PaO_2}{P_AO_2}$$

This value is used to assess patient oxygenation status. Clinically, values less than 0.60 are often believed to be an indication for oxygen administration. By the same token, values less than 0.15 are believed to indicate the presence of refractory hypoxemia, and usually the need for PEEP or CPAP therapy. The following pretest was developed to help the candidate become proficient in the above calculations and techniques.

1. Which of the following most accurately represents a patient's a/A ratio, given the following clinical data?

P_B	760 mm Hg
PCO_2	40 mm Hg
FIO_2	1.0
$P(A\text{–}a)O_2$	530 mm Hg
Respiratory exchange ratio (R)	0.8

A. 0.45
B. 0.20
C. 0.10
D. 0.15
E. 0.25

(1:183; 4:113)

2. Which of the following most accurately represents a patient's a/A ratio, given the following clinical data?

P_B	710 mm Hg
PaO_2	63 mm Hg
$PaCO_2$	47 mm Hg
FIO_2	0.70
Respiratory exchange ratio (R)	0.8

A. 0.15
B. 0.30
C. 0.10
D. 0.25
E. 0.33

(1:183; 4:113)

G. Respiratory Index Pretest (Advanced Level Only)

Questions in this category are designed to assess the practitioner's ability to calculate the so-called respiratory index. The formula for this is as follows:

$$\text{Respiratory index} = \frac{P(A-a)O_2}{PaO_2}$$

This value is used to assess patient oxygenation status. Clinically, a value greater than 1.0 is often believed to be an indication for oxygen administration. By the same token, values greater than 6.0 are believed to indicate the presence of refractory hypoxemia, and usually the need for PEEP or CPAP therapy. The following pretest was developed to help the candidate become proficient in the above calculations and techniques.

1. Which of the following choices most accurately represents a patient's respiratory index, given the following clinical data?

PaO_2	85 mm Hg
$PaCO_2$	50 mm Hg
Respiratory exchange ratio (R)	0.8
FIO_2	0.45
P_B	760 mm Hg

A. 1.8
B. 2.0
C. 2.2
D. 2.4
E. 3.1

(1:183; 4:113)

2. Which of the following choices most accurately represents a patient's respiratory index, given the following clinical data?

PaO_2	45 mm Hg
$PaCO_2$	65 mm Hg
Respiratory exchange ratio (R)	0.8
FIO_2	0.8
P_B	760 mm Hg

A. 3.0
B. 4.2
C. 5.3
D. 7.8
E. 10.2

(1:183; 4:113)

H. $C(a-\bar{v})O_2$ Pretest (Advanced Level Only)

Questions in this category are designed to assess the practitioner's ability to calculate the arterial minus venous oxygen content difference ($C(a-\bar{v})O_2$). To determine this value, the practitioner must have access to mixed venous blood from the pulmonary artery as well as to an arterial sample. This value is used to assess cardiovascular reserve and is a necessary part of the shunt equations. Among critically ill patients whose oxygen consumption is within normal limits *and* who have minimal peripheral arteriovenous shunting, $C(a-\bar{v})O_2$ values less than 4.0 vol% generally indicate the existence of good cardiovascular reserves, whereas values greater than 6.0 vol% are believed to indicate poor cardiovascular reserves. The following pretest was developed to help the candidate become proficient in calculating this value.

1. The respiratory therapy practitioner is monitoring a patient who is receiving continuous ventilatory support by way of a Servo 900 B ventilator. The following clinical data are obtained at this time from properly functioning central arterial and peripheral arterial lines:

Parameter	Arterial	Mixed Venous
PO_2	53 mm Hg	29 mm Hg
SO_2	85%	61%
Hb	9.7 g/dL	9.7 g/dL

Based on the above information, which of the following most accurately represents this patient's $C(a-\bar{v})O_2$ (use an O_2 carrying capacity of 1.34 mL O_2/g Hb)?

A. 4.6 vol%
B. 1.9 vol%
C. 2.8 vol%
D. 3.6 vol%
E. 3.2 vol%

(4:247–8)

2. Which of the following choices most accurately represents the $C(a-\bar{v})O_2$ for a patient on whom the following clinical data are collected?

PaO_2	46 mm Hg
SaO_2	80%
Hb concentration	19.1 g/dL
$P\bar{v}O_2$	26 mm Hg
$S\bar{v}O_2$	49%
O_2 carrying capacity	1.34 mL O_2/g Hb

A. 4.7 vol%
B. 9.2 vol%
C. 1.6 vol%
D. 7.3 vol%
E. 8.0 vol%

(4:247–8)

3. Which of the following choices most accurately represents the $C(a-\bar{v})O_2$ for a patient on whom the following clinical data are collected?

PaO_2	235 mm Hg
SaO_2	100%
Hb concentration	22.3 g/dL
$P\bar{v}O_2$	45 mm Hg
$S\bar{v}O_2$	76%
$PaCO_2$	29 mm Hg
P_B	745 mm Hg
FIO_2	0.8
O_2 carrying capacity	1.34 mL O_2/g Hb

A. 7.3 vol%
B. 6.7 vol%
C. 4.9 vol%
D. 5.2 vol%
E. 6.1 vol%

(4:247–8)

I. Fick Equation Pretest (Advanced Level Only)

Questions in this category are designed to assess the practitioner's ability to perform hemodynamic calculations using the Fick equation. This equation is as follows:

$$\text{Oxygen consumption} = (\text{Cardiac output})\ (C(a\text{-}\bar{v})O_2)$$

The units for this equation are as follows:

$$\frac{\text{mL Oxygen}}{\text{min}} = \frac{\text{mL Blood}}{\text{min}} \times \frac{\text{mL Oxygen}}{100\ \text{mL Blood}}$$

Thus, in a healthy, resting subject:

$$\frac{250\ \text{mL Oxygen}}{\text{min}} = \frac{5000\ \text{mL Blood}}{\text{min}} \times \frac{5.0\ \text{mL Oxygen}}{100\ \text{mL Blood}}$$

This equation can be rearranged to solve for cardiac output and C $(a\text{-}\bar{v})O_2$ as follows:

$$\text{Cardiac output} = \frac{\text{Oxygen consumption}}{C(a - \bar{v})O_2}$$

and

$$C(a - \bar{v})O_2 = \frac{\text{Oxygen consumption}}{\text{Cardiac output}}$$

The following pretest was developed to help the candidate become proficient in these calculations.

1. Given the following clinical data, which of the following represents the oxygen consumption ($\dot{V}O_2$) for a 50-kg patient?

Cardiac output ($\dot{Q}_T$)	3.9 L/min
$C(a\text{-}\bar{v})O_2$	6.8 vol%

   A. 310 mL/min
   B. 265 mL/min
   C. 250 mL/min
   D. 422 mL/min
   E. 235 mL/min

   (4:242; 5:188–9)

2. Given the following clinical data, calculate the oxygen consumption ($\dot{V}O_2$) for the following patient:

Cardiac output ($\dot{Q}_T$)	4.8 L/min
$C(a\text{-}\bar{v})O_2$	2.4 vol%

   Which of the following is the most correct choice?

   A. 115 mL/min
   B. 130 mL/min
   C. 96 mL/min
   D. 105 mL/min
   E. 200 mL/min

   (4:242; 5:188–9)

3. The respiratory therapy practitioner is monitoring the cardiopulmonary status of a patient who is receiving continuous ventilatory support. The following clinical data are made available at this time:

Cardiac output	9.8 L/min
$Pa O_2$	53 mm Hg
$P\bar{v}O_2$	29 mm Hg
$Sa O_2$	84%
$S\bar{v}O_2$	55%
Hb concentration	16.8 g/dL
O_2 carrying capacity	1.34 mL O_2/g Hb

   Based on the above information, which of the following most accurately represents this patient's oxygen consumption ($\dot{V}O_2$)?

   A. 560 mL/min
   B. 575 mL/min
   C. 600 mL/min
   D. 720 mL/min
   E. 637 mL/min

   (4:242; 5:188–9)

4. Given the following clinical information, calculate this patient's cardiac output ($\dot{Q}_T$):

Oxygen consumption ($\dot{V}O_2$)	250 mL/min
$C(a\text{-}\bar{v})O_2$	4.0 vol%

   A. 6.7 L/min
   B. 4.7 L/min
   C. 6.3 L/min
   D. 5.8 L/min
   E. 9.6 L/min

   (4:242; 5:188–9)

5. Given the following clinical information, calculate the $C(a\text{-}\bar{v})O_2$ for this 70-kg patient:

Cardiac output ($\dot{Q}_T$)	8.3 L/min
Oxygen consumption ($\dot{V}O_2$)	380 mL/min

   Which is the single best choice?

   A. 2.1 vol%
   B. 3.9 vol%
   C. 4.4 vol%
   D. 8.9 vol%
   E. 4.6 vol%

   (4:242; 5:188–9)

J. Pulmonary Vascular Resistance Pretest (Advanced Level Only)

Questions in this category are designed to assess the practitioner's ability to calculate pulmonary vascular resistance. This formula, like all resistance formulas, is derived from the Poiseuille and Ohm formulas. Therefore, just as the airway resistance formula asks one to divide the pressure drop across the conducting airways by the inspiratory flow rate, the pulmonary vascular resistance (PVR) formula asks that one divide the pressure drop across the pulmonary vascular circuit by the flow rate of blood through that circuit (i.e., the cardiac output). The following formulas represent two different ways to calculate PVR:

$$\text{Pulmonary vascular resistance (dyne-sec/cm}^{-5}\text{)} = \frac{\text{Mean PA pressure} - \text{PWP}}{\text{Cardiac output}} \times 80$$

The normal range for pulmonary vascular resistance (PVR) is 100–250 dyne sec/cm^{-5} or

$$\text{Pulmonary vascular resistance (mm Hg/L/min)} = \frac{\text{Mean PA pressure} - \text{PWP}}{\text{Cardiac output}}$$

The normal range for PVR in mm Hg/L/min is 1.5 to 3.0. For an individual with perfectly normal pulmonary arterial pressures, the calculation would be as follows:

$$\text{Mean PA pressure} = 15 \text{ mm Hg}$$

$$\text{PWP} = 9 \text{ mm Hg}$$

$$\text{Cardiac output} = 6.0 \text{ L/min}$$

$$\frac{15 - 9}{6} \times 80 = 53 \text{ dyne-sec/cm}^{-5}$$

or

$$\frac{15 - 9}{6} = 1.0 \text{ mm Hg/L/min}$$

These equations clearly show that the drop in pressure from the right to the left ventricle increases in direct proportion to the resistance to flow within that circuit.

Clinically, a reliable estimate of the pulmonary vascular resistance can be gathered by subtracting the pulmonary wedge pressure (PWP) from the pulmonary artery diastolic pressure (PAD). A PAD–PWP gradient greater than 5 mm Hg is believed to indicate abnormal resistance to right ventricular output (see reference 5). The following pretest was developed to help the candidate become proficient in this area.

1. The respiratory therapy practitioner is monitoring a critically ill patient in the intensive care unit. The following clinical data are collected from the patient's pulmonary artery catheter:

Pulmonary artery mean pressure	20 mm Hg
Cardiac output	6.0 L/min
Pulmonary wedge pressure	8 mm Hg

Which of the following choices most accurately represents this patient's pulmonary vascular resistance in dyne-sec/cm^{-5}?

A. 145
B. 200
C. 130
D. 160
E. 122

(5:158)

2. Given the following information, calculate the pulmonary vascular resistance in dyne-sec/cm^{-5}:

Pulmonary artery mean pressure	38 mm Hg
Cardiac output	3.9 L/min
Pulmonary wedge pressure	4 mm Hg

A. 697
B. 553
C. 450
D. 229
E. 326

(5:158)

3. Given the following information, calculate the pulmonary vascular resistance in mm Hg/L/min.

Pulmonary artery mean pressure	20 mm Hg
Cardiac output	3.0 L/min
Pulmonary wedge pressure	13 mm Hg

A. 2.7
B. 1.8
C. 2.3
D. 1.3
E. 3.5

(13:697–8)

PART 5

Calculations Used in Pulmonary Function Testing

Contents

A. Lung Volume and Capacity Pretest

Questions in this category are designed to assess the practitioner's ability to calculate the various lung volumes and capacities given appropriate laboratory data. These calculations and their solutions are all derived from the familiar lung volume and capacity diagram for a 70-kg patient that appears below:

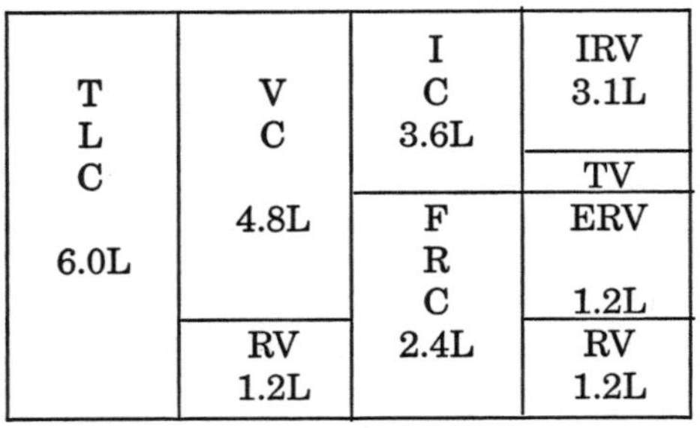

<table>
<tr><td rowspan="4">T
L
C

6.0L</td><td rowspan="3">V
C

4.8L</td><td rowspan="2">I
C
3.6L</td><td>IRV
3.1L</td></tr>
<tr><td>TV</td></tr>
<tr><td rowspan="2">F
R
C
2.4L</td><td>ERV

1.2L</td></tr>
<tr><td>RV
1.2L</td><td>RV
1.2L</td></tr>
</table>

The following pretest was developed to help the candidate become proficient in these techniques.

1. In response to a physician's order, the respiratory therapy practitioner gathers the following laboratory data:

IRV	2150 cc
TV	480 cc
ERV	2340 cc
RV	1470 cc

Based on the above information, which of the following most accurately represents this patient's total lung capacity?

A. 5830 cc
B. 7220 cc
C. 6260 cc
D. 6440 cc
E. 7000 cc

(3:178; 6:15–18)

2. Based on the following laboratory data, which of the choices most accurately represents the patient's vital capacity?

IRV	1725 cc
TV	355 cc
FRC	1630 cc
RV	920 cc

A. 2790 cc
B. 4230 cc
C. 3660 cc
D. 2940 cc
E. 3920 cc

(3:178; 6:1–4)

3. Given the following information, calculate the ERV.

IRV	3940 cc
FRC	2680 cc
TV	555 cc
RV	1175 cc

A. 2135 cc
B. 1175 cc
C. 1205 cc
D. 1675 cc
E. 1505 cc

(3:178; 6:1–4)

4. Given the following information, calculate the inspiratory reserve volume.

VC	1350 cc
FRC	1030 cc
RV	675 cc
TV	135 cc

A. 740 cc
B. 690 cc
C. 820 cc
D. 910 cc
E. 860 cc

(3:178; 6:1–4)

5. Given the following information, calculate the RV/TLC ratio.

IRV	1050 cc
TV	330 cc
FRC	1905 cc
VC	2670 cc

A. 19%
B. 13%
C. 32%
D. 10%
E. 25%

(3:178; 6:19)

B. Spirometry Pretest (Advanced Level Only)

Clinical spirometry is an area from which many different types of questions may be drawn. Some of these are as follows:

1. Percent Predicted Question
   To determine the value, the following formula is used:

$$\% \text{ Predicted} = \frac{\text{Observed value}}{\text{Predicted value}}$$

2. Bell Factor Question
   A spirometer's "bell factor" is the number of cc's of gas that must be displaced in order to move the bell and pen assembly 1.0 mm. For instance, if a particular spirometer has a factor of 41.27 cc/mm, a 25-mm vertical excursion noted on the recording paper will be generated each time 1030 cc is moved in or out of the bell. This volume, like all recorded volumes, must be expanded from ATPS to BTPS.
3. Percent Improvement After Bronchodilation (BD) Question
   The formula for this is:

$$\% \text{ Improvement after BD} = \frac{\text{Value observed after BD} - \text{Value observed before BD}}{\text{Value observed before BD}}$$

The following pretest was developed to help the candidate become proficient in these calculations and techniques.

1. From the following information, calculate the $FEV_1/FVC\%$.

FVC	4.12 L
FEV_1	3.06 L
$FEF_{200-200}$	6.53 L/sec
FEF_{25-75}	3.82 L/sec

A. 83%
B. 80%
C. 74%
D. 72%
E. 68%

(6:49–50)

2. From the following information, calculate the $FEV_3/FVC\%$.

Measured excursion of FVC	42 mm
Measured excursion of FEV_3	36 mm
Bell factor	41.27 cc/mm
ATPS to BTPS correction factor	1.096

A. 74%
B. 90%
C. 53%
D. 86%
E. 94%

(6:49–50)

3. The practitioner has just performed an FVC test on a patient with obstructive lung disease. In calculating the results of this effort, he/she makes hatch marks at points that are equal to 25% and 75% of the volume measured by the FVC tracing. The practitioner then draws a line through these two points, making sure the line crosses two vertical time lines representing 1 sec. The tangent crosses the first time line at a volume of 11,300 cc and the second time line at 8250 cc. Subsequently, the following data are noted:

ATPS to BTPS correction factor	1.102
Predicted FEF_{25-75}	4.95 L/sec

Based on the above data, what percent of predicted is this patient's observed FEF_{25-75}?

A. 72%
B. 68%
C. 85%
D. 60%
E. 42%

(6:49–50)

4. Following administration of 0.5 cc of 1:200 isoproterenol, a patient's $FEF_{25\text{-}75}$ is noted to increase from 1.35 L/min to 1.90 L/ min. Which of the following choices most accurately represents the percent improvement experienced by this patient?

A. 40%
B. 50%
C. 25%
D. 35%
E. 15%

(6:51–4)

C. Residual Volume Pretest (Advanced Level Only)

Questions in this category are designed to assess the practitioner's ability to calculate a patient's residual volume, functional residual capacity, or total lung capacity by open circuit nitrogen washout or closed circuit helium dilution methods. These volumes must also be converted to BTPS. The formulas for these are as follows:

1. Open-Circuit Nitrogen Washout Formula for determination of FRC

$$\text{FRC} = \frac{[\text{Final nitrogen \%} \times (\text{VE} + \text{VD})] - (\text{T} \times \text{Nitrogen correction})}{0.75}$$

VE = volume expired
VD = deadspace ventilation
T = test time
N_2 correction = 0.04 L/min (blood/tissue nitrogen washout factor)

2. Closed-Circuit Helium Dilution Formula

$$\text{FRC} = \left(\frac{\text{Initial He \%} - \text{Final He \%}}{\text{Final He \%}}\right) \times \left(\begin{matrix}\text{Initial volume} \\ -\text{He correction}\end{matrix}\right)$$

$$\text{Initial volume} = \frac{\text{He added}}{\text{Initial He \%}}$$

He absorption correction = 0.1 L

The following pretest was developed to help the candidate become proficient in these calculations.

1. The physician's order reads: "Patient to go to Pulmonary Function Lab for determination of all lung volumes and capacities." The following information is obtained by the respiratory therapy practitioner:

Spirometer Data

VC at ATPS	5240 cc
TV at ATPS	950 cc
IRV at ATPS	3110 cc
Correction factor from ATPS to BTPS	1.102

Data from 7-Minute Nitrogen Washout

Volume in Douglas bag	38.5 L
Concentration of final N_2 in Douglas bag	8.2%
Alveolar N_2 concentration	75%

Based on the above information, which of the following choices most correctly represents this patient's residual volume?

A. 1.8 L
B. 2.4 L
C. 3.5 L
D. 1.6 L
E. 2.9 L

(6:4–11)

2. A patient is seen in the pulmonary function laboratory for determination of his total lung capacity. From the following information, calculate its value.

Spirometric Data

IRV at ATPS	1.52 L
TV at ATPS	0.32 L
VC at ATPS	2.66 L
Correction factor from ATPS to BTPS	1.085

Data from 7-Minute Nitrogen Washout

Volume in spirometer	41.8 L
Concentration of N_2 in spirometer	6.7%
Alveolar N_2 concentration	75%

Based on the above data, which of the following most accurately represents this patient's TLC?

A. 6.05 L
B. 5.2 L
C. 4.8 L
D. 3.8 L
E. 5.6 L

(6:1–4)

3. Data were obtained from a closed-circuit helium dilution study. The subject was a 63-year-old woman with an 80 pack/year history:

Original volume in spirometer	2.8 L
Original concentration of helium	10.6%
Final concentration of helium	4.3%
Temperature correction factor	1.102

Based on the above information which choice most accurately represents this patient's FRC?

A. 3.6 L
B. 4.1 L
C. 4.6 L
D. 2.7 L
E. 2.3 L

(6:9 377–8)

PART 6

Calculations Used in Pharmacology

Contents

A. Units of Measurement Pretest

Questions in this category are designed to assess the practitioner's understanding of the various units of measurement commonly used in respiratory pharmacotherapeutics.

The following pretest was developed to help the candidate become proficient in these techniques.

1. Which of the following most accurately represents the weight of a volume of water 1 cc in size?

   A. 1.0 g
   B. 2.0 g
   C. 1000 mg
   D. 100 mg
   E. A and C are correct.

(7:75–81)

2. Which of the following most accurately represents the weight of a volume of water 1 mL in size?

   A. 1.0 g
   B. 1000 mg
   C. 10 g
   D. 1.0 μg
   E. A and B are correct.

(7:75–81)

3. Approximately how many milliliters are contained in a sample of water that occupies 1000 cc?

   A. 1.0
   B. 1000
   C. 50
   D. 5000
   E. 500

(7:75–81)

4. How many milligrams are there in 0.016 g?

   A. 160
   B. 16
   C. 1.6
   D. 320
   E. 640

(7:75–81)

5. How many micrograms are there in 1.0 mg?

   A. 1000
   B. 10,000
   C. 100,000
   D. 10
   E. 100

(7:75–81)

6. How many standard drops does it take to equal 1 mL of H_2O?

   A. 65
   B. 125
   C. 64
   D. 32
   E. 16

(7:75–81)

B. Percent and Ratio Solution Pretest

To understand these concepts, it is best to start by defining the following terms:

- *Solute*—the solid drug that is dissolved in the solvent.
- *Solvent*—the liquid media into which the drug (solute) is dissolved. Most drugs are dissolved in an aqueous solvent (H_2O). It is important to remember that 1.0 mL of H_2O weighs almost exactly 1 g. Thus, 100 mL of water will weigh 100 g.
- *Solution*—the mixture of solid solute and aqueous solvent.

Interestingly enough, when relatively small quantities of solute are dissolved in an aqueous medium, the total *volume* of the solution does not change appreciably. Thus, if 1000 mg of a drug is added to 100 mL of the H_2O, the resulting solution would weigh 101 g but still occupy 100 mL.

There are basically two types of solutions that the respiratory therapy practitioner will encounter:

1. Percent Solutions

$$\text{Solution percentage} = \frac{\text{Weight of solution}}{\text{Volume of solvent}} \times 100$$

   Thus, in the previous example 1000 mg of a given drug added to 100 mL of H_2O will result in a 1.0% solution. Percent solutions are sometimes called weight-to-volume (W/V) solutions.
2. Ratio Solutions
   A ratio solution is defined by the following formula, which indicates the ratio of solute weight to solvent weight:

$$\text{Solution ratio} = \text{Weight solute} + \text{Weight solvent}$$

   Thus, in the continuing example, 1000 mg of a given drug added to 100 mL of aqueous solution will result in a 1:100 solution. Ratio solutions are sometimes referred to as weight-to-weight (W/W) solutions.

- *Concentration*—When applied to pharmacologic agents this refers to the quantity of solute per unit of final solution. The most commonly used units for concentration are mg/mL. Thus, both a 1.0% (W/V) solution and a 1:100 (W/W) solution have a concentration of 10 mg/mL.

The following pretest was designed to test the candidate's understanding of these concepts and computations.

1. The respiratory therapy practitioner is asked to add 1.0 g of metaproterenol to 100 mL of aqueous solvent. This will result in which of the following concentrations?

   I. 1:1000
   II. 0.1%
   III. 1:100
   IV. 1.0%
   V. 0.01%

   A. I and II
   B. III only
   C. I and IV
   D. III and IV
   E. V only

(7:81–3)

2. If 250 mg of solute is added to 100 mL aqueous solvent, the result will be which of the following solutions?

   I. 0.4%
   II. 1:400
   III. 0.25%
   IV. 1:200
   V. 1:250

   A. II and III
   B. III and IV
   C. III only
   D. I and II
   E. I and V

(7:81–3)

3. If the practitioner adds 100 mg of a drug to 100 mL aqueous solvent, the result will be which of the following solutions?

   I. 0.1%
   II. 0.01%
   III. 1.0%
   IV. 1:1000
   V. 1:10,000

   A. II and IV
   B. I and IV
   C. II and V
   D. III and IV
   E. I and III

(7:81–3)

4. If the practitioner adds 2.0 g solute to 100 mL of aqueous solution, the result will be which of the following solutions?

   I. 1:250
   II. 1:50
   III. 2%
   IV. 1:400
   V. 4%

   A. II and III
   B. I and III
   C. II and V
   D. IV only
   E. I and V

(7:81–3)

5. The practitioner is asked to administer 1.0 mL of a 1.0% solution of isoetharine to an asthmatic patient. How many milligrams of drug does this represent?

   A. 10
   B. 20

C. 100
D. 1000
E. 1.0

(7:85–91)

6. The respiratory therapy practitioner is asked to administer 0.5 mL of a 1:200 solution of isoetharine. How many milligrams of drug does this represent?

A. 5.0
B. 2.5
C. 10
D. 4.0
E. 1.0

(7:85–91)

7. The respiratory therapy practitioner is asked to administer 3.0 mL of a 0.17% solution of bronchodilator to an asthmatic patient. Approximately how many milligrams of drug does this represent?

A. 1.0
B. 2.5
C. 5
D. 10
E. 24

(7:85–91)

8. The physician's order reads: "Administer 5 mg metaproterenol via hand-held nebulizer." How many milliliters of a 1:100 solution should be used?

A. 0.5
B. 1.0
C. 1.5
D. 2.0
E. 2.5

(7:85–91)

9. The physician's order reads: "Administer 75 mg Decadron® via hand-held nebulizer." How many milliliters of a 2.5% solution should be used?

A. 2.2
B. 0.5
C. 3.0
D. 1.5
E. 4.5

(7:85–91)

10. The physician's order reads: "Administer 15 mg metaproterenol via hand-held nebulizer." How many milliliters of a 2% solution should be used?

A. 1.0
B. 1.5
C. 0.75
D. 1.75
E. 0.5

(7:85–91)

C. Drug Dilution Pretest

Questions in this category are designed to assess the candidate's ability to dilute various pharmacologic agents from an original concentration to a desired concentration in accordance with a physician's order. The formula for this is as follows:

$$\text{Volume of diluent to be added} = \text{Total or new drug vol.} - \text{Original drug vol.}$$

$$\text{Total (new) volume} = \frac{\text{(Original volume) (Original concentration)}}{\text{New (desired) concentration}}$$

Thus, if the physician wants a 5% solution of acetylcysteine made up, and 20 mL of a 20% solution is all there is, the calculation is as follows:

$$\frac{(20\text{ mL }(20\%)}{5\%} = 80\text{ mL}$$

It is therefore known that the total volume of the new solution is 80 mL. Inserting this value into the original formula reveals the following:

Volume of diluent to be added = 80 mL – 20 mL = 60 mL

Thus, 60 mL of diluent (H_2O) must be added to 20 mL of a 20% solution in order to yield a 5% solution. The following pretest was developed to help the candidate become proficient in these calculations and techniques.

1. The respiratory therapy practitioner is asked to dilute 100 mL of a 2% solution of beclomethasone to a 1.0% concentration. How many milliliters of water must be added to the original mixture to obtain the desired concentration?

A. 100
B. 50
C. 200
D. 150
E. 10

(7:85–91)

2. How many milliliters of water must be added to 10 mL of a 20% solution of acetylcysteine to dilute it to a 5% concentration?

A. 40
B. 30
C. 50
D. 20
E. 10

(7:85–91)

3. The physician's order reads: "Instill 5 mL 5% $NaHCO_3$ q. 4h and p.r.n." All that is on hand are 50-mL ampules of an 8.4% solution. How many milliliters of distilled water must be added to obtain a 5% solution?

   A. 10
   B. 21
   C. 34
   D. 42
   E. 84

(7:85–91)

4. The medical director requests that a large quantity of 35% ETOH be made up. Using 500 mL of a 95% solution, approximately how much of the new solution can be made up?

   A. 1250 mL
   B. 1360 mL
   C. 1400 mL
   D. 1500 mL
   E. 1175 mL

(7:85–91)

Answer Key

Part I

A. 1. D 2. A 3. D 4. D 5. B
B. 1. B 2. D 3. E 4. E
C. 1. E 2. D
D. 1. B 2. C 3. C
E. 1. A 2. C 3. A
F. 1. A 2. E 3. D 4. C 5. B 6. C
G. 1. E 2. C
H. 1. D 2. B 3. C

Part II

A. 1. C 2. B 3. C 4. C 5. A 6. B 7. A 8. D
B. 1. A 2. B 3. D
C. 1. D 2. B 3. D
D. 1. B 2. A
E. 1. E 2. D

Part III

A. 1. C 2. D 3. B 4. A 5. E 6. A
B. 1. C 2. E 3. D 4. B 5. C 6. A
C. 1. E 2. D 3. D 4. B 5. B
D. 1. A 2. E 3. C 4. B 5. C 6. C 7. A
E. 1. B 2. C

Part IV

A. 1. B 2. D 3. E
B. 1. A 2. C 3. B 4. C 5. A
C. 1. A 2. A 3. D 4. D
D. 1. A 2. B 3. C
E. 1. E 2. B 3. E 4. A 5. D
F. 1. B 2. A
G. 1. B 2. E
H. 1. E 2. E 3. A
I. 1. B 2. A 3. E 4. C 5. E
J. 1. D 2. A 3. C

Part V

A. 1. D 2. A 3. E 4. E 5. A
B. 1. C 2. D 3. B 4. A
C. 1. E 2. E 3. C

Part VI

A. 1. E 2. E 3. B 4. B 5. A 6. E
B. 1. D 2. A 3. B 4. A 5. A 6. B 7. C 8. A 9. C 10. C
C. 1. A 2. B 3. C 4. B

EXPLANATIONS

Unit I

Part I

A.

1. D. There are 28.316 liters of oxygen in one cubic foot of gaseous oxygen.
2. A. A full E cylinder of oxygen contains 622 L.
3. D. A full H cylinder of oxygen contains 6900 L.
4. D. One cubic foot of liquid oxygen = 860.6 cubic feet of gaseous oxygen at ambient pressure and temperature.
5. B. Cylinder factor

$$= \frac{\text{cubic feet in a full cylinder x 28.3}}{\text{pressure of a full cylinder (psig)}}$$

or

$$\frac{\text{L of gas in a full cylinder}}{\text{pressure of a full cylinder (psig)}}$$

Cylinder factor = 356/2200 = 0.16

B.

1. B. Cylinder duration

$$= \frac{\text{pressure in cylinder} \times \text{cylinder factor}}{\text{delivered liter flow}}$$

Cylinder duration

$$= \frac{2200 \times 0.28}{3} = 205.3 \text{ min}/60 = 3.42 \text{ hours}$$

3.42 hours = 3 hr 25 min (.42 × 60)

2. D. Cylinder duration $= \frac{1600 \times 2.41}{5}$

$$= 771 \text{ min}/60 = 12.85 \text{ hours}$$

12.85 hr = 12 hr 51 min (0.85 × 60)

3. E. Cylinder duration $= \frac{2200 \times 3.14}{4}$
$= 1727$ min/60 = 28.78 hr

28.78 hr = 28 hr 47 min (0.78×60)

4. E. Cylinder duration $= \frac{700 \times 3.14}{7}$
$= 314$ min/60 = 5.2 hr

5.2 hr = 5 hr 12 min (0.2×60)

C.

1. E. $FIO_2 = \frac{(0.21 \times 9) + (1.0 \times 6)}{15} = \frac{1.89 + 6}{15} = \frac{7.89}{15} = 0.526$

2. D. $FIO_2 = \frac{(0.21 \times 15) + (1.0 \times 5)}{20} = \frac{3.15 + 5}{20} = \frac{8.15}{20} = 0.40$

D.

1. B. $PIO_2 = 0.21(760 - 47) = 149.7 = 150$ mm Hg
2. C. $PIO_2 = 0.40(727 - 47) = 272$ mm Hg
3. C. $PIO_2 = 0.70(420 - 47) = 261$ mm Hg

E.

1. A. $PAO_2 = 0.21(760 - 47) - (40 \times 1.25) = 150 - 50 = 100$ mm Hg
2. C. $PAO_2 = 1.0(640 - 47) - 30$ (remember, with $FIO_2 > 0.60$, R can be eliminated) $= 593 - 30 = 563$ mm Hg
3. A. $PAO_2 = 0.4(730 - 47) - (55 \times 1.25) = 273 - 69 = 204$ mm Hg

F.

1. A. Air:oxygen $= \frac{100 - 40}{40 - 20} = \frac{60}{20} = \frac{\text{3 L air for each}}{\text{1 L oxygen}}$
2. E. Air:oxygen $= \frac{100 - 60}{60 - 20} = \frac{40}{40} = \frac{\text{1 L air for each}}{\text{1 L oxygen}}$
3. D. Air:oxygen $= \frac{100 - 24}{24 - 21} = \frac{76}{3} = \frac{\text{25 L air for each}}{\text{1 L oxygen}}$

   Remember to use 0.21 for $FIO_2 \le 0.30$.

4. C. Air:oxygen $= \frac{100 - 40}{40 - 20} = \frac{60}{20} = \frac{\text{3 L air for each}}{\text{1 L oxygen}}$

   Total flow = 4 L (3 L air + 1 L oxygen) × 8 L/min = 32 L/min

5. B. Air:oxygen $= \frac{100 - 65}{65 - 20} = \frac{35}{45} = \frac{\text{0.8 L air for each}}{\text{1 L oxygen}}$

   Total flow = 1.8 L (0.8 L air + 1 L oxygen) × 12 L/min = 21.6 L/min = 22 L/min

6. C. Air:oxygen $= \frac{100 - 24}{24 - 21} = \frac{76}{3} = \frac{\text{25 L air for each}}{\text{1 L oxygen}}$

   Total flow = 26 L (25 L air + 1 L oxygen) × 4 L/min = 104 L/min

G.

1. E. Because the density of helium-oxygen mixtures is lower than the density of oxygen, and because oxygen flowmeters depend on the metered gas's kinetic support of a float, correction factors must be used in order to calculate flow rates for helium-oxygen mixtures. The correction factor for 80% He-20% O_2 mixtures is 1.8.

   $10 \times 1.8 = 18$ L/min

2. C. The correction factor for 70% He-30% O_2 mixtures is 1.6.

   $10 \times 1.6 = 16$ L/min

H.

1. D. Each atmosphere (ATA) above sea level is equivalent to 33 feet of sea water (FSW): 2 ATA = 33 FSW; 3 ATA = 66 FSW; 4 ATA = 99 FSW, etc. Thus, a diver submerged 100 feet deep experiences a pressure of approximately 4 ATA.
2. B. 2 ATA = 760 × 2 = 1520 mm Hg
   P sample $O_2 = FIO_2(PB - H_2O \text{ press.}) = 0.21(1520 - 47) = 1473 \times 0.21 = 309.3$ mm Hg
3. C. 1.5 ATA = 1140 mm Hg
   $PAO_2 = 1.0(1140 - 47) - 40 \times 1.25$
   = 1093 − 40 (Again, R may be eliminated because the FIO_2 is > 0.60.)
   = 1053 mm Hg

Part II

A.

1. C. STPD represents the conditions of a gas volume at 0° Centigrade, at 760 mm Hg, without water vapor (0 mm Hg).
   - 760 mm Hg = 14.7 psig = 1 ATA = 1034 g/cm^2
   - 0° C = 273° Kelvin
2. B. ATPD represents the condition of a gas volume at ambient temperature, ambient pressure, without water vapor (0 mm Hg).
3. C. ATPS represents the condition of a volume of gas at ambient temperature and pressure, saturated with water vapor. Relative humidity (RH) = content/capacity; when water vapor is saturated, content = capacity, and RH is 100%.
4. C. BTPD represents the condition of a gas volume at body temperature (37° C or 310° K), ambient pressure, without water vapor (0 mm Hg).
5. A. BTPS represents the condition of a gas volume at body temperature (37° C or 310° K), ambient pressure, saturated with water vapor (47 mm Hg).
6. B. Alveolar gas exerts a pressure of 47 mm Hg at BTPS.
7. A. Regardless of FIO_2, ABG values, or barometric pressure, alveolar gas exerts a pressure of 47 mm Hg.
8. D. Alveolar gas exists at BTPS; contains 44 mg of water vapor per liter of gas; and is saturated (100% RH and 100% body humidity).

B.

1. A. At BTPS, 1 L of gas contains 44 mg of water vapor.
2. B. Alveolar gas exists at BTPS; contains 44 mg of water vapor per liter of gas; and is saturated (100% RH and 100% body humidity).
3. D. STPD describes the condition of a gas without water vapor (0 mm Hg, 0 mg/L).

C.

1. D. RH = content/capacity (at body temperature) = 31/44 = 0.70 or 70%
2. B. RH = 9/44 = 0.20 or 20%
3. D. RH = 4/28 = 0.14 or 14%

D.

1. B. % body humidity = 14/44 = 0.32 or 32%
2. A. Percent body humidity is equivalent to RH at BTPS. Because RH = 50% at body temperature, % body humidity is also equal to 50%.

E.

1. E. Humidity deficit = 44 (absolute humidity of alveolar gas) – absolute humidity of inspired gas
   Humidity deficit = 44 – 23 = 21 mg/L
2. D. 0.65 (RH) = x/44, where x = content or absolute humidity of inspired gas
   $x = 0.65 \times 44$
   $x = 29$
   Humidity deficit = 44 – 29 = 15 mg/L

Part III

A.

1. C. Flow rate (L/sec) = Tidal volume (l)/Inspiratory time (sec)
   Flow rate = 0.85 L/0.65 sec
   = 1.3 L/sec or 78 L/min (1.3 × 60)
2. D. Flow rate = 0.5 L/1.1 sec
   = 0.45 L/sec × 60 = 27 L/min
3. B. Flow rate = 0.075 L/0.6 sec
   = 0.125 L/sec × 60 = 7.5 L/min
4. A. Inspiratory time = Tidal volume/Flow rate
   Inspiratory time = 650 mL/500 mL/sec
   = 1.3 sec
5. E. Inspiratory time = 950 mL/583 mL/sec (35 L/min × 1000/60)
   = 1.6 sec
6. A. Tidal volume = Flow rate × Inspiratory time
   Tidal volume = 0.83 L/sec (50 L/min/60) × 1.2 sec
   = 0.996 or 1 L

B.

1. C. I + E = Inspiratory Flow Rate (L/min) / Minute ventilation (L/min)
   I + E = 60 L/min/20 L/min
   = 3
   Because I must always = 1, the I:E must be 1:2.
2. E. I + E = 40 L/min/14.3 L/min (13 breaths/min × 1.1 L V_T)
   = 2.8
   I:E = 1:1.8
3. D. I + E = 4.5 L/min (0.75 × 60)/1.05 (0.25 × 42)
   = 4.3
   I:E = 1:3.3
4. B. Flow rate = Minute ventilation × (I + E)
   Flow rate = 18.4 (0.8 × 23) L/min × (1 + 2)
   = 18.4 L/min × 3
   = 55 L/min
5. C. Flow rate = 9.9 (0.3 × 33) L/min × (1 + 3)
   = 9.9 L/min × 4
   = 40 L/min
6. A. In order to deliver 150 breaths per minute, the ventilator must deliver 2.5 breaths every second (150/60). This equates to 1 breath every 0.4 seconds (1/2.5). If the ventilator has 0.4 seconds to complete I and E, and I = 0.2, then E must also = 0.2 (0.4 – 0.2). Thus, the I:E is 1:1.

C.

1. E. System compliance (cc/cm H_2O) = Test volume (cc) / Plateau pressure (cm H_2O)
   System compliance = 200 cc/61 cm H_2O
   = 3.3 cc/cm H_2O
2. D. In order to determine tidal volume, multiply flow rate and inspiratory time.
   Tidal volume = 0.05 L/sec (3.0 L/min / 60) × 1 sec
   = 0.05 L or 50 cc
   System compliance = 50 cc/56 cm H_2O)
   = 0.9 cc/cm H_2O
3. D. Compressed volume = (Pressure – PEEP) × Compliance factor
   = 52 × 2.1
   = 110 cc/cm H_2O
   Delivered tidal volume = Set tidal volume – Compressed volume
   Delivered tidal volume = 890 – 110 = 780 cc
4. B. Compressed volume = (Pressure – PEEP) × Compliance factor
   = (73 – 18) × 3.8
   = 55 cm H_2O × 3.8 cc/cm H_2O
   = 210 cc
   Delivered tidal volume = 1100 – 210 = 890 cc
5. B. Compressed volume = 58 cm H_2O × 0.6 cc/cm H_2O
   = 35 cc
   Delivered tidal volume = 45 cc – 35 cc = 10 cc

D.

1. A. EDC = Corrected tidal volume (cc)/Corrected peak pressure (cm H_2O)
   EDC = 730/38
   = 19 cc/cm H_2O
2. E. ESC = Corrected tidal volume (cc)/Corrected plateau pressure (cm H_2O)
   ESC = 620/42
   = 15 cc/cm H_2O
3. C. ESC = 880/53 cm – 14 cm PEEP
   = 880/39
   = 23 cc/cm H_2O
4. B. Corrected tidal volume = 1200 – (56 × 4.2)
   = 1200 – 235
   = 965 cc
   ESC = 965/56
   = 17 cc/cm H_2O

5. C. Corrected tidal volume = 920 – (44 – 16)2.4
= 920 – 67
= 853 cc
ESC = 853/44 – 16
= 853/28
= 30 cc/cm H_2O

6. C. Effective airway resistance = Proximal airway pressure – Plateau pressure (cm H_2O)/Inspiratory flow rate (L/sec)
Airway resistance = 45 – 33/1 L/sec (60 L/min/60)
= 12/1 = 12 cm H_2O/L/sec

7. A. Effective airway resistance = (58 – 47)/0.58 (35 L/min/60)
= 11/0.58
= 19 cm H_2O/L/sec

E.

1. B. ESC = Corrected tidal volume/Plateau pressure – PEEP
The LOWEST number divided into the corrected tidal volume, will yield the highest ESC. Of the choices listed, 9 cm PEEP subtracted from a plateau pressure of 37 cm H_2O, gives the lowest number (28). Values greater than 28 used in the denominator of the above equation would yield a lower ESC.

2. C. Again, in order to achieve the highest ESC, the lowest pressure must be divided into the tidal volume (550 cc). When each level of PEEP is subtracted from its corresponding plateau pressure, 15 cm H_2O gives the lowest number (49 – 15 = 34 cm H_2O).

Part IV

A.

1. B. $V_A = V_T - V_D$
= 950 – 180
= 770 cc

2. D. Minute V_A = RR × ($V_T - V_D$)
= 17 × (820 – 230)
= 17 × 590
= 10,030 mL/min or 10 L/min

3. E. Minute V_D = RR × ($V_T - V_A$)
= 42 × (420 – 260)
= 42 × 160
= 6720 mL/min or 6.7 L/min

B.

1. A. $V_D/V_T = Paco_2 - P\bar{E}co_2/Paco_2$
V_D/V_T = (53 – 31)/53
= 22/53
= 0.42

2. C. V_D/V_T = (40 – 28)/40
= 12/40
= 0.30

3. B. V_D/V_T = (85 – 33)/85
= 52/85
0.61

4. C. Minute V_A = RR × (V_T)(1 – V_D/V_T)
= 27 × 0.83(1 – 0.45)
= 27 × 0.83(0.55)
= 27 × 0.46
= 12.3 L/min

5. A. Minute V_A = 29 × 1.13(1 – 0.74)
= 29 × 1.13(0.26)
= 29 × 0.29
= 8.5 L/min

C.

1. A. Oxygen content disolved in plasma
= Po_2 × 0.003
= 570 × 0.003
= 1.7 vol%

2. A. Blood oxygen content = ([Hb] × 1.34 × Hb sat.) + (Po_2 × 0.003)
= (13.9 × 1.34 × .89) + (61 × 0.003)
= 16.6 + 0.18
= 16.8 vol%

3. D. Blood O_2 content = 22.4 × 1.34 × 0.85
= 25.5 vol%

4. D. PAO_2 = 1.0[1900 (760 × 2.5) – 47] – 35
= 1853 – 35
= 1818
$Pao_2 = P(A\text{-}a)o_2 - PAO_2$
= 1818 – 240
= 1578
Blood O_2 content = (3.6 × 1.34 × 1.0) + (1578 × 0.003)
= 4.8 + 4.7
= 9.5 vol%

D.

1. A. PAO_2 = 0.40(760 – 47) – (40/0.8)
= 285 – 50
= 235
$P(A\text{-}a)o_2$ = 235 – 88
= 147 mm Hg

2. B. PAO_2 = 0.85(710 – 47) – 73
= 564 – 73 (Remember that R need not be used when FIo_2 > 0.60.)
= 491
$P(A\text{-}a)o_2$ = 491 – 148
= 343 mm Hg

3. C. PAO_2 = 0.80(760 – 47) – 40
= 573 – 40
= 533
Pao_2 = 533 – 486
= 47 mm Hg

E.

1. E. $\dot{Q}_S/\dot{Q}_T = (P(A\text{-}a)o_2)(0.003)/[C(a\text{-}\bar{v})o_2] + [(P(A\text{-}a)o_2)(0.003)]$
PAO_2 = 1.0(760 – 47) – 40
= 713 – 40
= 673
$P(A\text{-}a)o_2$ = 673 – 265 = 408
$\dot{Q}_S/\dot{Q}_T$ = 408 × 0.003 / [2.3 + (408 × 0.003)]
= 1.22/(2.3 + 1.22)
= 1.22/3.52
= 0.34 or 34%

2. B. $PAO_2 = 1.0(760 - 47) - 40$
$= 713 - 40 = 673$
$P(A\text{-}a)O_2 = 673 - 150 = 523$
$CaO_2 = 15 \times 1.34 \times 1$
$= 20$ vol%
$C(a\text{-}\bar{v})O_2 = 20 - 16.3 = 3.7$ vol%
$\dot{Q}_S/\dot{Q}_T = 523(0.003) / [3.7 + 523(0.003)]$
$= 1.6/(3.7 + 1.6)$
$= 1.6/5.3$
$= 0.30$ or 30%
3. E. $\dot{Q}_S/\dot{Q}_T = 500(0.003) / [8 + 500(0.003)]$
$= 1.5/9.5$
$= 0.16$ or 16%
4. $\dot{Q}_S/\dot{Q}_T = 500(0.003) / [2.5 + 500(0.003)]$
$= 1.5/4$
$= 0.38$ or 38%
5. D. $\dot{Q}_S/\dot{Q}_T = (cc'O_2 - CaO_2)/(cc'O_2 - CvO_2)$
$= (20.6 - 19.8) / (20.6 - 16.3)$
$= 0.8/4.3$
$= 0.19$ or 19%

F.
1. B. $PAO_2 = 1.0(760 - 47) - 40$
$= 713 - 40$
$= 673$
$PaO_2 = 673 - 530 = 143$
a/A ratio $= PaO_2/PAO_2$
$= 143/673$
$= 0.21$
2. A. $PAO_2 = 0.70(710 - 47) - 47$
$= 464 - 47$
$= 417$
a/A ratio $= 63/417$
$= 0.15$

G.
1. B. $PAO_2 = 0.45(760 - 47) - (50 \times 1.25)$
$= 321 - 63$
$= 258$
$P(A\text{-}a)O_2 = 258 - 85 = 173$
Respiratory index $= P(A\text{-}a)O_2/PaO_2$
$= 173/85$
$= 2.0$
2. E. $PAO_2 = 0.8(760 - 47) - 65$
$= 570 - 65 = 505$
$P(A\text{-}a)O_2 = 505 - 45 = 460$
Respiratory index $= P(A\text{-}a)O_2/PaO_2$
$= 460/45$
$= 10.2$

H.
1. E. $CaO_2 = 9.7 \times 1.34 \times .85 = 11.1$ vol%
$CvO_2 = 9.7 \times 1.34 \times .61 = 7.9$ vol%
$C(a\text{-}\bar{v})O_2 = 11.1 - 7.9 = 3.2$ vol%
2. E. $CaO_2 = 19.1 \times 1.34 \times .80 = 20.5$ vol%
$CvO_2 = 19.1 \times 1.34 \times .49 = 12.5$ vol%
$C(a\text{-}\bar{v})O_2 = 20.5 - 12.5 = 8.0$ vol%
3. A. $CaO_2 = 22.3 \times 1.34 \times 1.0 = 30$ vol%
$CvO_2 = 22.3 \times 1.34 \times .76 = 22.7$ vol%
$C(a\text{-}\bar{v})O_2 = 29.9 - 22.7 = 7.3$ vol%

I.
1. B. Oxygen consumption = Cardiac output (C.O.) $\times C(a\text{-}\bar{v})O_2$
= 3900 mL/min × 6.8 mL O_2/100 mL Blood
= 26,520 mL/min/100 mL blood
= 265 mL/min
2. A. Oxygen consumption = 4800 mL/min × 2.4 mL O_2/100 mL blood
= 11,520 mL/min/100 mL blood
= 115 mL/min
3. E. $CaO_2 = 16.8 \times 1.34 \times 0.84 = 18.9$ vol%
$CvO_2 = 16.8 \times 1.34 \times 0.55 = 12.4$ vol%
$C(a\text{-}\bar{v})O_2 = 6.5$ vol%
O_2 consumption = 9800 mL/min × 6.5 mL O_2/100 mL blood
= 63,700/100
= 637 mL/min
4. C. C.O. = O_2 consumption/$C(a\text{-}\bar{v})O_2$
= 0.25 L/min/4 mL × 100 mL blood
= 6.3 mL
5. E. $C(a\text{-}\bar{v})O_2$ = O_2 consumption/C.O.
= 380 mL/min/8300 mL/min
= 0.046 mL × 100 mL blood = 4.6 vol%

J.
1. D. PVR = Mean PAP − PWP/C.O.
PVR = (20 − 8) / 6
PVR = 12/6
PVR = 2 Hg/L/min or
2 × 80 = 160 dyne-sec/cm^{-5}
2. A. PVR = (38 − 4) / 3.9
= 34/3.9
= 8.72 Hg/L/min or
= 8.72 × 80 = 697 dyne-sec/cm^{-5}
3. C. PVR = (20 − 13) / 3
= 7/3
= 2.3 Hg/L/min

Part V

A.
1. D. TLC = IRV + TV + ERV + RV
= 2150 + 480 + 2340 + 1470
= 6440 cc
2. A. VC = IRV + TV + ERV (FRC − RV)
= 1725 + 355 + (1630 − 920)
= 1725 + 355 + 710
= 2790 cc
3. E. ERV = FRC − RV
= 2680 − 1175
= 1505 cc
4. E. IRV = VC − ERV (FRC − RV) − VT
= 1350 − (1030 − 675) − 135
= 1350 − 355 − 135
= 860 cc
5. A. TLC = IRV + TV + FRC
= 1050 + 330 + 1905
= 3285 cc

RV = TLC − VC
= 3285 − 2670
= 615
RV/TLC ratio = 615/3285
= 0.19 or 19%

B.

1. C. FEV_1/FVC = 3.06 L/4.12 L
= 0.74 or 74%
2. Bell factor = 41.27
41.27 × 36 mm (FEV_3 excursion) = 1486 cc or 1.49 L
41.27 × 42 mm (FVC excursion) = 1733 cc or 1.73 L
FEV_3/FVC = 1.49 × 1.096(BTPS conversion)/1.73 × 1.096
= 1.63/1.9
= 0.86 or 86%
3. B. FEF_{25-75} = 11,300 − 8250
= 3050 × 1.102 (BTPS conversion)
= 3361 cc or 3.36 L
% predicted FEF_{25-75} = actual FEF_{25-75} − pred. FEF_{25-75}
= 3.36/4.95
= 0.68 or 68% predicted
4. A. % Improvement after BD = value after BD − value before BD/value before BD
= 1.9 − 1.35/1.35
= 0.55/1.35
= 0.40 or 40% improvement

C.

1. E. FRC = [Final N_2 % × (VE + VD)] − (T × N_2 correction)/0.75
FRC = (0.082 × 38.5) − (7 × 0.04/0.75)
= 3.16 − (0.28/0.75)
= 2.88/0.75
= 3.84 × 1.102 = 4.23
RV = (FRC + IRV + VT) − VC
= [4.23 + (3.11 × 1.102) + (.95 × 1.102)] − (5.24 × 1.102)
= (4.23 + 3.43 + 1.05) − 5.77
= 8.71 − 5.77
= 2.94 L
2. E. FRC = (0.067 × 41.8) − (7 × 0.04/0.75)
= (2.8 − 0.28) /0.75
= 2.52/0.75
= 3.36 × 1.085 = 3.65
RV = (FRC + IRV + VT) − VC
= [3.65 + (1.52 × 1.085) + (0.32 × 1.085)] − (2.66 × 1.085)
= (3.65 + 1.65 + 0.35) − 2.89
= 5.65 − 2.89
= 2.76
TLC = VC + RV
= 2.89 + 2.76
= 5.55 L
3. C. FRC = [(Initial He % − Final He %) / Final He %] × Initial volume − (He correction)
= (0.11 − 0.043/0.043) × 2.8 L − (0.1)
= (1.56 × 2.8) − 0.1
= 4.37 − 0.1 = 4.27
4.27 L × 1.085 = 4.6 L

Part VI

A.

1. E. 1 cc of water weighs 1 gram, or 1000 mg.
2. E. Because 1 cc = 1 mL, 1 mL of water also weighs 1 gram or 1000 mg.
3. B. 1000 cc = 1000 mL
4. B. 1 gram = 1000 mg. Thus, 0.016 grams × 1000 = 16 mg.
5. A. There are 1000 micrograms in 1 mg.
6. E. 1 mL of water contains 16 drops.

B.

1. D. Solution % = weight of solution/weight of solvent × 100
= 1/100
1:100 or 0.01, which equals 1%
2. A. Solution % = 0.25 g (always remember to use equivalent units—grams and mL)/100 mL
= 0.0025 or 0.25%
0.25:100 must be manipulated so that the first number in the ratio is 1. Multiplying by 4 yields a 1:400 solution.
3. B. Solution % = 0.1 g/100 mL
= 0.001 or 0.1%
Multiply 0.1:100 by 10, so that the first number in the ratio = 1; 1:1000 solution.
4. A. Solution % = 2 g/100 mL
= 0.02 or 2%
Divide by 2, so that the first number in the ratio = 1; 1:50.
5. A. 1.0 % = x g/1 mL
0.01 = x g/1 mL
x = 0.01 × 1 mL
x = 0.01 g = 10 mg
6. B. 1:200 = x g/0.5 mL
0.005 (1/200) = x g/0.5 mL
x = 0.005 × 0.5 mL
x = .0025 g = 2.5 mg
7. C. 0.0017 = x g/3 mL
x = 0.0017 × 3
x = 0.005 g = 5 mg
8. A. 1/100 = 0.01
0.01 = 0.005 g/x mL
x = 0.005/0.01
x = 0.5 mL
9. C. 0.025 = 0.075 g/x mL
x = 0.075/0.025
x = 3 mL
10. C. 0.02 = 0.015 g/x mL
x = 0.015/0.02
x = 0.75

C.

1. A. Total (new) volume = Original volume × Original concentration/New, or desired, concentration
Total (new) volume = 100 mL × 2/1
= 200 mL
Volume of diluent = Total or new drug vol. − Original drug volume
Volume of diluent = 200 mL − 100 mL
= 100 mL

2. B. New volume $= 10 \times 20/5$
$= 40$ mL
Volume of diluent $= 40$ mL $- 10$ mL
$= 30$ mL
3. C. New volume $= 8.4 \times 50/5$
$= 420/5$
$= 84$ mL
Volume of diluent $= 84 - 50$
$= 34$ mL
4. B. New volume $= 95 \times 500/35$
$= 47{,}500/35$
$= 1357$ mL or approximately 1360 mL

UNIT II

Situational Set Pretest (Entry Level Only)

Several questions on the NBRC Entry Level Examination are presented in the situational set format. This design is similar to the more sophisticated latent image branching-logic problems presented on the NBRC Clinical Simulation Examination. These "situational sets" or case presentations assess the candidate's ability to manage a patient and/or respiratory care equipment within the clinical setting. The situational set begins with a short scenario. This narrative typically contains pertinent clinical data such as blood gas results, cardiopulmonary vital signs, results of chest radiography, and so on. By analyzing this information carefully, the candidate will be able to solve the problem that is presented. The scenario is followed by several questions that test the candidate's ability to assess the nature and extent of the clinical problem and to make appropriate decisions regarding respiratory care. The following section contains 22 of these situational sets.

Set 1
Chronic Obstructive Pulmonary Disease I

A 59-year-old patient with a history of COPD is brought to the emergency department after several days of increasing respiratory distress. Baseline blood gases are drawn and the patient is placed on 1 L oxygen via nasal cannula. Data from the original and a subsequent arterial sample appear below:

	Room Air Sample	1 Liter Nasal O_2
Pao_2	36 mm Hg	46 mm Hg
$Paco_2$	84 mm Hg	80 mm Hg
pH	7.24	7.30
HCO_3^-	32 mEq/L	34 mEq/L

1. Based on the above data, the most appropriate recommendation for the respiratory therapy practitioner to make at this time would be:

   A. Increase oxygen flow to 2 L/min
   B. Make no change in therapy
   C. Intubate and place patient on continuous ventilatory support
   D. Place patient on 35% air entrainment mask
   E. Decrease oxygen to 0.5 L/min

   (9:136–8)

2. Conservative and supportive therapy is the general rule in managing acute respiratory insufficiency superimposed on COPD. This statement is justified by all of the following statements except:

   A. Poor tolerance of continuous mechanical ventilation
   B. General success of respiratory therapy
   C. Favorable response to oxygen therapy in this group
   D. Reversible nature of bronchospasm
   E. Rarity of severe and life-threatening distress in these patients

   (9:136–8)

3. Physical examination of the patient reveals a loose cough productive of moderate quantities of rusty-colored secretions. Which of the following is likely to be responsible for this finding?

   A. Bronchial asthma
   B. Pseudohemoptysis
   C. Pneumococcal pneumonia
   D. *Pseudomonas* pneumonia
   E. Anaerobic lung abscess

   (9:68)

4. Which of the following is not considered part of the conservative supportive approach to the management of the COPD patient who requires hospitalization?

   A. IPPB
   B. Antibiotic therapy
   C. Continuous ventilatory support
   D. Chest physical therapy
   E. Oxygen therapy

   (9:136–8)

5. The decision to intubate and initiate continuous ventilatory support in patients with severe chronic obstructive pulmonary disease is made on demonstration of all of the following *except*:

   A. $Paco_2$ greater than 70 mm Hg
   B. Inability to protect the airway
   C. Sudden onset of severe cardiovascular symptomatology
   D. Progressive acidosis despite controlled oxygen administration
   E. Worsening fatigue and sensorium

   (9:135–6)

Set 2
Epiglottitis

A 3-year-old girl in severe respiratory distress is brought to the emergency department by her parents. Physical signs include a loud barking cough and high-pitched inspiratory stridor. She is unable to swallow and is noted to be drooling profusely. Her mother says that she became ill approximately 4 hours prior to admission. Arterial blood gas analysis on 3 L oxygen via cannula reveals the following data:

Pao_2	53 mm Hg
$Paco_2$	27 mm Hg
pH	7.48
HCO_3^-	20 mEq/L
Base excess	–3.0 mEq/L

1. Which of the following is the correct interpretation of this patient's arterial blood gas data?

   A. Fully compensated respiratory acidosis
   B. Partially compensated respiratory alkalosis
   C. Metabolic acidosis with respiratory alkalosis
   D. Fully compensated metabolic alkalosis
   E. Partially compensated metabolic acidosis

   (8:255)

2. The clinical presentation of epiglottitis differs from that of croup in which of the following respects?

   I. The onset of symptoms is more rapid.
   II. It usually affects a neonatal population.

III. It is a more common presentation.
IV. Distress is generally more severe.

A. I, III, and IV
B. II, III, and IV
C. I, II, III, and IV
D. I and IV
E. I and III

(8:255)

3. Which of the following pathogens is most frequently associated with epiglottitis?

A. Viral agents
B. *Escherichia coli*
C. *Pseudomonas*
D. *Haemophilus influenzae*
E. *Bacillus fragilis*

(8:254)

4. Examination of the pharynx in patients with epiglottitis:

I. May result in complete upper airway obstruction
II. Will typically reveal a cherry-red epiglottis
III. Should include suctioning

A. I and III
B. I, II, and III
C. II and III
D. I and II
E. I only

(8:257)

5. Which of the following are treatments for epiglottitis?

I. Establishing an adequate airway
II. Appropriate antibiotic therapy
III. Cool aerosol mist
IV. Immediate hospitalization

A. I, II, and III
B. I, II, III, and IV
C. I, II, and IV
D. I and IV

(8:256–7)

Set 3
Chronic Obstructive Pulmonary Disease II

A 34-year-old woman with advanced cystic fibrosis is admitted to the emergency department. The patient is cyanotic, febrile, and confused. Arterial blood is drawn just prior to and 20 minutes after she is placed on 3 L oxygen via nasal cannula. These data are reported below:

	Room Air Sample	3 L Nasal Oxygen
Pao_2	35 mm Hg	46 mm Hg
$Paco_2$	73 mm Hg	97 mm Hg
pH	7.31	7.17
HCO_3^-	37 mEq/L	32 mEq/L

1. Based on the foregoing information, which of the following recommendations should the respiratory therapy practitioner make at this time?

A. Increase oxygen to 4 L/min
B. Decrease oxygen to 1 L/min
C. Intubate and place on a ventilator with an FIo_2 of 0.35
D. Intubate and place on an FIo_2 of 0.35 via T tube
E. Make no change in therapy

(9:351)

2. In most patients suffering from chronic hypercapnia who require oxygen therapy, the hazard of CO_2 retention can usually be minimized by keeping the Pao_2 between ___ mm Hg.

A. 30–40
B. 40–50
C. 50–70
D. 60–80
E. 70–90

(9:138)

3. Which of the following statements regarding the use of the continuous ventilatory support in the management of COPD is not true?

A. Barotrauma is a known complication.
B. Worsening of V/Q relationships is common.
C. The patient's work of breathing frequently increases following placement on continuous ventilatory support.
D. Ventilator dependence may occur.
E. Nosocomial infections may prolong course.

(9:361–4)

Set 4
Pulmonary Function Testing

A 71-year-old patient is admitted to the hospital for a cholecystectomy. Preoperative lung function tests are performed on this 65-kg patient with the following results:

	Observed	% Predicted
$\frac{FEV_1}{FVC}$ %	31%	
$FEF_{200-1200}$	1.89 L/sec	31

1. On the basis of the foregoing data, which of the following pulmonary mechanical defects is most likely present?

   A. Restrictive lung disease
   B. Normal study
   C. Upper airway obstruction only
   D. Mild obstructive pulmonary disease
   E. Severe obstructive pulmonary disease

(6:39–48)

2. Which of the following best describes this patient's risk of developing postoperative pulmonary complications?

   A. No risk
   B. Low risk
   C. Moderate risk
   D. High risk
   E. Not enough information available

(6:39–48)

3. Which of the following is considered the best test for detecting early obstructive changes in the smaller airways?

   A. $FEF_{200-1200}$
   B. MVV
   C. $FEF_{25-75}\%$
   D. FEV_1
   E. $FEV_1\%$ FVC

(6:46–7)

4. In this patient, the elevated FRC is suggestive of all but which of the following abnormalities?

   A. Loss of pulmonary elastic recoil
   B. Emphysema
   C. Air trapping
   D. Diffuse parenchymal consolidation
   E. Obstruction to expiratory airflow

(6:39–40)

Set 5
Flail Chest

A 16-year-old, 60-kg automobile accident victim is rushed to the emergency department by ambulance. The victim is unconscious, deeply cyanotic, and in life-threatening distress. Respirations are extremely labored and paradoxical breathing is noted on the right anterior chest. Multiple lacerations and contusions are present from which the patient is bleeding profusely. As paramedics bring him into the trauma room, he is noted to be receiving 10 L oxygen via simple oxygen mask.

1. Which of the following actions should the respiratory therapy practitioner take at this time?

   A. Palpate the carotid pulse
   B. Assist in hemostasis
   C. Establish an airway
   D. Assess level of consciousness
   E. Begin external cardiac compressions

(9:296)

2. Which of the following statements is (are) true regarding flail chest?

   I. Double fractures of several adjacent ribs may be etiologic.
   II. Lung contusion is a rare accompanying pathology.
   III. Continuous ventilatory support is always indicated.

   A. II and III
   B. I and II
   C. I only
   D. I, II, and III
   E. I and III

(9:294–7)

3. Following successful intubation, the physician asks the respiratory therapy practitioner to place the patient on a volume ventilator. Which of the following therapies (in addition to mechanical ventilation) is (are) believed to aid in stabilization of the chest wall?

   I. Pharmacologic sedation and/or paralysis
   II. Strapping of the chest
   III. Traction of the appropriate thoracic segment
   IV. Bronchial hygiene therapy

   A. I and III
   B. II and III
   C. III only
   D. I and II
   E. I and IV

(9:296–7)

4. Continuous ventilatory support in the patient with flail chest:

   I. May be necessary for 1 or more weeks
   II. May be helpful in preventing hypoxia
   III. May be complicated by pulmonary barotrauma

   A. I, II, and III
   B. II and III
   C. I and II
   D. I only
   E. I and III

(8:171)

Set 6
Bronchiectasis

A 45-year-old patient was admitted to the respiratory service 2 weeks ago. His relevant history began in childhood with a pneumonia that did not receive adequate medical attention. Since that time his pulmonary symptomatology has become increasingly pronounced. This is his sixth hospitalization, but it is the first time he has been examined by a pulmonary specialist.

1. The chief complaint of the patient with bronchiectasis is:

   A. Orthopnea
   B. Easy fatigability
   C. Dyspnea
   D. Sleep apnea
   E. Cough and sputum production

   (8:102)

2. In general, sputum produced by the patient with bronchiectasis is:

   I. Mucoid
   II. Copious
   III. Purulent
   IV. Scanty

   A. II and IV
   B. I and III
   C. I and IV
   D. II and III
   E. I and II

   (8:102)

3. Definitive diagnosis of bronchiectasis is made on the basis of which of the following?

   A. History and physical examination
   B. Sputum culture and sensitivity
   C. Bronchography
   D. Angiography
   E. Pulmonary tomography

   (8:105)

4. Pulmonary function and arterial blood studies on a bronchiectasis patient typically reveal:

   I. Decreased expiratory flow rates
   II. Increased inspiratory capacity
   III. Hypoxemia
   IV. Massive intrapulmonary shunting

   A. II and III
   B. I and II
   C. III and IV
   D. I and III
   E. I, II, III, and IV

   (8:103–4)

5. All of the following have a place in this patient's home care program. Which is believed to be the most indispensable aid to maintaining bronchial hygiene?

   A. Aerosol therapy
   B. Hyperinflation therapy
   C. Pulmonary drainage techniques
   D. Antibiotic therapy
   E. Breathing exercises

   (9:162–3)

Set 7
Ventilator Emergency

The respiratory therapy practitioner is assigned to a ventilator patient in the cardiac care unit. While making rounds the therapist hears the ventilator's high pressure alarm sounding. Although unconscious, the patient is diaphoretic, cyanotic, and in respiratory distress.

1. What is the first thing that must be done to alleviate this patient's distress?

   A. Check the ventilator to see if it is malfunctioning
   B. Take the patient off the ventilator and ventilate manually
   C. Go to the nurses' station and get help
   D. Have a physician paged
   E. Measure the patient's blood pressure

   (9:362)

2. Following the action outlined in the previous question, which *two* of the following actions must be taken simultaneously?

   I. Call for a stat chest roentgenogram
   II. Check the ventilator for malfunction
   III. Have a partner bag the patient with 100% O_2
   IV. Examine the patient's chest to determine the cause of distress
   V. Check the patient's blood pressure

   A. I and III
   B. IV and V
   C. III and IV
   D. III and V
   E. II and III

   (9:362)

3. Percussion at this time reveals sharply diminished aeration on the left side and a hyperresonant percussion note on the right side. Which of the following disorders may be responsible for this finding?

   I. Intubation of the right mainstem bronchus
   II. Right-sided pneumothorax
   III. Right-sided atelectasis
   IV. Left-sided pneumothorax

   A. I and II
   B. II and IV
   C. I and III
   D. II and III
   E. I, II, and IV

(9:288)

4. While waiting for the physician to arrive, the practitioner notes that the patient is becoming increasingly cyanotic. Soon, the carotid pulse is not palpable. Over the past 2 min the cardiac rate has dropped from 200 to approximately 20. Based on this information, the therapist should:

   A. Draw a stat arterial blood gas sample
   B. Insert a 16-gauge needle in the second or third interspace of the affected side
   C. Advance the airway slightly
   D. Auscultate the chest
   E. Begin external cardiac compressions

(8:182-3)

Set 8
Myasthenia Gravis

A 28-year-old woman suffering from myasthenia gravis presents to the emergency room in myasthenia crisis, following an upper respiratory infection lasting approximately 3 days. She states that she is beginning to experience some difficulty breathing.

1. The most appropriate action for the respiratory therapist would be:

   A. Intubate and institute mechanical ventilation
   B. Administer high-dose corticosteroids
   C. Measure the patient's vital capacity and MIP or NIF
   D. Administer 100% FIo_2

(9:311–12)

2. Diagnosis of myasthenia gravis is supported by all but which of the following?

   A. Demonstration of fatigue following repetitive or sustained contraction of certain muscles
   B. Regaining of strength after a period of rest
   C. Regaining of strength following administration of Tensilon
   D. Ascending paralysis
   E. All of the above support the diagnosis of myasthenia gravis

(9:311–12)

3. Myasthenia crisis may be precipitated by:

   I. Exposure to certain allergens
   II. Emotional upset
   III. Respiratory infection
   IV. An excessive amount of anticholinesterase drugs

   A. I, II, III, and IV
   B. I, II, and III
   C. I, III, and IV
   D. II, III, and IV

(9:312)

Set 9
Guillain Barré Syndrome

A 52-year-old man is brought to the emergency department. For the past 2 days he has been experiencing progressive numbness and weakening of the extremities. When several hours ago he became short of breath and could not walk when rising from his chair, he had a neighbor drive him to the hospital. Physical findings include tachypnea, dysphagia, and slurred speech. Antecedent history was unremarkable except for an upper respiratory tract infection in the past 2 weeks. Arterial blood gases drawn on room air just prior to direct admission to the intensive care unit were:

Pao_2	81 mm Hg
$Paco_2$	52 mm Hg
pH	7.30
Base excess	–3.9 mEq/L
HCO_3^-	20 mEq/L

1. True statements regarding the patient's blood gas and acid-base status include:

   I. Respiratory acidosis exists.
   II. A widened $P(A\text{-}a)o_2$ exists.
   III. Physiologic shunting is evident.
   IV. Metabolic acidosis is present.

   A. I and IV
   B. II and III
   C. I, II, and IV
   D. I, III, and IV
   E. II and IV

(8:273)

2. Which of the following statements regarding the Guillain-Barré syndrome is (are) true?

   I. It may lead to respiratory muscle paralysis.
   II. It is considered an obstructive disorder.
   III. Its primary pathology involves neuromuscular blockade.

IV. Its primary pathology involves the neuromuscular junction.

A. I, II, and IV
B. III and IV
C. I only
D. I, II, III, and IV
E. I, III, and IV

(8:271)

3. Which of the following statements regarding the clinical picture of patients with Guillain-Barré syndrome is (are) true?

I. Loss of vital capacity is a consistent finding.
II. Pulmonary edema is frequently severe.
III. Increased anteroposterior diameter is a common radiologic finding.
IV. Cough with sputum is the chief complaint.

A. I and III
B. II, III, and IV
C. I, III, and IV
D. I only
E. II and III

(9:315)

4. True statements regarding the use of mechanical ventilation in patients with Guillain-Barré syndrome include:

I. PEEP therapy is usually required.
II. It is indicated when the vital capacity is less than 20% of predicted.
III. Mechanical hyperventilation is indicated to reduce intracranial pressure.
IV. It may be required for several weeks or longer.

A. I and IV
B. II, III, and IV
C. III and IV
D. II and IV
E. I, II, III, and IV

(8:274)

Set 10
Croup

A 13-month-old, well-nourished infant is brought to the emergency department in respiratory distress. His mother says that he has had a cold for the past 2 days. About 18 hr ago he developed a loud barking cough and began making crowing sounds on inspiration. Symptoms slowly continued to deteriorate, necessitating his admission.

1. All of the following physical findings were seen in this patient. Which is the most characteristic of the pediatric croup syndrome?

A. Tachycardia
B. Fever
C. Inspiratory stridor
D. Tachypnea
E. Productive cough

(8:254–5)

2. Which of the following is the most common causative agent in episodes of croup?

A. *Hemophilus influenzae*
B. *Bacillus pneumoniae*
C. Viral organisms
D. *Escherichia coli*
E. *Bordetella pertussis*

(8:254)

3. Which of the following statements regarding croup is (are) true?

I. It is also known as laryngotracheobronchitis.
II. The underlying pathology involves pharyngeal edema.
III. It is known to respond to aerosol therapy.

A. I and II
B. II and III
C. I and III
D. II only
E. III only

(8:254)

4. Which of the following statements regarding croup as compared with epiglottitis is (are) true?

I. Symptoms are generally more severe.
II. Onset of symptoms is more rapid.
III. An emergency airway is required less frequently.

A. I and III
B. II and III
C. I and II
D. I only
E. III only

(8:254–5)

Set 11
Pediatric Cardiopulmonary Resuscitation

A 6-year-old boy is brought to the emergency department after being struck by an automobile while riding his bicycle. On admission he is comatose and cyanotic. As he is rushed in by paramedics, it is noted that he is receiving 8 L oxygen via mask and that an overly large oropharyngeal airway has been taped in place. Gross inspection at this time also reveals multiple lacerations and contusions over his thorax, abdomen, and legs. Rapid assessment of this patient reveals the absence of air movement and ventilatory efforts.

1. Based on the above information, the practitioner would now:

   A. Check the carotid pulse
   B. Assess pupillary response
   C. Give two slow breaths
   D. Give several quick breaths
   E. Give four back blows

(10:20–23)

2. Use of an improperly sized oropharyngeal airway in conjunction with an oxygen mask is particularly hazardous for which of the following reasons?

   A. It can lead to an increased mechanical deadspace.
   B. It will lower the effective FIO_2.
   C. It can cause airway obstruction.
   D. It may cause reflex tachycardia.
   E. It may impinge on the soft palate.

(10:69–71)

3. True statements about rescue breathing in the child include:

   I. The side effect of gastric distention is more common than it is in the adult.
   II. When accompanying external cardiac compressions, the rate should be 25/min.
   III. Mouth-to-nose ventilation is generally preferred.
   IV. It should be administered during the downstroke of every fifth compression.

   A. II, III, and IV
   B. I, III, and IV
   C. II and III
   D. I only
   E. I, II, and IV

(13:299)

4. Which of the following statements regarding airway obstruction in children is (are) true?

   I. It is more common than in adults.
   II. It is commonly caused by toys and peanuts.
   III. The emergency procedure does not include back blows.

   A. I and II
   B. I, II, and III
   C. III only
   D. II and III
   E. I and III

(10:23–5)

5. Emergency cardiac compressions in the child:

   I. Should be administered at a rate of 100/min
   II. Should compress the sternum 1½ to 2 inches
   III. Can frequently be performed with the heel of one hand

   A. I and III
   B. II and III
   C. I, II, and III
   D. II only
   E. I and II

(13:299)

Set 12
Sleep Apnea

The respiratory therapist has been asked to perform polysomnography on a 55-year-old man who presents with daytime sleepiness and frequent, loud snoring at night (as reported by his spouse). The patient is obese, and reports that he wakes up tired each morning, with a headache. A diagnosis of sleep apnea syndrome is suspected.

1. Which of the following are included in the polysomnography?

   I. Ear oximetry
   II. EEG/EOG
   III. ECG
   IV. Monitoring airflow at the patient's mouth and nose

   A. I, II, III, and IV
   B. II and III
   C. I, III, and IV
   D. I and IV

(8:289)

2. Based on the above presentation, this patient probably suffers from which type of sleep apnea?

   A. Central
   B. Obstructive
   C. Mixed
   D. Non-REM

(8:286–7)

3. When may a diagnosis of sleep apnea be made?

   A. Greater than 200 episodes of apnea in an 8-hr period of sleep
   B. Greater than 30 episodes of apnea over a 6-hr period of sleep
   C. When patient reports difficulty sleeping through the night
   D. When patient demonstrates a reduced FRC, combined with tiredness

(9:331)

4. Management of obstructive sleep apnea may include:

   I. Weight reduction
   II. Oxygen therapy
   III. CPAP
   IV. Central nervous system stimulants

A. I, II, III, and IV
B. II and III
C. I and IV
D. I, II, and III

(8:292–3)

5. Management of central sleep apnea may include:

I. CPAP
II. Weight reduction
III. Phrenic nerve pacemaker
IV. Negative pressure ventilation

A. I, II, III, and IV
B. I, III, and IV
C. III and IV
D. II and III

(8:292–3)

Set 13
Upper Airway Emergency

The respiratory care practitioner is paged to the cardiac care unit to check the equipment storeroom. As he walks by the adjacent visitor's waiting room, he notices an elderly woman slump over in her chair and fall to the floor.

1. All of the following are steps that are followed in performing basic cardiopulmonary resuscitation. Please place them in correct order.

I. Check for pulse
II. Give two slow breaths
III. Establish unconsciousness
IV. Tilt the head and lift the chin and check for breathing
V. Begin external cardiac compressions
VI. Call for help

A. III, VI, IV, I, II, and V
B. III, VI, IV, II, I, and V
C. III, VI, II, I, IV, and V
D. VI, IV, III, I, V, and II
E. VI, II, I, III, IV, and V

(10:23–4)

2. Single-rescuer cardiopulmonary resuscitation of the adult victim consists of:

A. 15 compressions followed by two ventilations
B. 10 compressions followed by two ventilations
C. 5 compressions followed by one ventilation
D. 5 compressions followed by two ventilations
E. 15 compressions followed by four ventilations

(10:20–4)

3. The therapist attempts to deliver two slow breaths to this victim but is unable to move air into the lungs. All of the following are steps in the procedure to relieve complete airway obstruction in the unconscious adult victim. Please place them in proper order.

I. Give four abdominal or chest thrusts.
II. Sweep the mouth with your fingers.
III. Reposition the head and neck and try to ventilate.

A. II, I, and III
B. III, II, and I
C. I, II, and III
D. I, III, and II
E. III, I, and II

(10:23–4)

4. According to the American Heart Association, the chest thrust may be preferable to the abdominal thrust in which of the following cases?

I. Comatose victims
II. Pregnant victims
III. Very obese victims
IV. Infants
V. Children

A. I, III, IV, and V
B. II, III, and IV
C. II, III, and V
D. I, II, III, IV, and V
E. II, III, IV, and V

(10:236)

5. After several repetitions of the above procedure, the therapist is able to dislodge a large piece of food from the victim's airway. By this time help has arrived. Place the following lifesaving steps in their proper order.

I. Give two slow breaths.
II. Check for pulse.
III. Begin two-rescuer cardiopulmonary resuscitation.

A. III, II, and I
B. II, III, and I
C. I, III, and II
D. I, II, and III
E. III, I, and II

(10:23–4)

Set 14
Cystic Fibrosis

An infant is admitted to the seventh floor pediatric ward with a tentative diagnosis of "failure to thrive." Four months ago this patient was sent home with her mother following an uneventful delivery. Since then she has had several upper respiratory tract infections and a persistent cough. Her main problem at this time has been an inability to gain weight despite apparently normal feeding habits. Abdominal distention and bulky, foul-smelling stools are pertinent features of this infant's clinical picture.

1. True statements regarding cystic fibrosis include:

   I. It is a chronic, restrictive pediatric pulmonary disorder.
   II. It may also be called mucoviscidosis.
   III. It is a hereditary disorder of the body's endocrine system.
   IV. It is rarely fatal.
   V. Primary pulmonary pathology involves hypersecretion of mucus.

   A. I, II, IV, and V
   B. I, III, IV, and V
   C. II and V
   D. III and V
   E. I, II, III, and V

(9:167)

2. Which of the following is most helpful in establishing the diagnosis of cystic fibrosis?

   A. Pulmonary tomography
   B. Measurement of sweat electrolytes
   C. Angiograms
   D. Lung biopsy
   E. Sputum culture and sensitivity

(9:168)

3. Retained pulmonary secretions in the patient with cystic fibrosis *least* frequently leads to:

   A. Atelectasis
   B. Pneumonia
   C. Left ventricular failure
   D. Increased work of breathing
   E. Blood gas abnormalities

(9:262–4)

4. Pulmonary function testing in the patient with cystic fibrosis usually shows evidence of:

   I. Decreased FEF_{25-75}
   II. Increased $\frac{FEV_1}{FVC}\%$
   III. Increased residual volume
   IV. Decreased inspiratory flow rates

   A. I and III
   B. I, III, and IV
   C. I only
   D. I, II, and IV
   E. III and IV

(9:262–3)

5. Oxygen administration to the patient with cystic fibrosis:

   I. May eliminate the hypoxic drive in the patient with chronic ventilatory failure.
   II. Will have no effect on arterial hypoxemia.
   III. Is rarely necessary.

   A. I and III
   B. I, II, and III
   C. II and III
   D. I only
   E. II only

(9:266)

Set 15
Drug Overdose

A 15-year-old is brought by paramedics to the emergency department with an esophageal obturator airway in place. She is being ventilated by a manual resuscitator that is connected to supplemental oxygen. Her height is average and her weight is well in excess of 100 kg. Spontaneous respirations are 6/min and shallow. Skin color is ashen but not cyanotic. Pulse is 130, the blood pressure is 70/40, and the patient does not respond to painful stimuli.

1. Which of the following should the respiratory therapy practitioner recommend at this time?

   A. Pass a nasogastric tube
   B. Intubate and support ventilation
   C. Obtain stat arterial blood gas analysis
   D. Begin hemodialysis
   E. Remove the esophageal obturator airway

(9:321)

2. Which of the following best describes this patient's sensorium?

   A. Alert and oriented
   B. Restless and agitated
   C. Lethargic and confused
   D. Light coma
   E. Deep coma

(9:320)

3. An arterial blood sample is drawn while the patient is breathing room air. The results appear below:

Pa_{O_2}	35 mm Hg
Pa_{CO_2}	65 mm Hg
pH	7.20
HCO_3^-	24 mEq/L
Base excess	–4.0 mEq/L

   Based on the above information, the patient's hypoxemia is most likely due to:

   A. Hypoventilation
   B. Shunting
   C. Low V/Q
   D. High V/Q
   E. A and C are correct.

(9:321)

4. Regarding this patient's acid-base status:

   A. A mixed respiratory and metabolic acidosis exists.
   B. A mixed respiratory and metabolic alkalosis exists.
   C. Respiratory acidosis alone exists.
   D. Partially compensated metabolic alkalosis exists.
   E. A partially compensated respiratory acidosis exists.

(1:191)

Set 16
Adult Respiratory Distress Syndrome

The respiratory therapy practitioner is monitoring a 25-year-old man who was admitted after an industrial accident involving inhalation of chlorine gas. Eight hours post admission the patient has tachycardia, tachypnea, and hypertension. Auscultation of the chest reveals diminished breath sounds bibasally and scattered inspiratory rales. Arterial blood sampled with the patient breathing 8 L oxygen via simple oxygen mask yields the following data:

$Pa{O_2}$	34 mm Hg
$Pa{CO_2}$	23 mm Hg
pH	7.50
HCO_3^-	18 mEq/L

1. Which of the following is most likely to be responsible for this patient's arterial hypoxemia?

   A. Low V/Q
   B. High V/Q
   C. Diffusion defect
   D. Intrapulmonary shunting
   E. Hypoventilation

(9:209–10)

2. Administration of 100% oxygen to this patient at this time would most likely have which of the following effects?

   I. Widening of the $P(A\text{-}a)O_2$
   II. Dramatic increase in the PaO_2
   III. Narrowing of the $P(A\text{-}a)O_2$

   A. III only
   B. I only
   C. II and III
   D. II only
   E. I and II

(9:209–10)

3. The physician wants to place the patient on the level of PEEP that will yield the highest systemic oxygen transport. Which of the following is believed to be the best indicator of this?

   A. PaO_2
   B. Cardiac output
   C. $P(A\text{-}a)O_2$
   D. $S\bar{v}O_2$
   E. Effective static compliance

(1:864–5)

4. In an attempt to determine the optimal therapeutic level of PEEP, the following information is gathered:

Level of PEEP ($cm\ H_2O$)	SaO_2(%)	$S\bar{v}O_2$(%)
0	74	40
3	74	47
6	76	53
9	78	58
1125	8706	50

Based on the above information the best level of PEEP for the patient is:

   A. 3 cm H_2O
   B. 6 cm H_2O
   C. 9 cm H_2O
   D. 12 cm H_2O
   E. 15 cm H_2O

(1:866)

5. Four days later, the patient is on an FIO_2 of 0.6 with 10 cm H_2O PEEP. Arterial blood gas data obtained at this time with the patient in the assist/control mode are as follows:

PaO_2	151 mm Hg
$PaCO_2$	32 mm Hg
pH	7.46
HCO_3^-	22 mEq/L

Based on the above information, which of the following setting changes should the respiratory therapy practitioner recommend at this time?

   A. Decrease the PEEP to 5 cm H_2O and add 100 cc mechanical deadspace
   B. Decrease the FIO_2 to 0.5
   C. Decrease the FIO_2 to 0.5 and add 500 cc mechanical deadspace
   D. Decrease the PEEP to 8 cm H_2O and place patient on intermittent mandatory ventilation
   E. Decrease the FIO_2 to 0.3 and raise the PEEP to 12 cm H_2O

(1:863–8)

Set 17
Status Asthmaticus

A 50-year-old man is brought to the emergency department in severe respiratory distress. The patient is dusky but not cyanotic, and his wheezing can be heard across the room. This admission was preceded by an upper respiratory infection that had increased in severity over the past week, requiring increased use of the patient's MDI bronchodilator. The patient is immediately placed on 3 L nasal oxygen and an arterial blood sample is drawn. The following arterial gas and acid-base data are obtained at this time:

$Pa{O_2}$	68 mm Hg
$Pa{CO_2}$	29 mm Hg
pH	7.50
HCO_3^-	22 mEq/L
Base excess	+ 1.0 mEq/L

1. Which of the following is the correct interpretation of the above acid-base status?

   A. Partially compensated respiratory alkalosis
   B. Partially compensated metabolic acidosis
   C. Uncompensated respiratory alkalosis and uncompensated metabolic acidosis
   D. Uncompensated metabolic acidosis and partially compensated respiratory alkalosis
   E. Uncompensated respiratory alkalosis

   (9:155–6)

2. Which of the following statements regarding the management of the status asthmaticus patient is *not* true?

   A. The patient should be hospitalized immediately.
   B. Systemic corticosteroids should be administered via IV.
   C. Sedatives are indicated to calm the patient.
   D. Intubation and mechanical ventilation are often necessary.
   E. Patients must be adequately hydrated.

   (9:155–6)

3. Two hours later, the patient has become severely obtunded. Sinus tachycardia with frequent premature ventricular contractions is noted on the monitor. Auscultation reveals sharply diminished air entry bilaterally. All of the following actions are believed to be indicated at this time. Which is the number one priority?

   A. Drawing an arterial blood sample
   B. Initiation of continuous ventilatory support
   C. Insertion of a Swan-Ganz catheter
   D. Obtaining a chest roentgenogram
   E. Monitoring blood pressure

   (9:155–6)

Set 18
Aspiration Pneumonia

A 19-year-old woman is intubated and placed on a Bennett 7200 ventilator subsequent to having aspirated gastric contents during obstetric surgery. She is receiving an $FI{O_2}$ of 1.0 with no PEEP and a V_T of 10 cc/kg. Arterial blood gas and acid-base data obtained with the ventilator in the assist/control mode are as follows:

$Pa{O_2}$	56 mm Hg
$Pa{CO_2}$	47 mm Hg
pH	7.47
HCO_3^-	17 mEq/L
Base excess	– 4.9 mEq/L

1. Which of the following is the most correct interpretation of this patient's acid-base status?

   A. Metabolic acidosis with respiratory alkalosis
   B. Mixed respiratory and metabolic acidosis
   C. Fully compensated respiratory acidosis
   D. A laboratory error exists.
   E. Metabolic acidosis alone exists.

   (1:189–91)

2. Episodes of aspiration that occur while the patient is in a supine position are known to most frequently involve which of the following areas of the lung?

   A. Right lower lobe, superior segment
   B. Right lower lobe, medial support
   C. Right lower lobe, anterior segment
   D. Right lower lobe, lateral segment
   E. Right lower lobe, posterior segment

   (9:235)

3. Methods used to minimize the incidence of gastric aspiration include all but which of the following?

   A. Keeping patient NPO
   B. Administering narcotic agents
   C. Applying nasogastric suction
   D. Administering antacids
   E. Administering cimetidine

   (9:235–7)

4. Four days later, the patient is alert and is receiving an $FI{O_2}$ of 0.6 with 10 cm H_2O PEEP and a V_T of 12 cc/kg in the assist/control mode. At that time the following blood gas data are reported:

$Pa{O_2}$	183 mm Hg
$Pa{CO_2}$	27 mm Hg
pH	7.44
HCO_3^-	20 mEq/L

   Based on the above information, which of the following would be the most appropriate recommendation for the respiratory therapy practitioner to make at this time?

A. Lower the PEEP and add mechanical deadspace
B. Lower the FIO_2 and place the patient on SIMV
C. Increase the tidal volume and lower the FIO_2
D. Increase the tidal volume and lower the PEEP
E. Place the patient on SIMV with other settings unchanged

(1:611–22)

Set 19
Tension Pneumothorax

A 19-year-old man is brought to the emergency department after experiencing sharp chest pain while playing basketball. Gross observation reveals a tall, thin man in severe distress. Despite receiving 10 L oxygen via simple oxygen mask, the patient is deeply cyanotic. Percussion of the chest yields a dull note on the right side and a hyperresonant note on the left. Additionally, a distinct shift in the trachea toward the right side is noted. Cardiac leads are attached and the monitor shows multifocal premature ventricular contractions and sinus tachycardia. The blood pressure is measured at this time to be 40/0.

1. Which of the following should the respiratory therapy practitioner recommend at this time?

   A. Obtaining stat arterial blood sample
   B. Obtaining stat chest roentgenogram
   C. Inserting a needle in the eighth interspace of the left chest wall
   D. Administration of intermittent positive pressure breathing
   E. Inserting a needle in the third interspace of the left chest wall

   (8:182–3)

2. Which of the following is the most correct diagnosis?

   A. Open pneumothorax
   B. Traumatic tension pneumothorax
   C. Bronchopulmonary dysplasia
   D. Spontaneous tension pneumothorax
   E. Open tension pneumothorax

   (8:175–7)

3. Which of the following is the most probable cause of this patient's cyanosis?

   A. Decreased cardiac output
   B. Capillary shunting
   C. Anemia
   D. Ventilation in excess of perfusion
   E. A and B are correct.

   (8:16, 180)

Set 20
Respiratory Complications in AIDS

The main causes of morbidity and mortality in patients suffering from Acquired Immune Deficiency Syndrome are pulmonary in nature. A 36-year-old male, known to be HIV positive, presents to the ER with a fever, cough, and shortness of breath. The patient exhibits oral thrush, cachexia, and generalized lymphadenopathy.

1. Based on the above clinical presentation, the most likely diagnosis is:

   A. Aspiration pneumonia
   B. Pneumocystis carinii pneumonia (PCP)
   C. Pneumococcal pneumonia
   D. Epiglottitis

   (9:102–3)

2. Clinical tests that will assist in making a definitive diagnosis include:

   I. Sputum culture and sensitivity
   II. Bronchoscopy
   III. Arterial blood gas
   IV. Chest x-ray

   A. I, II, III, and IV
   B. I and IV
   C. II, III, and IV
   D. I and II

   (9:103)

3. Aerosolized pentamidine:

   A. Is approved by the FDA for both primary and secondary prophylaxis against PCP.
   B. Is indicated when the patient's CD4-positive lymphocyte count is $< 200\ mm^3$.
   C. Dosage is 300 mg in 6 mL of sterile water.
   D. B and C
   E. All of the above.

   (9:104)

4. Side effects associated with the administration of aerosolized pentamidine include:

   A. Cough and wheezing
   B. Worsening dyspnea
   C. Chest pain
   D. Hemoptysis

   (9:103–4)

5. The patient is a previous IV drug user, and has exhibited a positive reaction to tuberculin skin tests, but has previously showed no symptoms of the disease. Five days after his current hospital admission, the patient is producing bloody sputum and complaining of shortness of breath and drenching night sweats accompanied by a high fever. CXR reveals pulmonary lesions in the lower lung fields, and hilar and mediastinal lymphadenopathy. The most likely cause of the patient's distress is:

   A. Kaposi's sarcoma
   B. Cytomegalovirus
   C. Tuberculosis
   D. Viral pneumonia

(9:105–6)

6. Treatment includes:

   I. Broad-spectrum antibiotics
   II. Isoniazide
   III. Rifampin
   IV. Pyrazinamide

   A. I, II, III, and IV
   B. I only
   C. II, III, and IV
   D. II and III

(9:106)

Set 21
Pulmonary Rehabilitation and Home Care

A 60-year-old patient newly diagnosed with COPD (emphysema and chronic bronchitis) is preparing for hospital discharge. She will be going home on oxygen at 2 L/min via oxygen concentrator.

1. All but which of the following should be included in her discharge planning?

   A. Instructions on notifying local emergency medical company and electric company of her status
   B. Delivery and maintenance of oxygen equipment
   C. Hazards associated with oxygen use
   D. Instructions for calculation of $P(A-a)O_2$

(11:121–30)

2. This patient will be ready to begin outpatient pulmonary rehabilitation in the near future. What assessment(s) should be made prior to this patient's involvement in a pulmonary rehabilitation program?

   I. Patient interview/clinical history
   II. Physical examination
   III. Pulmonary Function Testing
   IV. Evaluation of exercise capacity

   A. I, II, III, and IV
   B. I and II
   C. II, III, and IV
   D. III and IV

(12:106–19)

3. Components of comprehensive pulmonary rehabilitation include all but which of the following?

   A. Breathing retraining
   B. Exercise
   C. Nutrition analysis/education
   D. Psychiatric evaluation

(12:201–13)

Set 22
Home Ventilator Care

A 22-year-old male patient with a history of muscular dystrophy has been in a subacute care unit in your hospital for the past several months on a ventilator. He is able to breathe spontaneously for approximately 4 hr at a time during the day, but requires full ventilatory support overnight. This patient will be able to leave the hospital as soon as arrangements can be made for a portable ventilator at his home. His parents are very supportive and are able to assist him with his care.

1. As the primary respiratory therapist, it is your responsibility to conduct a physical assessment of the home environment. This includes:

   A. Evaluation of cleanliness
   B. Determination of adequate space for respiratory care/nursing equipment and supplies
   C. Assessment of electrical outlets
   D. B and C
   E. All of the above

(11:114–19)

2. Patient and family education should include which of the following:

   I. Ventilator setup, maintenance, troubleshooting
   II. Sterile technique
   III. Equipment cleaning
   IV. Psychosocial concerns

   A. I, II, III, and IV
   B. I, II, and III
   C. II, III, and IV
   D. I, II, and IV

(11:117–21)

3. In the event that this patient is able to be weaned from the ventilator at night, the most plausible

alternative to continuous mechanical ventilation is:

A. IPPB
B. BiPAP
C. PCV
D. Aminophylline

(13:358–9)

4. Another mode of noninvasive ventilation that is sometimes used in the home environment, for patients with neuromuscular disease, is:

A. ECMO
B. Esophageal obturator
C. Oropharyngeal ventilation
D. Negative pressure ventilation

(13:359)

Answer Key

Set 1

1. A. Although the PaO_2 has responded slightly to oxygen at 1 L/min, severe hypoxemia still exists (the patient's oxygen needs to be increased). Baseline ABGs, along with clinical history, indicate that the patient is a CO_2 retainer, breathing on a hypoxic drive. Conservative management is the standard approach to COPD patients—increase the oxygen to 2 L/min.
2. E. Severe and life-threatening respiratory distress are not at all rare in the COPD patient—this statement is the only false one.
3. C. Pneumococcal pneumonia typically produces rusty-colored sputum.
4. C. Continuous ventilatory support is an aggressive approach to treatment of the patient in respiratory distress—all of the other treatments listed are conservative and supportive.
5. A. Because patients with severe COPD may often demonstrate $PaCO_2$ values of 70 mm Hg or greater, this is not an indication for intubation and mechanical ventilation in this patient population.

Set 2

1. B. pH of 7.48 reveals alkalosis. $PaCO_2$ is decreased; this indicates respiratory alkalosis ($PaCO_2$ and pH are indirectly proportional). HCO_3^- is slightly out of normal range, but the pH has not yet returned to normal. This indicates partial compensation.
2. D. Epiglottitis typically affects children ages 2 to 4, and is characterized by an abrupt onset, difficulty swallowing, fever, and drooling. Its incidence is less than that of croup.
3. D. Epiglottitis is always caused by *Haemophilus influenzae.*
4. D. Examination of the pharynx of patients with epiglottitis will reveal a cherry-red epiglottis. Because epiglottitis is life-threatening, and examination of the pharynx may cause airway obstruction, the pharynx should be examined only if intubation equipment is at hand.
5. C. Antibiotic therapy is begun to treat *Haemophilus influenzae*; hospitalization is required due to the life-threatening nature of epiglottitis; establishing an adequate airway is necessary so that the patient can be ventilated.

Set 3

1. C. This patient exhibits acute respiratory failure based on her ABGs and requires intubation and mechanical ventilation support.
2. C. If the PaO_2 is kept too low, tissue hypoxia will occur; if it is kept too high, CO_2 retention will occur. It is generally accepted that maintaining the PaO_2 between 50 and 70 mm Hg is the safest range.
3. C. Often, COPD patients exhibit an increased work of breathing when they are placed on continuous mechanical ventilation due to air trapping and increased ventilatory pressures.

Set 4

1. E. The PFT results indicate severe obstructive pulmonary disease: flow rates are markedly decreased, while FRC is increased above normal.
2. D. Due to the severity of this patient's disease, he is at high risk for developing pulmonary complications.
3. C. FEF_{25-75} is considered to be the most sensitive test for determining early small airways obstruction.
4. D. Increased FRC indicates air trapping, caused by loss of elastic recoil, typically seen in emphysema; because the air is trapped, it is unable to be exhaled, indicating obstruction. Consolidation would not result in increased FRC.

Set 5

1. C. Because the patient is unconscious, cyanotic, and in life-threatening distress, the respiratory therapist's first concern should be to establish an airway.
2. C. Flail chest is defined as double fractures of three or more adjacent ribs, fracture of several ribs with separation from their cartilage, or fracture of the sternum. Flail chest is frequently accompanied by lung contusions. Mechanical ventilation is indicated only if the patient's ventilation is impaired; flail chest is often managed without it.
3. E. Sedation and/or paralysis may be necessary in order to prevent excessive movement of the flail segment; bronchial hygiene therapy will assist in the prevention of secretion accumulation. Traction

and strapping of the chest were used in the past as treatment for flail chest, but are rarely, if ever, used today.

4. A. Continuous ventilatory support may help to prevent hypoxemia, and may be necessary until the flail segment is healed. This may take a week or more, depending on the size of the segment. A well-documented complication associated with mechanical ventilation is pneumothorax (barotrauma).

Set 6

1. E. Patients suffering from bronchiectasis typically report increased cough productive of copious amounts of foul-smelling sputum.
2. D. See number 1 above.
3. C. Bronchography is a diagnostic test that requires the injection of opaque contrast material into the lungs, so that the outline of the bronchi/bronchioles can be seen. This test is diagnostic for bronchiectasis, also illustrating the extent of tracheobronchial involvement.
4. D. Decreased flow rates, hypoxemia, and hypercapnea are characteristic findings associated with bronchiectasis.
5. C. While all of the therapies listed should be included in this patient's treatment regimen, bronchial drainage is crucial for the removal of secretions, so that they do not become infected.

Set 7

1. B. Whenever there is a problem with a mechanical ventilator, the patient should be removed from the machine and ventilated via manual resuscitation bag.
2. C. Once the patient is no longer on the ventilator, the most appropriate action is to examine the patient's chest (auscultation, palpation, percussion, observation), while a second therapist provides manual ventilation with 100% oxygen.
3. A. If the endotracheal tube has advanced into the right mainstem, percussion will be hyperresonant on the right (because all of the tidal volume is being delivered here), with decreased or no aeration on the left. The same results are typical of a right-sided pneumothorax.
4. E. With a cardiac rate of 20 bpm, the only choice for the therapist is to begin external cardiac compressions.

Set 8

1. C. Because the course of myasthenia crisis is unpredictable, close monitoring of the patient's ventilatory status is very important. Maximum Inspiratory Pressure (MIP), or Negative Inspiratory Force (NIF), are commonly used indicators of diaphragmatic strength.
2. D. Myasthenia gravis is characterized by descending, not ascending, paralysis. Other statements about the disease are true.
3. D. Myasthenia crisis may be brought on by emotional upset, infection, or an excessive amount of anticholinesterase drugs. Exposure to allergens precipitates asthma, but not myasthenia crisis.

Set 9

1. A. The patient's pH is acidotic (7.30); caused by a combined problem: Pa_{CO_2} is high, and HCO_3^- is low.
2. C. Guillain-Barré Syndrome is a disease of the peripheral motor neurons that may lead to paralysis of the diaphragm, requiring intubation and continuous ventilatory support.
3. D. As the respiratory muscles weaken, the VC of Guillaine-Barré patients will decrease.
4. D. When the VC drops to 20% predicted or less, intubation and mechanical ventilation are indicated. Treatment for Guillaine-Barré is symptomatic and may require several weeks of ventilatory support before the disease runs its course.

Set 10

1. C. Loud inspiratory stridor is a classic symptom of pediatric croup.
2. C. Croup is almost always caused by a virus.
3. C. Another name for croup is laryngotracheobronchitis. Treatment for croup involves cool mist aerosol therapy and/or racemic epinephrine.
4. E. Croup is generally less severe than epiglottitis; onset of symptoms occurs more gradually; and it usually does not require intubation.

Set 11

1. C. In the absence of air movement and ventilatory effort, current American Heart Association (AHA) recommendation is to give two slow breaths (to minimize the incidence of gastric distension).
2. C. Using an oropharyngeal airway that is not the right size may actually cause obstruction of the airway.
3. D. Gastric distension is more common in the child (than in the adult) during rescue breathing. Rescue breathing in the child should occur at a rate 20 breaths per minute; mouth-to-nose ventilation is appropriate only for the infant; rescue breaths should be administered during the upstroke of cardiac compressions.
4. A. Airway obstruction is more common in children than in adults; children commonly aspirate small toys or parts of toys or peanuts; back blows are an integral part of the emergency procedure for dislodging the foreign body.
5. A. Emergency cardiac compressions performed on the child can often be done with the heel of one hand and should be administered at a rate of 100

per minute. The sternum should be compressed 1 to 1½ inches.

Set 12

1. A. Polysomnography includes EEG, ECG, monitoring airflow at the patient's mouth, pulse oximetry, and impedance pneumography or intercostal electromyography (to measure ventilatory effort).
2. B. Loud snoring, daytime sleepiness, obesity, and morning headache are characteristic symptoms of obstructive sleep apnea.
3. B. A diagnosis of sleep apnea may be made when a patient suffers 30 or more episodes of apnea over a 6-hr period of sleep. Many patients with sleep apnea suffer from as many as 200 such episodes per night.
4. D. Management of obstructive sleep apnea includes weight reduction, oxygen therapy, and CPAP (to hold the airways open).

Set 13

1. B. The American Heart Association recommends the following sequence for basic cardiac life support: Establish unconsciousness; call for help; check for breathing; give two slow breaths; check for pulse; begin cardiac compressions.
2. A. Single-rescuer CPR consists of 15 compressions followed by two ventilations.
3. C. Complete airway obstruction may be relieved by performing four abdominal or chest thrusts; finger sweep; and repositioning of the head to attempt ventilation.
4. B. Chest thrust may be preferable to the abdominal thrust in obese victims, infants, or patients in the advanced stages of pregnancy.
5. D. The therapist should give two slow breaths, check for pulse, and begin two-rescuer CPR.

Set 14

1. C. Cystic fibrosis is a hereditary disease of the exocrine glands characterized by hypersecretion of mucous, pancreatic insufficiency, and abnormal sweat electrolyte concentrations. Also known as mucoviscidosis, it is a chronic, obstructive pulmonary disease that is terminal.
2. B. Measurement of sweat electrolyte concentrations contributes to the diagnosis of cystic fibrosis.
3. C. Retained secretions may lead to atelectasis, pneumonia, increased work of breathing, and hypoxemia, but not to left ventricular failure.
4. A. Typical PFT results in the patient with cystic fibrosis include decreased expiratory flow rates; increased RV and FRC.
5. D. The hypoxic drive to breathe may be dulled due to the administration of high concentrations of oxygen in those cystic fibrosis patients who are chronic CO_2 retainers.

Set 15

1. B. Because the patient exhibits ventilatory (shallow respirations at 6/min) and circulatory (HR 130; BP 70/40) distress, she should be intubated and placed on a mechanical ventilator.
2. E. Because the patient does not respond to painful stimuli, she may be categorized as in a deep coma.
3. E. The patient's hypoxemia is likely to be due to hypoventilation ($Paco_2$ 65 mm Hg), which results in a low V/Q.
4. C. Respiratory acidosis alone exists. The HCO_3^- is normal, signifying that no renal compensation has occurred yet.

Set 16

1. D. Due to the inhalation of the noxious gas, the cause of this patient's hypoxemia is most likely due to intrapulmonary shunting.
2. B. Administration of 100% oxygen would only widen the $P(A\text{-}a)o_2$. Shunting is not responsive to oxygen therapy (the oxygen-enriched gas is merely passing by the unventilated alveoli).
3. B. The best indicator of systemic oxygen transport is the cardiac output (liters of blood pumped by the heart each minute). If the cardiac output is diminished, less blood, carrying less oxygen, will be delivered to the tissues.
4. C. Nine centimeters PEEP yields the highest venous and arterial blood saturations.
5. B. FIo_2 greater than 0.5 puts the patient at risk for oxygen toxicity, so the best choice is to decrease the delivered oxygen to a safe level.

Set 17

1. E. The pH (7.5) indicates alkalosis; $Paco_2$ indicates respiratory cause (29 mm Hg); no compensation has occurred because the HCO_3^- is within normal limits.
2. C. Sedatives are contraindicated in the patient with status asthmaticus (or any patient experiencing an asthma attack). These drugs may diminish the drive to breathe.
3. B. The patient needs to be intubated and provided with continuous ventilatory support. He is obtunded, is unable to adequately ventilate, and is experiencing serious ventricular dysrhythmias.

Set 18

1. D. The reported alkalosis (7.47) is not consistent with either the $Paco_2$ (it should be low in the case of respiratory alkalosis), or the HCO_3^- (it should be high in the case of metabolic alkalosis). In this scenario, the opposite is true of both the $Paco_2$ and HCO_3^- values.
2. A. Because the patient was supine at the time of aspiration, the gastric contents will most likely go to the superior segment of the right lower lobe.
3. B. Administration of narcotic agents increases the likelihood of aspiration. Damage to the lungs as a

result of gastric contents aspiration depends upon amount and pH of those contents. Keeping patients NPO minimizes the amount; antacids and cimetidine make the gastric contents less acidic.

4. B. Due to the risk of oxygen toxicity, this patient's FIO_2 should be lowered to a safe level. She should also be placed on SIMV to encourage eucapneic ventilation and weaning.

Set 19

1. E. This patient is suffering from a spontaneous tension pneumothorax on the left side. Treatment for this life-threatening disorder is insertion of a needle in the third interspace of the left chest.
2. D. Spontaneous pneumothorax typically occurs for no reason in tall thin males. Diagnosis of tension pneumothorax may be made based on tracheal shift, cyanosis, and decreased blood pressure.
3. E. This patient is cyanotic due to decreased cardiac output (the air in the pleural space puts pressure on the heart, and it is unable to empty efficiently). Capillary shunting occurs due to atelectasis (air continues to enter the affected side, putting pressure on the opposite lung, ultimately causing atelectasis).

Set 20

1. B. PCP is common in HIV-positive patients and is consistent with the symptoms typified by this patient.
2. D. Pneumocystis carinii present in sputum or lung tissue is necessary to make a definitive diagnosis. This may be obtained either via sputum sample or bronchoscopy biopsy specimen.
3. E. Aerosolized pentamidine has been approved by the FDA for treatment in PCP; usual dose is 300 mg in 6 mL of sterile water; it is indicated for use in HIV-positive patients whose CD4-positive lymphocyte count is 200 mm^3.
4. A. Cough and wheezing have been reported by patients and some caregivers associated with aerosolized pentamidine administration.
5. C. Patient is exhibiting the classic signs and symptoms of reinfection tuberculosis. This is not uncommon in AIDS patients.
6. C. Treatment for tuberculosis is a 9-month regimen of isoniazide, rifampin, and pyrazinamide.

Set 21

1. D. It is not necessary for the patient to be able to calculate an A-a gradient. She does, however, need to notify the local electric company and EMS of her status, so that her electricity can be restored as soon as possible in case of a power outage, or so she can be transported to a place where there is electrical power in the event that her compressed gas supply runs out. The therapist should also help the patient arrange for oxygen equipment delivery and maintenance, and should educate the patient about the hazards associated with oxygen.
2. A. Before a patient begins a structured pulmonary rehabilitation program, he/she should be evaluated for exercise tolerance, have a complete PFT evaluation, undergo a physical examination, and be interviewed (initial clinical assessment/intake) so that an appropriate rehab program can be designed for the patient.
3. D. Nutrition, breathing retraining, and exercise are all necessary components of a comprehensive pulmonary rehabilitation program. Patients may be assessed for psychosocial status (this usually involves talking with the patients and/or having them complete a questionnaire about how the disease affects various aspects of their life), but a psychiatric evaluation is not routinely completed.

Set 22

1. E. Before arrangements for equipment can be made with a DME, the respiratory therapist should assess the home for adequate space, cleanliness, and adequate type and number of electrical outlets.
2. A. Comprehensive patient and family education should include instruction and/or demonstration concerning the following topics: sterile technique for both suctioning and equipment cleaning (to minimize the occurrence of infection); ventilator setup, maintenance, troubleshooting, circuit change; and psychosocial concerns.
3. B. Patients with neuromuscular disease have been shown to do well on BiPAP, to provide noninvasive ventilatory support through the night.
4. D. Another noninvasive approach to continuous positive pressure ventilation is negative pressure ventilation in the form of a chest cuirass, pneumobelt, or similar devices.

UNIT III

Hemodynamics Review and Pretest

It has been well documented that respiratory care practitioners play an important role in the management of patients with cardiovascular disorders. These individuals frequently require procedures such as continuous ventilatory support and arterial blood gas analysis.

Increasingly, the management of these patients is being guided by valuable information obtained from flow-directed, balloon-tipped pulmonary artery catheters. Information from these devices is extremely important to the respiratory therapy practitioner since it allows therapeutic modalities such as pressure control, PEEP, and oxygen to be administered in precise dosages.

A common clinical problem is the management of those patients with large physiologic shunts complicated by marginal cardiovascular reserves. In many instances, these patients would be likely to benefit from PEEP therapy. Unfortunately, pronounced cardiovascular depression is often seen with this modality. Cardiovascular support with fluids and inotropic agents is frequently indicated to minimize these side effects.

However, these support agents may also produce undesirable effects. For example, excessive fluid administration may increase intrapulmonary shunting, and sympathomimetics can worsen ventricular ectopy.

Unfortunately, when one system is treated, another often gets worse. This pathophysiologic standoff has stumped clinicians since Hippocrates' day and continues to do so. Consequently, it is not difficult to see how the ability to monitor cardiac output, pulmonary wedge pressure, and $S\bar{v}O_2$ can simplify matters greatly.

This section reviews the important concepts that are necessary in order to understand the clinical assessment of central and peripheral vascular hemodynamics. To help make this material more manageable, this outline is followed:

- I. Understanding Congestive Heart Failure
- II. The Pulmonary Circulation
  - A. Pulmonary Wedge Pressure (PWP)
    - 1. Physiology
    - 2. Increased PWP
      - a. Left ventricular failure
      - b. Left ventricular failure versus hypervolemia
    - 3. Decreased PWP
    - 4. Effect of PEEP on PWP measurements
  - B. Pulmonary Arterial Pressures
    - 1. Pulmonary hypertension
    - 2. Pulmonary vascular resistance
    - 3. Pulmonary hypotension
  - C. Other Measurements Available with Pulmonary Artery Catheterization
    - 1. $C(a-\bar{v})O_2$ and cardiac output measurements
    - 2. $S\bar{v}O_2$ and $P\bar{v}O_2$ measurements

3. Central Venous Pressure/Right Atrial Pressures
4. Elevated CVP

III. Peripheral Circulation
   A. Arterial Hypertension
      1. Chronic hypertension
      2. Acute hypertension
   B. Arterial Hypotension (shock)
      1. Decreased cardiac output
      2. Decreased peripheral vascular resistance

IV. Hemodynamics Cases and Discussions

PART 1

Understanding Congestive Heart Failure

It is the function of the powerful left ventricle to perfuse the **high pressure, high resistance peripheral circulation.** Concurrently, the considerably less muscled right ventricle pumps an identical output through the **low pressure, low resistance pulmonary vasculature.**

A healthy 70-kg subject has a circulating blood volume of approximately 6 L. At rest, roughly two thirds (4 L) of this volume is in the venous system and another fourth (1.5 L) is in the arterial system. The remaining 10% (0.5 L) is in the pulmonary vasculature.

In conceptualizing the body's circulatory system, it is important to remember that (under normal circumstances) the right and left sides of the heart are parallel circuits with *exactly* the same output. Should these outputs not match one another down to the smallest fraction of a milliliter, right- or left-sided congestive heart failure is inevitable. The following scenario illustrates this fact.

Consider a 70-kg patient with a cardiac rate of 100 beats/min. If the stroke volume of this patient's right and left ventricles is 70 mL, then both sides of the heart will have an identical output of 7 L/min. What would happen if the left ventricle suffered an ischemic episode and its stroke volume decreased 0.1 mL to 69.9 mL? **Within 1 hr the volume of blood within the pulmonary vasculature would have doubled (to 1200 mL) and the patient would be in left-sided congestive heart failure,** i.e., .1 mL × 100 beats = 10/mL/beats/min × 60 min = 600 mL.

Clinically, this patient would display signs of increased cardiorespiratory workloads, and should a pulmonary artery catheter be in place, a substantial increase in the pulmonary wedge pressure (PWP) would be noted. Oxygen administration, inotropic stimulation, diuresis, and pharmacologic reduction of venous return all have their place in correcting myocardial workload/demand imbalances such as this, and would undoubtedly be of great benefit to this patient.

PART 2

The Pulmonary Circulation

The pulmonary circulation begins with the right atrium and ends at the aortic valve. **It is characterized as a low pressure, low resistance system.** This is due to the presence of an extensive vascular bed.

It is perhaps best thought of as an enormous sheet of blood with a surface area equal to roughly two thirds of the alveolar septum (45 m^2). This is the reason postpneumonectomy patients may not develop pulmonary hypertension. This, unfortunately, is not the case with many critically ill patients. Hypoxemia, hypercarbia, and acidosis are all potent constrictors of pulmonary arterioles, and are all common occurrences in critically ill patients. It is this fact that is responsible for the widespread use of pulmonary artery catheters.

The following concept must be understood from the outset if one is to grasp the clinical significance of pulmonary artery catheterization:

> In a patient with normal pulmonary vascular resistance and a healthy right ventricle, the central venous pressure (CVP), measured in the right atrium, will accurately represent left ventricular filling or preloading pressures. However, if the pulmonary vascular resistance is increased or if the right heart is compromised, the CVP cannot be relied on to assess left ventricular or volemic status.

Here lies the problem with CVP measurement. The patients on whom it is accurate usually do not need it. The clinical importance of pulmonary artery catheterization can be summed up as follows.

> Pulmonary artery catheterization allows for measurement of the PWP. This value is not affected by changes in pulmonary vascular resistance. Thus, under most clinical circumstances it accurately reflects left ventricular filling pressures. This means that it can be used to assess the left ventricular function as well as the volemic status of the patient.

A. Pulmonary Wedge Pressure (PWP)

Physiology

The normal range of values for the PWP is either 4–12 mm Hg, or 5–15 mm Hg, depending upon the source. When a pulmonary artery catheter is in the "wedge" position, the pressure transducer, mounted on the patient's bed, measures vascular system backpressure under conditions of no blood flow. By inflating the catheter's balloon and stopping blood flow through that particular pulmonary artery branch, the clinician eliminates the component of pulmonary vascular resistance: no flow, no resistance.

The respiratory therapy practitioner employs this principle every time he or she occludes a ventricular's exhalation valve to obtain a plateau pressure. By stopping flow at end inspiration, the component of airway resistance is eliminated. The resulting static pressure is actually a reflection of alveolar pressure, and thus is not influenced by changes in airway resistance characteristics. By the same token, when the clinician inflates a pulmonary artery catheter's balloon and measures the PWP, he or she is actually getting a reflection of left atrium pressure.

In the absence of blood flow, the catheter's transducer "reads" the pressure of a static column of blood extending from the pulmonary capillaries into the pulmonary vein, and finally into the left atrium. The mean left atrial pressure is the filling pressure or **preload** of the left ventricle. This left ventricular end diastolic pressure (LVEDP) is a major determinant of stroke volume and, therefore, cardiac output.

The LVEDP is a reflection of the relationship between the volume within the left ventricle and the elastic forces of the myocardium. This (the Frank-Starling relationship) is expressed most clearly by constructing a myocardial compliance/performance curve (Figure 1).

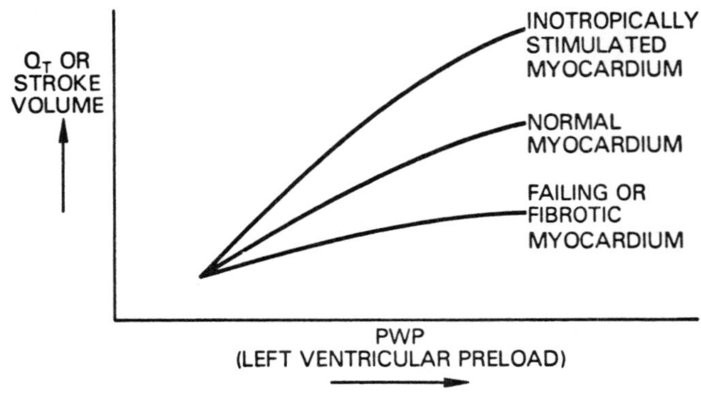

Figure 1.

From this illustration, it is not hard to see that either a low PWP (hypovolemia) or a loss of myocardial muscle tone (such as occurs following infarction) will lead to a decrease in cardiac output.

Increased PWP

The most important clinical problem associated with increases in the PWP is the development of pulmonary edema. This is believed to be inevitable whenever the pressure rises above 25 mm Hg.

Among critically ill and malnourished patients, significant edema often develops at considerably lower pressures. Lacking an adequate protein source, the serum albumin levels of these patients may drop to dangerously low levels. This and other serum proteins are responsible for maintaining intravascular volume because of the colloidal osmotic pressure they exert.

Also at risk of developing pulmonary edema at relatively low PWPs are those patients with adult respiratory distress syndrome (ARDS). These patients have experienced alveolar capillary damage through one mechanism or another (e.g., liquid aspiration or gram-negative sepsis). Because of this damage, the inflamed parenchyma becomes extremely edematous, even in the presence of normal serum protein and PWP levels.

Many clinical conditions have been associated with increases in the PWP. Fortunately, most of these are rare. Thus, we need concern ourselves mainly with the following two disorders as illustrated by the preceding Frank-Starling curve. Left ventricular dysfunction and hypervolemia are, by far, the most common and clinically significant disorders associated with increased PWP. The two most common causes of left heart failure are acute myocardial infarction and mitral regurgitation.

Consider the following self-study question:

Question

Which of the following disorders are known to cause the PWP to become elevated?

I. Adult respiratory distress syndrome
II. Left ventricular failure
III. Right ventricular failure
IV. Hypervolemia
V. Increased pulmonary vascular resistance

A. I, III, and IV
B. II, III, and IV
C. I and V
D. II and V
E. II and IV

Answer: E

Only left ventricular failure and hypervolemia lead to increased PWP. PWP does not reflect changes in pulmonary vascular resistance.

Right ventricular failure will not increase PWP, and neither will adult respiratory distress syndrome. Patients with right ventricular failure or adult respiratory distress syndrome often have increased PWPs, but it is almost always due to concurrent left ventricular dysfunction or hypervolemia. **Left ventricular failure is the most common clinical cause of right ventricular failure.**

Left Ventricular Failure

The left ventricle is a pump. Failure of this pump will cause blood to back up into the left atrium, and eventually into the pulmonary vasculature. One of the major indications for PWP measurement is the early detection of left ventricular dysfunction. Because it directly reflects left-sided heart activity, analysis of the PWP waveform is considered the most sensitive indicator of impending left ventricular failure. Left ventricular failure is commonly caused by an acute ischemic episode, such as a myocardial infarction. It may also result from increased myocardial workloads, noted when mitral valve disease leads to acute "regurgitation." Fortunately, mitral stenosis, aortic valvular disorders, and cardiac tamponade are much rarer.

Therapy for left ventricular failure includes increasing myocardial contractile force and decreasing venous return. The former may be accomplished by using pharmacologic agents such as dopamine and dobutamine, both of which have a positive inotropic effect.

Venous return (the PWP or preload) is usually reduced pharmacologically by administering diuretics and/or morphine. Morphine has a potent dilatory effect on the venules.

When arterial hypertension is present, IV nitroglycerine is indicated. Conversely, cardiogenic shock may require high doses of dopamine to maintain blood pressure. The following self-study question illustrates these points.

Question

The following data were collected on a 70-kg patient in the cardiac care unit:

Pulmonary artery systolic	53 mm Hg
Pulmonary artery diastolic	39 mm Hg
PWP	32 mm Hg
Cardiac output	3.4 L/min
$C(a-\bar{v})O_2$	7.3 vol%
Temperature	36.8° C

Which of the following pharmacologic agents would the respiratory therapy practitioner be *least* likely to recommend for this patient?

A. Dopamine
B. Morphine
C. Oxygen
D. Propranolol
E. Furosemide

Answer: D

Propranolol is used to treat the hyperdynamic left ventricle (decreasing heart rate and increasing strength of contraction), and is not indicated for the treatment of left ventricular failure. Dopamine is indicated for its positive inotropic effect; morphine, for its dilatory effect; O_2 to treat the increased $C(a-\bar{v})O_2$; and furosemide (Lasix) to decrease venous return.

Left Ventricular Failure versus Hypervolemia

Increased PWP due to left ventricular failure can usually be differentiated from increased PWP caused by hypervolemia, if the cardiac output $C(a-\bar{v})O_2$ is known. The following self-study question illustrates this fact.

Question

The following data were collected on a 70-kg patient in the cardiac care unit:

Pulmonary artery systolic	53 mm Hg
Pulmonary artery diastolic	34 mm Hg
PWP	28 mm Hg
Cardiac output	10.6 L/min
$C(a-\bar{v})O_2$	2.7 vol%
Oxygen consumption ($\dot{V}O_2$)	285 mL/min

Based on the above information, which of the following is most likely to be responsible for this patient's elevated PWP?

A. Hypervolemia
B. Hypovolemia
C. Left ventricular failure
D. Adult respiratory distress syndrome
E. Right ventricular failure

Answer: A

The reasoning for this becomes a matter of common sense if you remember that it is impossible for a patient in left ventricular failure to have a cardiac output nearly twice the normal.

Left ventricular failure leads to a decreased cardiac output. In examining the Frank-Starling curve, the reader will notice that as the PWP goes up, the cardiac output increases. Eventually, a point is reached at which output falls dramatically, but initially output increases.

Again, note the relationship between the cardiac output and the $C(a-\bar{v})O_2$. Because of the very large Q_T and the narrow $C(a-\bar{v})O_2$, this patient's cardiovascular reserves must be excellent.

Decreased PWP

The PWP is considered to be decreased whenever if falls below approximately 5 mm Hg. **By far, the most common cause of this is hypovolemia.** The following case history represents a typical patient.

Question

The following data were collected on a 70-kg patient seen in the intensive care unit:

Pulmonary artery systolic	22 mm Hg
Pulmonary artery diastolic	6 mm Hg
PWP	2 mm Hg
$C(a-\bar{v})O_2$	7.9 vol%
Temperature	37° C

Which of the following assessments regarding the above patient are most likely to be true?

I. The patient is hypovolemic.
II. Left ventricular failure exists.
III. The cardiac output is probably decreased.
IV. Pulmonary edema is inevitable.

A. I and III
B. I and IV
C. I and II
D. I, II, and III
E. I, III, and IV

Answer: A

The patient's low PWP indicates the probable presence of hypovolemia. Regarding the patient's cardiovascular reserves, they are anything but excellent. With few exceptions (massive catabolism and hyperthyroidism among them), a $C(a-\bar{v})O_2$ of 7.9 vol% in a normothermic patient indicates the existence of a severely decreased cardiac output. Left ventricular failure would be accompanied by increased pulmonary artery pressure. If pulmonary edema were pending, PWP would be increased.

Effect of PEEP on PWP Measurements

If the catheter is properly placed in the pulmonary artery, the effect of mild to moderate doses of PEEP on PWP measurements is usually minimal. It has been suggested that, on average, the PWP will increase approximately 1 mm Hg for each 5 cm H_2O of PEEP or mean airway pressure. Thus, if a patient's mean airway pressure was 40 cm H_2O, their end expiratory PWP would be approximately 8 mm Hg higher than if measured off the ventilator.

Ways of reducing PEEP-induced and respiratory artifacts include the use of strip rather than digital recorders, as well as taking measurements at end expiration.

B. Pulmonary Arterial Pressures

The following table lists the normal values for the pressures within the pulmonary artery:

Pressure	Range of Clinical Normals	Laboratory Normals
PA systolic	20–35	25
PA diastolic	5–15	8
PA mean	10–20	15

When the pulmonary artery catheter balloon is deflated, the transducer will record pulmonary arterial systolic and diastolic pressures. Electronic instrumentation will derive the pulmonary arterial mean pressure from this information. Consider the following self-study question:

Question

The respiratory therapy practitioner is monitoring a patient in the intensive care unit. The following clinical data are gathered:

PA systolic	24 mm Hg
PA diastolic	8 mm Hg
PA mean	15 mm Hg
PWP	28 mm Hg
Cardiac output	6.9 L/min

Which of the following is the most appropriate assessment regarding the above information?

A. The data are in error.
B. Left ventricular dysfunction exists.
C. The pulmonary vascular resistance is elevated.
D. The patient is hypervolemic.
E. The above represents a normal study.

Answer: A

Since it is the function of the right ventricle to deliver blood to the left ventricle and not the other way around, it is impossible for the PWP to exceed the PA systolic pressure. It would be equally impossible for peripheral venous pressures to exceed peripheral arterial pressure. Blood flows forward, not backward. The PWP is usually slightly lower than the PA diastolic pressure, unless the pulmonary vascular resistance is increased; then it is *considerably* lower.

Pulmonary Hypertension

Pulmonary hypertension exists whenever the pressures in the pulmonary arterial circuit are greater than 35/15. This occurs most commonly as the result of one of three disorders:

1. Left ventricular dysfunction
2. Hypervolemia
3. Increased pulmonary vascular resistance (PVR)

Since left ventricular failure and hypervolemia were discussed in the section on increased PWP, only PVR will be discussed here.

Pulmonary Vascular Resistance

Clinically, the PVR is considered to be elevated whenever the gradient between PA diastolic and PWP (PAD – PWP) is greater than 5 mm Hg. This may be also calculated more by using the following equation:

$$PVR = \frac{\text{Mean pulmonary artery pressure} - PWP}{\text{Cardiac output}} \times 80$$

In this case, PVR is reported in dyne/sec/cm^{-5}.

The PVR may be increased either by factors that constrict the pulmonary arterioles or by factors that destroy or obstruct the pulmonary vascular bed. Acidosis, hypercarbia, and particularly hypoxemia all have a profound effect on pulmonary arteriolar smooth muscle tone; these are the most common causes of increased PVR seen clinically.

Pulmonary embolization, alveolar septal destruction, and surgical removal of lung tissue, although less common and usually less severe, will also increase the PVR.

One of the major values of PWP measurement is that pulmonary hypertension due to increased PVR may be differentiated from pulmonary hypertension caused by left ventricular problems and hypervolemia. The following case history illustrates this.

Question

The following data were collected on a 50-kg patient seen in the intensive care unit:

PA systolic	43 mm Hg
PA diastolic	21 mm Hg
CVP	12 mm Hg
PWP	3 mm Hg
Cardiac output	3.9 L/min
$C(a-\bar{v})O_2$	7.2 vol%

Which of the following statements regarding this patient is (are) most likely to be true?

I. Left ventricular failure exists.
II. The patient is probably hypovolemic.
III. Cardiovascular reserves are excellent.
IV. The pulmonary vascular resistance is increased.

A. I, II, and III
B. II and IV
C. I and III
D. II and III
E. I only

Answer: B

Since the PAD – PWP gradient is 18 mm Hg, the PVR is considerably elevated. By looking at the CVP or the pulmonary artery pressures, the clinician would have had little idea that hypovolemia existed. In fact, just the opposite might have occurred. The clinician, faced with elevated pressures and signs of diminished perfusion, might have believed left ventricular dysfunction to be the chief problem. Had this erroneous assessment led to the decision to administer a diuretic, the result could conceivably have been catastrophic.

Pulmonary Hypotension

For all practical purposes, there is only one cause of decreased central vascular pressures, and that is hypovolemia. This holds true for all the pulmonary arterial pressures as well as the PWP and the CVP.

C. Other Measurements Available with Pulmonary Artery Catheterization

$C(a-\bar{v})O_2$ and Cardiac Output Measurements

The $C(a-\bar{v})O_2$ is believed to be a reliable indicator of cardiac output whenever the oxygen consumption is relatively normal and constant. Fortunately, this is frequently the case. The following table relates cardiac output, cardiac index, and $C(a-\bar{v})O_2$, to the cardiovascular reserves of a 70-kg critically ill patient with normal oxygen consumption:

Cardiovascular Reserves	Excellent	Good	Marginal	Poor	Failure
Cardiac Output	10 L/min	7.5 L/min	5.5 L/min	↓4.5 L/min	3.5 L/min
$C(a-\bar{v})O_2$	2.5 vol%	3.5 vol%	5.0 vol%	↑ 6.0 vol%	8.0 vol%
Cardiac Index ($L/min/m^2$)	6.2	4.7	3.5	2.8	2.2

It must be emphasized that the above values are for a critically ill patient. Among the critically ill, an average $C(a-\bar{v})O_2$ is 3.5 vol%. This is in contrast to the laboratory normal of 5.0 vol%, which is measured on a healthy subject at rest.

The most common method of obtaining C.O. in the hospital is with the use of a PA catheter, employing the thermodilution method. A bolus of saline (typically 10 cc) either iced or at room temperature is rapidly injected into the RA (proximal port of the PA catheter). The change in temperature that occurs between the RA (proximal port) and the PA (distal port), is reported as C.O., and is accurate to plus or minus 10%. Usually, 3 or 4 measurements are made, and an average is calculated and reported as the patient's C.O. These measurements should ideally be within 5% of each other.

Normal C.O. is from 4 to 8 L/min. It is calculated by multiplying HR (beats/min) and SV (mL/beat).

$S\bar{v}O_2$ and $P\bar{v}O_2$ Measurements

These are believed to be the most reliable indicators of tissue oxygenation status. The following table illustrates this:

Tissue Oxygenation Status	$P\bar{v}O_2$	$S\bar{v}O_2$
Normal	35–45 mm Hg	65–75%
Mild to moderate hypoxia	30–35 mm Hg	55–65%
Severe hypoxia	↓ 30 mm Hg	↓ 55%

From the above table it can be appreciated that because of the steepness of the oxyhemoglobin dissociation curve in this range, a drop in $P\bar{v}O_2$ of several millimeters of mercury may be of great significance.

The $S\bar{v}O_2$ is perhaps the more reliable of the two because it is not affected by changes in the positioning of the oxyhemoglobin dissociation curve.

The addition of an oximeter to the standard four- or five-channel pulmonary artery catheter allows for continuous readout of $S\bar{v}O_2$ at the patient's bedside. This is becoming an increasingly valuable tool to guide the administration of cardiorespiratory therapy.

Central Venous Pressure/Right Atrial Pressures

The central venous pressure (CVP) is measured within the right atrium. It can be measured with a CVP catheter (designed to measure only the CVP) or with three-, four-, or five-channel pulmonary artery catheters.

Among ICU/CCU patients, a very wide range of pressures from 2 mm Hg to 12 mm Hg are considered to be within "normal limits." The laboratory normal range is much lower and is usually stated to be within 2 mm Hg to 6 mm Hg. Patients with laboratory normal cardiovascular systems are in short supply in critical care units. Thus, a wider range of pressure is clinically accurate.

Elevated CVP

Like the PWP, the CVP is measured upstream from a ventricle. Thus, its value constitutes the filling pressure of the right ventricle. In addition, the same two major causes of elevated PWP cause elevated RA/CVP pressures. These causes are:

1. Hypervolemia
2. Right ventricular failure

Right ventricular failure can be the result of either a right ventricular infarct or pulmonary hypertension. As you will recall, pulmonary hypertension is the result of either:

1. Increased pulmonary vascular resistance
2. Left heart failure
3. Hypervolemia

PART 3

Peripheral Circulation

The peripheral circulation begins with the aortic valve and ends at the entrance to the right atrium. It is characterized as a high pressure, high resistance circulation. This is because its pressures and resistance to blood flow represent a fivefold to tenfold increase over those in the central circuit.

The normal arterial blood pressure is generally stated to be 120/80, but patients are generally not considered hypotensive or hypertensive until a wider range of 90/60 through 140/90, respectively, is exceeded. However, as is often the case, what is normal for one patient may not be normal for another.

A. Arterial Hypertension

In general, hypertension is not believed to exist until the peripheral arterial diastolic pressure exceeds 90 mm Hg. Mild to moderate elevations in this value (90 mm Hg to 100 mm Hg) are often unaccompanied by overt symptoms. Severe elevations (greater than 110 mm Hg) are usually the result of significant organic pathology, are generally symptomatic, and necessitate prompt intervention.

Chronic Hypertension

Unfortunately, chronic hypertension is a very common problem, but it can be managed adequately in most cases. Mild to moderate elevations in the *diastolic* blood pressure (90 mm Hg to 110 mm Hg) may be caused by nothing more than an overly stressful life-style. Severe hypertension (upwards of 110 mm Hg) usually indicates some degree of irreversible sclerotic changes in the arterial wall.

For the sake of completeness, it should be mentioned that peripheral arterial hypertension will increase left ventricular workload. Thus, hypertension is one of the risk factors associated with the development of congestive heart failure. Accordingly, peripheral arterial vasodilators, such as nitroglycerine, are frequently used in the management of chronic hypertensive patients who develop congestive heart failure. The use of vasodilators to decrease left ventricular afterload is frequently accompanied by an increase in cardiac output.

Acute Hypertension

Acute elevations in systemic blood pressure are part of the body's generalized response to stress of any kind. Physiologically, these elevations represent an attempt to shunt blood away from the tissue beds to the central organs and skeletal muscles, where it can be used for the fight or flight response. This response is mediated in large part by the release of norepinephrine from sympathetic fibers located in arteriolar smooth muscle fibers.

In general, elevations of greater than 30/15 from baseline are considered medically significant. Severe stress or illness may result in elevations of 60/30 from baseline.

For the sake of completeness, the so-called *Cushing Effect* should be mentioned here. Cushing was the first to describe the sudden, and often massive, increases in arterial blood pressure that occur following acute increases in intracranial pressure associated with neuropathology. This represents an autoregulatory mechanism designed to maintain *cerebral perfusion pressure* within its normal range of 60 mm Hg to 100 mm Hg. This relationship is shown as follows:

Cerebral perfusion pressure = (Mean arterial pressure) – (Intracranial pressure)

60–100 mm Hg = (70–110 mm Hg) – (10–20 mm Hg)

It is not uncommon for patients suffering from acute neurologic emergencies (e.g., cerebrovascular accident, neurotrauma) to present with blood pressures in excess of 200/150.

B. Arterial Hypotension (Shock)

A patient is not generally considered to be hypotensive until the arterial blood pressure falls below 90/60. When these episodes are prolonged or severe enough, circulatory failure or shock is said to exist. A good definition of shock is as follows: *a state of circulatory failure characterized by peripheral arterial hypotension and tissue hypoxia.*

From a pathophysiologic standpoint, there are two causes of shock:

1. Decreased cardiac output
2. Decreased peripheral vascular resistance

Decreased Cardiac Output

Decreased cardiac output is most commonly caused by left ventricular failure and hypovolemia. Differential diagnosis is accomplished most easily by measuring PWP. The following two self-study questions illustrate this clearly.

1. The following clinical data were gathered on a 70-kg adult patient in an intensive care unit:

Cardiac output	3.1 L/min
PWP	36 mm Hg
$C(a-\bar{v})O_2$	7.9 vol%
Oxygen consumption ($\dot{V}O_2$)	245 mL/min

Which of the following mechanisms is most likely responsible for this patient's low cardiac output?

A. Right ventricular failure
B. Left ventricular failure
C. Hypovolemia
D. Increased PVR
E. Adult respiratory distress syndrome

Answer: B

Elevated PWP, coupled with diminished cardiac output, indicates left ventricular failure.

2. The following clinical data were gathered on a 70-kg adult patient in an intensive care unit:

Cardiac output	3.1 L/min
PWP	3 mm Hg
$C(a-\bar{v})O_2$	7.9 vol%
Oxygen consumption ($\dot{V}O_2$)	245 mL/min

Which of the following mechanisms is most likely responsible for this patient's low cardiac output?

A. Right ventricular failure
B. Left ventricular failure
C. Hypovolemia
D. Adult respiratory distress syndrome
E. Increased PVR

Answer: C

The PWP is used clinically to approximate left ventricular filling pressures. It is well known medically that the cardiac output is largely dependent on the filling pressure of the left ventricle. This is, of course, the Frank-Starling relationship, and it is illustrated in Figure 2.

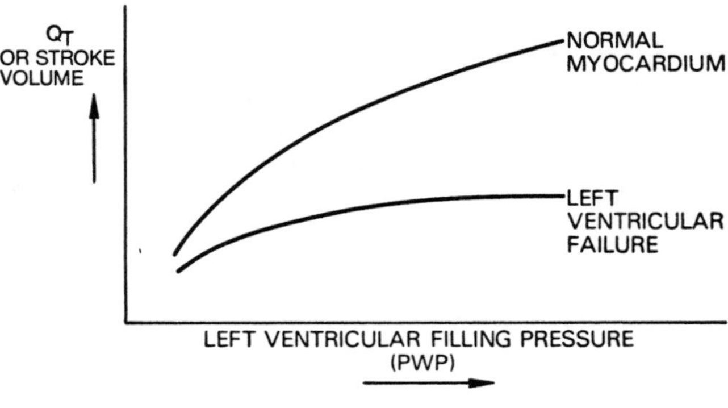

Figure 2.

The graph clearly shows that the cardiac output is low at low pressures. Clinically, a low PWP in conjunction with a low cardiac output usually indicates hypovolemia.

Decreased Peripheral Vascular Resistance

Septic, anaphylactic, and *neurogenic shock* all lead to circulatory failure via the same pathway: generalized peripheral vasodilation. This increase in the vascular space without an increase in vascular volume will lead to arterial hypotension.

When arterial hypotension is widespread, the heart becomes unable to mobilize the blood trapped in peripheral vessels. This stagnant blood becomes increasingly acidotic and, in severe cases, may begin to clot. When clotting is extensive, disseminated intravascular coagulation (DIC) is said to exist. One of the hallmarks of this condition is thrombocytopenia. In this way, these and other cellular factors are "used up."

Sepsis and anaphylaxis are known to cause vasodilation through the release of large quantities of the vasoactive chemicals histamine, serotonin, and bradykinin. These inflammatory mediators are not only powerful vasodilators, but also play important roles in activating complement and clotting mechanisms.

Neurogenic shock is the result of the loss of sympathetic (alpha) innervation to the periphery. Loss of sympathetic innervation may be traumatic or anoxic in origin. Cervical spine transection and low brain (hypothalamic) death are good representative examples. It must be pointed out, however, that hypotension is an uncommon manifestation of neuropathology. Hypertension is, in fact, seen much more frequently. An increased arterial blood pressure is necessary in order to maintain adequate cerebral perfusion pressure.

PART 4

Hemodynamics Cases and Discussions

The following four case studies are designed to assess your understanding of the hemodynamic concepts just discussed. Each case is followed by a brief discussion designed to reinforce these concepts. As you read through these, if you have additional questions, please refer to the appropriate section of this unit.

Hemodynamics Case I

An unconscious 70-kg patient is brought to the emergency department by paramedics. Barbiturate intoxication is suspected. The patient is immediately intubated and placed on continuous ventilatory support. Because profound hypotension exists, a large quantity of crystalloid is administered. The patient is then transferred to the intensive care unit where she is placed on a volume ventilator with an FIO_2 of 0.4.

Eight hours later, the patient's chest roentgenogram shows evidence of alveolar and interstitial edema. The following data are gathered at this time, with the patient on an FIO_2 of 0.6 in the assist/control mode:

PaO_2	34 mm Hg
$PaCO_2$	34 mm Hg
pH	7.28
HCO_3^-	14 mEq/L
Base excess	−7.8 mEq/L
Oxygen consumption ($\dot{V}O_2$)	250 mL/min
$C(a\text{-}\bar{v})O_2$	2.9 vol%
PWP	27 mm Hg
$P\bar{v}O_2$	24 mm Hg
$S\bar{v}O_2$	46%

1. Which of the following is most likely to be responsible for this patient's base deficit?

   A. Renal insufficiency
   B. Gastric hyperactivity
   C. Anaerobic metabolism
   D. Metabolic compensation
   E. Normocarbia

Answer: C

2. Assessment of which one of the above parameters would lead the practitioner to rule out left ventricular failure as the cause of this patient's acute pulmonary edema?

   A. $C(a\text{-}\bar{v})O_2$
   B. PWP
   C. PaO_2
   D. Arterial pH
   E. Base deficit

Answer: A

3. Which of the following should the respiratory therapist recommend at this time?

   I. Increase FIO_2 to 1.0
   II. Administer diuretics
   III. Begin PEEP therapy
   IV. Administer 1/4 normal saline intravenously

   A. II and IV
   B. I, III, and IV
   C. II and III
   D. III only
   E. I only

Answer: C

4. If the patient's effective static compliance had been monitored over the past few hours, which of the following would most likely have been noted?

   A. Widening of the gradient between peak and plateau pressures
   B. Increase in plateau pressure and increase in peak pressure
   C. Decrease in plateau pressure
   D. No change in peak pressure and increase in plateau pressure
   E. Decrease in pulmonary elastance

Answer: B

Case I Discussion

Question 1

The tip-off in this question is the critically low $P\bar{v}O_2$. This indicates the presence of severe tissue hypoxia. The resultant production of lactic acid is most likely responsible for this patient's metabolic acidosis.

Question 2

The very low $C(a-\bar{v})O_2$ coupled with the normal oxygen consumption ($\dot{V}O_2$) indicates a high cardiac output, thus ruling out left ventricular failure. An elevated PWP without a diminished cardiac output is associated with uncomplicated hypervolemia.

Question 3

The presence of refractory hypoxemia in the presence of an increased cardiac output is a clear indication for PEEP therapy. Diuretics are needed to lower the PWP and reduce pulmonary edema. Increasing the FIO_2 to 1.0 would probably not be of significant benefit since the hypoxemia is due to physiologic shunting.

Question 4

Peak and plateau pressure monitoring is often an effective method of anticipating the need for therapeutic intervention. In this case, gradual increases in both peak and plateau pressures would have alerted the practitioner that alveolar filling pathology was worsening.

Hemodynamics Case II

A comatose 63-year-old man with a long history of drug and ETOH abuse presents to the emergency department with massive G.I. bleeding. After successful resuscitation, he is transferred to the intensive care unit, where he is placed on a volume ventilator with an FIO_2 of 0.8 and 10 cm H_2O PEEP. Arterial blood gas analysis at this time reveals the following information:

PaO_2	58 mm Hg
$PaCO_2$	43 mm Hg
pH	7.26
HCO_3^-	13.6 mEq/L
Base excess	−9.7 mEq/L
Hb	6.3 gm %

1. The physician believes that the patient's hypoxia would be easier to manage if a pulmonary artery catheter were present. The respiratory therapy practitioner is asked to assist in its placement. During the procedure, the therapist notes the waveforms shown in Figure 3 on the monitor.

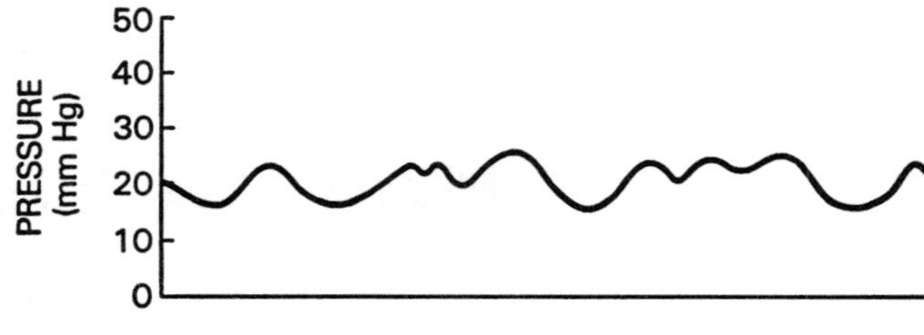

Figure 3.

Which of the following statements about the above is (are) true?

I. A pulmonary arterial tracing is noted.
II. The catheter should be retracted.
III. The catheter is in the wedge position.
IV. The catheter should be flushed with a heparin solution.

A. I and IV
B. I only
C. III and IV
D. II and III
E. III only

Answer: E

2. Following successful placement and calibration, the following values were obtained:

PA systolic	56 mm Hg
PA diastolic	41 mm Hg
PWP	30 mm Hg
CVP	8 mm Hg
$C(a-\bar{v})O_2$	7.2 vol%
Oxygen consumption ($\dot{V}O_2$)	280 mL/min

Based on the above information, the most likely cause for the above data is which of the following?

A. Right ventricular failure
B. Left ventricular failure
C. Adult respiratory distress syndrome
D. Hypervolemia
E. Hypovolemia

Answer: B

3. Based on the foregoing information, which of the following should the respiratory therapist recommend at this time?

A. Increase the level of PEEP
B. Administer inotropic agents
C. Administer dromotropic agents
D. Increase venous return
E. Increase FIO_2

Answer: B

4. Which of the following statements regarding this patient's pulmonary arterial pressures is (are) true?

   I. They are normal.
   II. Pulmonary hypertension exists.
   III. They are affected by the PVR.

   A. I only
   B. II and III
   C. III only
   D. I and III
   E. II only

Answer: B

Case II Discussion

Question 1

Based on the information presented, the catheter is in the wedge position.

Question 2

The presence of an elevated PWP with a severely widened $C(a\text{-}\bar{v})O_2$ greater than 6.0 vol% frequently indicates the presence of poor cardiovascular reserves.

Question 3

Of the alternatives presented, administration of inotropics is by far the best choice. Additionally, the medical staff would probably attempt to decrease venous return by considering a lower level of PEEP.

Question 4

Pulmonary arterial pressures greater than 35/15 are believed to indicate pulmonary hypertension. Pulmonary arterial pressures are affected by changes in PVR. Because the patient's PAD–PWP gradient is greater than 5 mm Hg, the PVR must be considered elevated.

Hemodynamics Case III

A 38-year-old patient was admitted to the emergency department in hemorrhagic shock following a motorcycle accident. Because of profound hypotension and arrhythmias, advanced cardiac life support measures were used. Following stabilization, the patient was transferred to the intensive care unit and placed on a volume ventilator with an FIO_2 of 0.6 in the control mode without PEEP. Blood gas data obtained at that time were as follows:

PaO_2	41 mm Hg
$PaCO_2$	45 mm Hg
pH	7.28
HCO_3^-	18.2 mEq/L

1. Based on the above information, which of the following modifications should the respiratory therapy practitioner make at this time?

   A. Increase the FIO_2 to 0.9
   B. Decrease the respiratory rate and increase the FIO_2
   C. Increase the tidal volume and the FIO_2
   D. Place on 10 cm H_2O PEEP with an FIO_2 of 0.6
   E. Place on 10 cm H_2O CPAP with an FIO_2 of 0.6

Answer: D

2. The physician believes that this patient's management should be guided by serial PWP measurements. After cutting down to the subclavian vein, a balloon-tipped catheter is inserted. During the procedure the tracing shown in Figure 4 was noted.

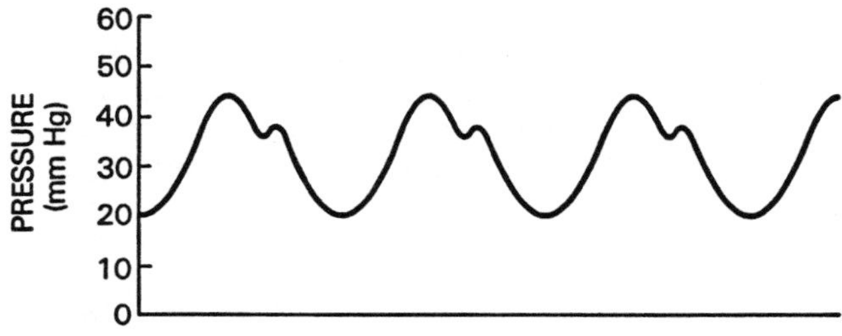

Figure 4.

Which of the following statements regarding the above waveform is (are) true?

   I. The catheter is in the pulmonary artery.
   II. The catheter may be advanced.
   III. The catheter is in the wedge position.
   IV. The catheter is in the left ventricle.

   A. I only
   B. I and II
   C. III only
   D. II only
   E. IV only

Answer: B

3. Following successful placement the following data were obtained:

PA systolic	48 mm Hg
PA diastolic	32 mm Hg
PWP	22 mm Hg
CVP	15 mm Hg
$C(a\text{-}\bar{v})O_2$	2.6 vol%

Based on the following information, the most likely assessment is which of the following?

   A. Hypovolemia
   B. Hypervolemia
   C. Left ventricular failure
   D. Acute pulmonary embolus
   E. Tension pneumothorax

Answer: B

4. Based on the foregoing information, which of the following should the therapist recommend?

   A. Increase venous return
   B. Administer diuretics
   C. Administer fluids
   D. Administer norepinephrine
   E. Wean from the ventilator

Answer: B

Case III Discussion

Question 1

Because refractory hypoxemia exists, the patient needs a trial of PEEP. CPAP is usually not appropriate during the acute phase of respiratory failure because of the increased work of breathing that may result from its application.

Question 2

The pulmonary arterial waveform can be recognized by the wide swings in pressure and by the presence of the dicrotic notch. This latter represents closure of the pulmonic valve. Because the balloon is inflated during catheter insertion, the catheter should be advanced until a PWP tracing is observed. The balloon should then be passively deflated.

Question 3

The presence of an increased PWP and an increased cardiac output is most suggestive of hypervolemia. A $C(a\text{-}\bar{v})O_2$ of less than approximately 4.0 vol% generally indicates the presence of good cardiovascular reserves.

Question 4

Diuresis is indicated to lower the PWP and treat pulmonary edema. The patient should not be weaned from the ventilator at this time.

Hemodynamics Case IV

A 68-year-old man is admitted to the intensive care unit after falling at a local nursing home. He is comatose and febrile and has a blood pressure of 40/0. The patient's appearance suggests protein malnutrition. The admission workup also shows a fractured right femur and swelling in the pelvic region, probably indicative of hemorrhage. Because of this, he is scheduled for emergency surgery. After successful control of bleeding, he is returned to the intensive care unit. Data obtained at that time include:

FIO_2	0.40 (via T tube system)
PaO_2	83 mm Hg
$PaCO_2$	65 mm Hg
pH	7.20
Base excess	–5.1 mEq/L
BP	130/90
CVP	20 mm Hg

1. True statements regarding the above information include which of the following?

   I. Refractory hypoxemia exists.
   II. Ventilatory support is indicated.
   III. Systemic hypotension exists.
   IV. The CVP is elevated.

   A. II and IV
   B. I and II
   C. I, II, and III
   D. I, III, and IV
   E. I, II, and IV

Answer: A

2. The CVP is elevated. Which of the following might be responsible?

   I. Right ventricular failure
   II. Hypervolemia
   III. Pulmonary hypertension

   A. II only
   B. I, II, and III
   C. II and III
   D. I and III
   E. I only

Answer: B

3. The physician believes the CVP does not accurately represent left heart filling pressures. To help guide this patient's therapy, he decides to place a pulmonary artery catheter. Subsequently, a 7 French catheter is inserted percutaneously into the subclavian vein. During the procedure, the waveform shown in Figure 5 is seen.

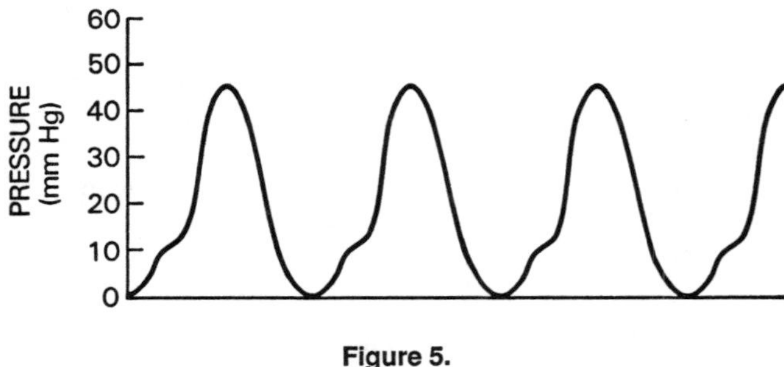

Figure 5.

Which of the following is the true statement regarding this tracing?

A. The catheter tip is in the right ventricle.
B. The catheter tip is in the wedge position.

C. The catheter tip should be retracted.
D. The catheter tip is in the pulmonary artery.
E. Artifact is present.

Answer: A

4. Following placement of the pulmonary artery catheter, the following data were obtained:

PA systolic	43 mm Hg
PA diastolic	26 mm Hg
PWP	3 mm Hg
CVP	20 mm Hg

Based on the above information, which of the following is the most likely cause of the above results?

A. Left ventricular failure
B. Hypervolemia
C. Hypovolemia with increased PVR
D. Adult respiratory distress syndrome
E. Aortic stenosis

Answer: C

Case IV Discussion

Question 1

The $Paco_2$ of 65 mm Hg in the presence of a severely acidotic pH is a clear indication for ventilatory support. The patient is not severely hypoxemic. The normal CVP is 5 mm Hg to 15 mm Hg.

Question 2

All of these may contribute to the increased CVP. Please see text for further discussion.

Question 3

A right ventricular waveform can be identified by wide swings in pressure and a diastolic pressure that falls to approximately 0 mm Hg. Also note the absence of the dicrotic notch.

Question 4

The PWP of 3 mm Hg most likely indicates the presence of hypovolemia. The PAD–PWP gradient is 23 mm Hg. Because this is considerably greater than the normal of less than 5 mm Hg, this patient's PVR must definitely be considered elevated.

UNIT IV

Examination Category Review and Pretest

NBRC Examinations have been carefully designed to determine whether candidates possess a level of competence that would allow them to practice respiratory therapy on an entry or an advanced practitioner level. The 1992 NBRC Job Survey painstakingly identified tasks that comprise the profession of respiratory therapy. The survey further delineated which of these tasks were performed by individuals just entering the field (entry level) and those by individuals who are recognized experts (advanced practitioners). The NBRC has designed examinations to assess the candidate's ability to perform these entry- and advanced-level tasks in a patient care setting.

For all its exhaustive specificity and detail, the 1992 NBRC Job Survey is built on the simple fact that much of the practice of respiratory care starts with a physician's written instructions, which may or may not have been recommended by the respiratory care practitioner. Once the order is transcribed, an appropriate health care practitioner is assigned to carry out its letter and intent. For the individual respiratory therapy practitioner, the NBRC indicates that this consists of three phases. These are listed below.

1. *Gather and analyze pertinent clinical data.* The respiratory therapy practitioner, once assigned to a particular patient, reviews the patient's chart and other pertinent records. He or she then collects and evaluates additional data at the patient's bedside. After analyzing that information, the practitioner may deem it appropriate to recommend that additional data be obtained. The therapist may be required to obtain or perform these additional studies himself/herself. Finally, the practitioner must assess the overall appropriateness of the therapeutic plan and, whenever necessary, participate in its development.
2. *Bring all appropriate respiratory care equipment to the patient's bedside.* After all appropriate clinical information has been gathered, the practitioner must then select the appropriate equipment for safe and proper performance of the diagnostic and therapeutic procedures ordered by the physician. Accordingly, the therapist must be able to assemble and check this equipment for proper function. Of course, should the equipment not operate properly, the practitioner must be able to correct any malfunctions. This latter statement is meant to include those actions necessary to ensure cleanliness and calibration of all equipment.
3. *Perform prescribed respiratory therapeutic procedures.* Finally, the practitioner must perform the therapeutic procedures that have been ordered by the physician. It is in the performance of these procedures that the analytical and judgmental skills of the practitioner are perhaps most considerable. Not only must the therapist be competent in initiating and performing these procedures, he or she must also be capable of assessing the patient's response to therapy. Should the patient experience an adverse reaction or if optimal therapeutic benefit is not being derived, the therapist must appropriately modify therapy. In the event that this modification requires a change in the physician's order,

the practitioner must then communicate his or her recommendations promptly and along established lines of communication.

The specifications of both the Entry Level and Advanced Practitioner Examinations were written around the above job description. Thus, each examination is divided into the above *three* major content categories. These three are divided into 13 entry-level, and 10 advanced-level subcategories, which on the 1992 Job Survey were broken down into 258 entry-level, and 387 advanced-level tasks. The questions in this book and on the NBRC Examinations are written specifically to assess the candidate's ability to understand the significance and to perform each one of these tasks. Therefore, in order to evaluate his or her proficiency in each one of these areas, the reader is asked to look up each exam content category in the Table of Contents and review the self-study examination questions contained therein.

PART 1

Clinical Data

Twenty-five percent of the questions on the Entry Level Examination and 20% of the questions on the Advanced Practitioner Examination are taken from this content category. These questions assess the candidate's ability to gather and analyze appropriate clinical information prior to selecting equipment or performing therapy. The NBRC 1992 Job Survey identifies four major competencies in this category for the Entry Level Examination:

A. Review patient records and recommend diagnostic procedures.
B. Collect and evaluate clinical information.
C. Perform procedures and interpret results.
D. Assess therapeutic plan.

and three major competencies for the Advanced Level Exam:

A. Review patient records and recommend diagnostic procedures.
B. Collect and evaluate clinical information.
C. Perform diagnostic procedures, interpret results, and assist in care plan.

Each one of these areas will be addressed in detail in the following pages.

A. Review Patient Records and Recommend Diagnostic Procedures

Questions in this category are designed to assess the candidate's ability to evaluate information found in the patient's chart prior to performing therapy. This information can often alert the practitioner to potential hazards. For instance, if in reading the patient's chart the practitioner notes that the patient has severe coronary artery disease and that this patient is also to receive a sympathomimetic aerosol, the practitioner would want to monitor this patient's cardiovascular status very carefully during therapy. Questions in this category will also test the candidate's ability to recommend the gathering of additional information through diagnostic testing that will contribute to the respiratory care plan.

Entry-Level Pretest

According to the NBRC, 4.3% of the questions on the Entry Level Examination are from the review patient records and recommend diagnostic procedures category. Candidates should be prepared to assess the following pertinent data:

1. Patient history, physical examination, and current vital signs
2. Admission and current respiratory care orders
3. Patient progress notes
4. Pulmonary function values and blood gas results
6. Results of chest x-rays
7. Results of respiratory monitoring (including tidal volume, minute volume, respiratory rate, I:E ratio, maximum inspiratory and expiratory pressures, vital capacity, pulse oximetry, lung compliance, and airway resistance)
8. Results of cardiovascular monitoring—blood pressure and heart rate

Candidates should also be able to recommend the following diagnostic tests as appropriate:

1. Chest x-ray
2. Blood gas analysis
3. Pre and post bronchodilator therapy
4. Pulse oximetry

The following self-study questions were developed based on the NBRC Composite Examination Matrix.

1. In reviewing the chart of a patient with cystic fibrosis, the respiratory therapy practitioner would most likely note that the patient's chief complaint is which of the following?

   A. Cough with copious sputum production
   B. Sleep apnea
   C. Nocturnal dyspnea
   D. Chest pain on exertion

   (8: Chap 20)

2. In reviewing a patient's chart prior to therapy, the respiratory therapy practitioner notes that a 30-year-old patient's peak expiratory flow rate is 10.2 L/sec. This value is most consistent with which of the following?

   A. Obstructive defect
   B. Restrictive defect
   C. Small airways disease
   D. Normal study

   (13:590)

3. In reviewing a patient's chart prior to therapy, the respiratory therapy practitioner notes that a 40-year-old patient's arterial blood pressure is 160/120. This value is most consistent with:

   A. Myocardial infarction
   B. Arterial hypertension
   C. Normotension
   D. Arterial hypotension

   (5:111)

4. Patient's respiratory rate is 20; tidal volume = 600 mL. Minute volume is:

   A. Normal
   B. Elevated
   C. Diminished
   D. Unable to be determined from the available data

   (13:588)

5. Which of the following represents the normal oxygen saturation of a healthy young adult?

   A. 90
   B. 97
   C. 80
   D. 75

   (19:64)

6. Calculate the patient's static compliance (in mL/cm H_2O), based on the following information. Ventilator settings: A/C 10; V_T = 500 mL; FIO_2 = 50%; PEEP = 10 cm H_2O; PIP = 55 cm H_2O; Plateau pressure = 40 cm H_2O.

   A. 12.5
   B. 17
   C. 25
   D. 40

   (15:628–9)

7. A patient suffering from a pneumothorax in the RUL would produce the following chest x-ray:

   A. Completely white on the right side
   B. Completely black on the left side
   C. RUL completely white
   D. RUL completely black

   (9:286–9)

8. The normal value for arterial blood HCO_3^- is approximately:

   A. 22–26 mEq/L
   B. 34–38 mEq/L
   C. 46–50 mEq/L
   D. 60–64 mEq/L

   (19:61–2)

9. In reviewing a patient's orders prior to performing therapy, the respiratory therapy practitioner notes that the physician wants spirometry before and after administration of a bronchodilator. From this information the therapist may safely assume that:

   A. The patient may be HIV positive.
   B. The patient may have tuberculosis.
   C. An anaerobic pneumonitis is suspected.
   D. The physician suspects asthma.

   (6:190–3)

10. Patient has fallen from the roof of his two-story house. He exhibits paradoxical breathing and mild respiratory distress. Flail chest is suspected. The RCP could confirm the diagnosis by recommending:

    A. Mixed venous blood gases
    B. Spirometry
    C. Chest x-ray
    D. Peak flow measurement

    (9:294–7)

11. Pulse oximetry is limited under the following conditions:

    A. Respiratory alkalosis
    B. Irregular breathing pattern
    C. Increased pigmentation of patient's skin
    D. All of the above

    (19:265–6)

Answer Key

1. A. The classic symptom reported by cystic fibrosis patients is cough that is productive of large amounts of thick sputum.
2. D. A normal healthy male can generate a PEFR of approximately 10 L/sec. This value is slightly lower in females.
3. B. Arterial hypertension is defined as systolic pressure of > 140 torr and a diastolic pressure > 90 torr.
4. B. Minute volume is calculated by multiplying RR by tidal volume, in this case, 20 × 0.6 L = 12 L/min. Normal minute volume is 5 to 10 L/min, so this represents an elevated value.
5. B. Normal adults have an oxygen saturation of approximately 97%.
6. B. Calculation of static compliance with PEEP is as follows: Static compliance = Tidal volume divided by (Plateau pressure – PEEP). In this case, 500 divided by (40 – 10); 500/30 = 16.7.
7. D. Because the RUL would contain excessive air, it would appear completely black.
8. A. The normal value for arterial blood HCO_3^- is approximately 22–26 mEq/L.
9. D. Reversibility of airways obstruction may be assessed by performing a before-and-after bronchodilator study. If the FEV_1 improves 12–15% from pre to post test, the airways obstruction is considered to be reversible.
10. C. Flail chest could be confirmed by observing sternal fracture, fractures of three or more adjacent ribs, or rib fracture with separation from cartilage, as seen on a CXR.

11. C. Pulse oximetry is limited by weak pulse, presence of hemoglobin moieties, and pigmentation.

Advanced Practitioner Pretest

According to the NBRC, 6% of the questions on the Advanced Practitioner Examination are from the review patient records and recommend diagnostic procedures category. In addition, the Composite Examination Matrix states that questions in this category will assess the candidate's ability to assess the following pertinent data:

1. Results of electrolytes, hemoglobin and hematocrit, CBC, and/or blood chemistries
2. Fluid balance (intake and output)
3. Results of cardiovascular monitoring [including cardiac output, pulmonary capillary wedge pressure, pulmonary artery pressures, central venous pressure, ECG, mixed venous O_2, $C(a\text{-}\bar{v})O_2$]
4. Results of respiratory monitoring (including V_D/V_T, shunt studies, capnography, inspiratory and expiratory flow and volume waveforms, transcutaneous O_2 and CO_2)
5. Sputum culture and sensitivity and Gram's stain results
6. Culture, sensitivity, and Gram's stain results from blood and other body fluids
7. Results of upper airway x-rays
8. Perinatal and neonatal test results (including maternal and perinatal histories, APGAR scores, gestational age, L/S ratio)
9. Results of other diagnostic tests including sleep studies and ventilation/perfusion scan, and pulmonary stress testing

Examination candidates are also expected to recognize when to recommend the following additional procedures:

1. Electrolytes
2. CBC
3. Sputum culture and sensitivity
4. Chest x-ray
5. Upper airway x-ray
6. Maximum voluntary ventilation (MVV)
7. Blood gas analysis
8. Insertion of arterial, umbilical, or central venous pressure monitoring lines
9. ECG
10. Cardiac output and shunt studies
11. Pulmonary stress testing
12. Pulmonary function tests (including flow-volume loops, spirometry before and after bronchodilator, diffusion capacity, FRC, nitrogen washout distribution, and total lung capacity)
13. V_D/V_T
14. Lung compliance and other mechanics
15. Bronchoscopy
16. Pulse oximetry and transcutaneous O_2/CO_2 monitoring

The following self-study questions were developed from the NBRC Composite Examination Matrix.

1. Normal deadspace to tidal volume ratio is:

   A. 10%
   B. 15%
   C. 30%
   D. 50%

   (19:116–7)

2. Which of the following statements is (are) true regarding pleural transudates?

   I. They may be caused by left ventricular failure.
   II. They are a thin, watery liquid.
   III. They are associated with lung abscess.
   IV. They have a very high protein content.

   A. II and III
   B. I and II
   C. I and IV
   D. III and IV
   E. III only

   (8: Chap 12)

3. On reading a 65-kg patient's chart prior to administering IPPB therapy, the respiratory therapy practitioner notes that the patient's FVC is 1 L. On the basis of this information, the therapist can safely assume that:

   A. A severe restrictive disorder exists.
   B. The patient would benefit more from incentive spirometry than from IPPB.
   C. A mild obstructive disorder exists.
   D. The patient should receive incentive spirometry in addition to IPPB.

   (4:89)

4. A patient in the ICU has a urine output of 500 mL over the past 24 hr. This indicates:

   A. Normal output
   B. Polyuria
   C. Anuria
   D. Oliguria

   (17:204)

5. Which of the following is true of APGAR scores?

   I. It is the only means of assessing a newborn's general condition at birth.
   II. It is recorded at 1 and 5 min after birth.
   III. A score of "7" is considered good.
   IV. Assessment is based on three signs.

   A. I and III
   B. IV only
   C. II and III
   D. I and IV

   (14:37)

6. In reading a patient's chart prior to performing IPPB, the respiratory therapy practitioner notes an electrophoresis study that indicates a very low serum concentration of the enzyme α-1-antitrypsin. The practitioner would expect the patient to have which of the following pulmonary disorders?

   A. Centrolobular emphysema
   B. Panlobular emphysema
   C. Collagen vascular disease
   D. Pancoast superior sulcus syndrome

(8:92–3)

7. The normal value for D_LCO for males when performed by the single breath method is:

   A. 12 mm Hg/mL/sec
   B. 15 mL/min/mm Hg
   C. 25 mL/min/mm Hg
   D. 8 mL/mm Hg/min

(17:245)

8. The RCP wants to assess arterial blood pressure and arterial blood gases. This can be done by insertion of which line?

   A. Central venous
   B. Pulmonary artery
   C. Arterial
   D. Any of the above

(5:101–2)

9. Which of the following most accurately represents an average $C(a\text{-}\bar{v})O_2$ for a critically ill patient with good cardiovascular reserves?

   A. 11.0 vol%
   B. 3.5 vol%
   C. 5 vol%
   D. 7.5 vol%

(4:247–8)

10. Normal value for pulmonary capillary wedge pressure is:

   A. 10 mm Hg
   B. 20 mm Hg
   C. 30 mm Hg
   D. 40 mm Hg
   E. 50 mm Hg

(5:147)

11. The respiratory therapy practitioner is reviewing a patient's chart prior to therapy. The practitioner notices that the bacteriology report on a sputum sample sent 24 hr previously states that the sample contained numerous squamous epithelial cells and a wide variety of gram-positive organisms. From this information the practitioner may safely conclude that:

   A. The patient has lung cancer.
   B. The laboratory report is in error.
   C. The sample contained excessive saliva.
   D. The patient has extrinsic asthma.

(9:27–8)

12. In reviewing a patient's chart prior to therapy, the respiratory therapist notices that the latest chest roentgenogram revealed a diffuse bilateral alveolar filling pattern with increased vascular markings and prominent Kerley-B lines. These findings are most consistent with:

   A. Pulmonary embolus
   B. Bronchiectasis
   C. Cardiogenic pulmonary edema
   D. Bronchial asthma

(9:264–8)

13. In reading a patient's chart prior to bronchodilator therapy, the respiratory therapy practitioner notes that the patient had a permanent pacemaker implanted several months ago. Development of which of the following arrhythmias would most likely have been responsible for pacemaker placement?

   A. Sinus tachycardia
   B. Sinus arrhythmia
   C. Third-degree (complete) heart block
   D. Multifocal premature ventricular contractions

(10:151)

14. A patient with chronic obstructive pulmonary disease who is on a volume-cycled ventilator has a pulmonary artery (Swan-Ganz) catheter in place. In reading the patient's chart, the respiratory therapy practitioner notes that the patient's mean pulmonary pressures have consistently been around 35 mm Hg. This value most likely represents:

   A. Pulmonary hypotension
   B. Pulmonary hypertension
   C. Normal study
   D. Adult respiratory distress syndrome

(5:147)

15. A patient in the intensive care unit is noted to have a serum potassium concentration of 2.6 mEq/L. This value most likely indicates the presence of:

   A. Metabolic alkalosis
   B. Hypocalcemia
   C. Hypokalemia
   D. Normal study

(17:212)

16. Which of the following is the most widely used method of obtaining cardiac output in the ICU?

A. Fick method
B. Dye indicator dilution
C. Thermodilution
D. Impedance cardiography

(5:190)

17. In order to calculate a dead space to tidal volume ratio (V_D/V_T), which of the following are necessary?

I. Arterial blood gas
II. End-tidal CO_2
III. Arterial oxygen content
IV. Mixed venous oxygen content

A. I and II
B. II and III
C. III and IV
D. I, II, and III

(19:118)

18. A ventilation-perfusion scan would be most likely to assist in diagnosing which of the following diseases/disorders?

A. Atelectasis
B. Pulmonary embolus
C. Pneumothorax
D. Hemothorax

(1:923)

19. Which of the following statements regarding the L/S ratio is/are true?

A. The higher the ratio, the greater the infant's chance of developing ARDS.
B. The L/S ratio accurately predicts lung maturity 98% of the time.
C. The lower the ratio, the greater the infant's chance of developing RDS.
D. B and C

(14:33–4)

20. Which of the following scoring systems are used to assess gestational age?

A. Dubowitz
B. APGAR
C. Ballard
D. A and C

(14:36–9)

21. A patient is breathing 100% oxygen. If the Pa_{O_2} is 200 mm Hg, the shunt can be estimated to be:

A. 5–10%
B. 10–15%
C. 15–20%
D. 20–25%

(1:953)

22. Which of the following are indications for capnography?

I. Polysomnography
II. Monitoring the adequacy of mechanical ventilation
III. Monitoring cardiopulmonary resuscitation
IV. Indirect calculation of cardiac output

A. I, II, III, and IV
B. I, II, and III
C. II, III, and IV
D. II and III

(1:712)

23. Which of the following statements regarding transcutaneous O_2/CO_2 monitoring is/are true?

A. Electrodes must be heated.
B. Monitoring is used mostly in neonates and small children.
C. Electrode sites should be changed every 8 hr.
D. A and B

(1:711)

24. Which of the following information can be gained by performing a 7-min nitrogen washout test?

A. Small airways disease
B. Thoracic gas volume
C. Distribution of gas in the lung
D. V_D/V_T

(6:87–9)

25. Which of the following are true statements about the flow-volume loop?

A. Subjects are instructed to inhale to TLC and exhale to FRC.
B. Obstructive lung disease reveals decreased flow.
C. Restrictive lung disease reveals decreased volume.
D. B and C

(6:57–60)

Answer Key

1. C. Normal dead space to tidal volume ratio is 20–40%.
2. B. Transudates are characterized by thin, watery fluid, with few blood cells and low protein counts. It may be caused by right or left heart failure.
3. B. This patient's FVC is > 15 mL/kg (15 × 65 = 975 mL), so IS is the preferred treatment.
4. D. Normal urine output is approximetely 1500 mL/day. Oliguria is defined as a decreased amount of urine output.
5. C. APGAR scoring is one of several assessments of the neonate's overall condition at birth. It evaluates 5 signs, is assessed at 1 and 5 minutes after birth, and is scored as follows: 0–3 = poor; 4–6 = fair; 7–10 = good.

6. B. Panlobular emphysema is associated with α-1 antitrypsin deficiency; centrilobular is associated with cigarette smoking.
7. C. Normal DLCO is 25 mL/min/mm Hg; in women the number is closer to 20 mL/min/mm Hg.
8. C. Only the arterial line can measure arterial blood pressure and arterial blood gases.
9. C. Normal $C(a-\bar{v})O_2$ for a critically ill patient with good cardiovascular reserves is 5.0 vol%.
10. A. Normal PWP is 4–12 mm Hg.
11. C. Squamous epithelial cells and gram-positive organisms in a sputum sample indicate that the secretions are from above the larynx.
12. C. Diffuse bilateral alveolar filling pattern with increased vascular markings and prominent Kerley-B lines are most consistent with cardiogenic pulmonary edema.
13. C. Third-degree (complete) heart block is an indication for replacement of a pacemaker. The other dysrhythmias listed are not indications.
14. B. Normal mean pulmonary artery pressure is 10–20 torr. Because the level is much greater than this, pulmonary artery hypertension is present.
15. C. Hypokalemia is defined as potassium levels < 3.5 mEq/L (normal values: 3.5–5.5 mEq/L).
16. C. Thermodilution is the most common method of obtaining C.O. in the ICU because serial measurements may be obtained quickly, without recirculation on any type of dye.
17. A. Calculation of dead space to tidal volume ratio is as follows: $PaCO_2 - (P\bar{E}CO_2/PaCO_2)$.
18. B. Ventilation/perfusion scans may be useful in diagnosing pulmonary embolus. Pulmonary angiography provides definitive diagnosis.
19. C. As the ratio of lecithin to sphyngomyelin drops below 2, incidence of RDS increases. The incidence of false negative results may be as high as 20–25%.
20. D. Ballard and Dubowitz scoring methods may both be used to assess gestational age: APGAR assesses the neonates overall condition.
21. D. If a patient is breathing 100% oxygen, there is a 5% shunt for every 100 mm Hg the PaO_2 is below expected. For a patient breathing 100% oxygen at sea level, normal PaO_2 would be approximately 600 mm Hg. A PaO_2 of 200 mm Hg is 400 below normal—400 × 0.05 = 20% shunt. Add to this the normal 3–4% shunt that everyone has, and the value is approximately 23%.
22. B. Applications for capnography include monitoring adequacy of mechanical ventilation and/or CPR; monitoring airflow during polysomnography; regulating hyperventilation; monitoring anesthesia; and verifying a steady-state before indirect calorimetry.
23. D. Transcutaneous monitoring is used most often in neonates and pediatrics; electrodes should be heated to 44–45° C; and the site of the electrode should be changed every 4 hours to prevent burning of the skin.
24. C. Distribution of gas in the lung is assessed by nitrogen washout.
25. D. The flow-volume curve of a patient with obstructive lung disease reveals decreased flow, while the curve of a patient with restrictive lung disease reveals decreased volume.

B. Collect and Evaluate Clinical Information

Questions in this category are designed to assess the candidate's ability to obtain additional pertinent clinical information prior to performing diagnostic or therapeutic procedures. In the clinic this information can be obtained in one of three ways:

1. By performing a chest physical examination (including inspection, palpation, and auscultation);
2. By interviewing the patient;
3. By inspecting the patient's chest roentgenogram.

Entry Level Pretest

According to the NBRC, 8.6% of the questions on the Entry Level Examination are from the collect and evaluate clinical information category. In addition, the Composite Examination Matrix states that the questions in this category will assess the previously mentioned competencies in order to obtain a comprehensive evaluation of the patient's cardiopulmonary status. The following self-study questions were developed based on the NBRC Composite Examination Matrix.

1. Which of the following signs and symptoms are typical of a patient admitted for an exacerbation of COPD?

   A. Asymmetrical chest movement
   B. Digital clubbing
   C. Diaphragmatic breathing
   D. Nasal flaring

   (9:129, 133–4)

2. A patient who is disoriented to time and place and is unable to cooperate with the respiratory care practitioner or follow directions would be *unable* to perform which of the following therapies?

   A. Incentive spirometry
   B. IPPB
   C. MDI
   D. A and C

   (4:68, 92–4)

3. Normal breath sounds that are heard over the lung periphery are termed:

   A. Bronchovesicular
   B. Vesicular
   C. Bronchial
   D. Amorphic

   (3:362–4)

4. Which of the following is (are) most frequently used to describe the sputum of patients with lung abscess?

   I. Mucoid
   II. Tenacious
   III. Copious
   IV. Purulent

   A. II and III
   B. I and IV
   C. III and IV
   D. I and II

(9:75–7)

5. Which of the following disorders is most frequently associated with the term *orthopnea?*

   A. Idiopathic respiratory distress syndrome
   B. Congestive heart failure
   C. Bronchial asthma
   D. Bronchiolitis

(9:267)

6. During auscultation of blood pressure, the beginning of Karotkoff sounds indicates which stage of the cardiac cycle?

   A. Ventricular systole
   B. Ventricular diastole
   C. Protodiastole
   D. Atrial contraction

(5:96–7)

7. The phrase "episodic shortness of breath in which sleep is interrupted" best defines:

   A. Orthopnea
   B. Paroxysmal nocturnal dyspnea
   C. Dyspnea
   D. Biot's breathing
   E. Sleep apnea

(9:267)

8. A patient presents to the pulmonary clinic with a history of emphysema. What physical findings are likely to be noted?

   A. Diaphragmatic breathing
   B. Cachectic appearance
   C. Increased A-P diameter
   D. B and C

(9:133–4)

9. The presence of which of the following chest physical findings suggests the presence of pulmonary consolidation?

   I. Increased vocal fremitus
   II. Vesicular breath sounds
   III. Bronchial breath sounds
   IV. Crackles (rales)

   A. I, III, and IV
   B. II, III, and IV
   C. III and IV
   D. I, II, III, and IV

(13:20–5)

10. Patients who are deeply comatose would be *least* likely to exhibit which one of the following signs and symptoms?

   A. Absence of tracheal or carinal reflexes
   B. Soft tissue obstruction of upper airway tissues
   C. Purposeful response to pain
   D. Abnormal peripheral muscle tone

(4:156)

11. Severe respiratory distress in the newborn may be characterized by which of the following?

   A. Nasal flaring
   B. Sternal retractions
   C. Expiratory grunting
   D. All of the above

(14:71–4)

12. Pink-tinged pulmonary secretions have been associated with:

   A. Asthma
   B. Left ventricular failure
   C. Cor pulmonale
   D. Use of albuterol

(8:134–43)

13. The decision to intubate and initiate continuous ventilatory support in patients with acute neuromuscular disorders is most reliably made on the basis of which of the following clinical determinations?

   A. Arterial blood gas analysis
   B. History and physical examination
   C. Serial vital capacity measurements
   D. Peak expiratory flow rates

(9: Chap 23)

14. Which of the following physical findings is (are) *most* likely to be seen in a patient with a large tension pneumothorax?

   I. Hyperresonant percussion note over the affected area
   II. Mediastinal shift away from the affected side
   III. Absent breath sounds over the affected area
   IV. Stridor

   A. I, II, and III
   B. I, III, and IV
   C. II, III, and IV
   D. I, II, III, and IV

(9:286–9)

15. The onset of harsh "barking" cough with inspiratory stridor over the past 1–2 days is characteristic of which of the following disorders?

    A. Epiglottitis
    B. Senile emphysema
    C. Bronchopulmonary dysplasia
    D. Croup

    (8:254–5)

16. Which of the following chest physical findings is most frequently associated with partial upper airway obstruction?

    A. Tracheal shift
    B. Inspiratory stridor
    C. Harsh dry cough
    D. Dullness to percussion

    (10:23)

17. Which of the following disorders is most likely to be associated with the presence of Kussmaul's type breathing?

    A. Postanoxic encephalopathy
    B. Damage to the medulla oblongata
    C. Pulmonary emphysema
    D. Diabetic acidosis

    (3:357)

18. The phrase "periods of hyperpnea that wax and wane and are frequently separated by apneic spells" most accurately describes:

    A. Hyperventilation
    B. Biot's breathing
    C. Obstructive breathing
    D. Cheyne-Stokes respirations
    E. Kussmaul's breathing

    (3:357)

19. For which of the following disorders is the presence of very large quantities of putrid-smelling sputum a common clinical finding?

    A. Anaerobic lung abscess
    B. Extrinsic asthma
    C. Pulmonary emphysema
    D. Pulmonary interstitial fibrosis

    (8:192)

20. Which of the following signs and symptoms may be observed in a patient presenting to the emergency room suffering a severe acute asthma attack?

    I. Diaphoresis
    II. Use of accessory muscles
    III. Peripheral edema
    IV. Bilateral expiratory wheezing

    A. I, III, and IV
    B. II, III, and IV
    C. I, II, and IV
    D. I, II, and III

    (9: Chap 9)

21. Patients with which of the following conditions would be most likely to exhibit cyanosis?

    I. Anemia
    II. Low cardiac output
    III. Polycythemia
    IV. High cardiac output

    A. I and IV
    B. II only
    C. I and II
    D. II and III

    (13:580)

22. Which of the following is *least* likely to occur following slippage of a patient's endotracheal tube into the right mainstem bronchus during continuous ventilatory support?

    A. Left-sided pneumothorax
    B. Increased aeration on the right side
    C. Increased ventilator plateau pressure
    D. Dull percussion note on the left side

    (1:272)

23. The presence of which of the following is *least* likely to be associated with the term *hyperventilation?*

    A. Bradypnea and hypopnea
    B. Hyperpnea and tachypnea
    C. Hyperpnea with a normal V_D/V_T
    D. Arterial hypocapnia

    (1:219)

Answer Key

1. B. Digital clubbing is a typical physical finding associated with COPD, as are cyanosis, use of accessory muscles of ventilation, and barrel chest.
2. D. Performance of both MDI and IS require a cooperative and alert patient. IPPB may be given to unconscious patients by using a mask or mouthseal and noseclips.
3. B. Breath sounds heard over the lung periphery are termed vesicular.
4. C. Lung abcess typically produces large amounts of foul-smelling sputum.
5. B. Orthopnea is a common symptom of heart failure (dyspnea on lying down).
6. A. During auscultation of blood pressure, the beginning of Karotkoff sounds indicates ventricular systole, while diastole is characterized by the disappearance of Karotkoff sounds.
7. B. Episodic shortness of breath in which sleep is interrupted defines paroxysmal nocturnal dyspnea.
8. D. Patients with emphysema are likely to have increased A-P diameter (barrel chest), and have a thin, wasted appearance (cachexia).
9. A. Consolidation (such as occurs in pneumonia) typically produces bronchial breath sounds over the lung

periphery; crackles over the large airways; and increased fremitus (fluid transmits sound).

10. C. Patients in a deep coma do not respond purposefully to pain. Only a small percentage of these patients, however, will lose their carinal reflex.
11. D. Severe respiratory distress in the newborn may be characterized by nasal flaring, sternal retractions, and expiratory grunting.
12. B. Pulmonary edema caused by left ventricular failure produces characteristic frothy pink sputum.
13. C. The decision to intubate and initiate continuous ventilatory support in patients with acute neuromuscular disorders is most reliably made on the basis of serial measurements of vital capacity.
14. A. In patients with tension pneumothorax, a hyperresonant percussion note may be heard over the affected area; trachea and mediastinum shift away from the affected side; and breath sounds are absent over the affected side.
15. D. Croup develops over 24–48 hr and is characterized by a barking cough and the presence of stridor. In epiglottitis, stridor is muffled, onset is sudden, and cough is usually absent.
16. B. Inspiratory stridor is a classic finding associated with partial upper airway obstruction.
17. D. Kussmaul's breathing is characteristic of metabolic acidosis.
18. D. Irregular breathing that increases and decreases in rate and depth with periods of apnea is termed Cheyne-Stokes.
19. A. Very large quantities of putrid-smelling sputum is a common clinical finding of lung abscess (anaerobic).
20. C. Patients suffering from a severe asthma attack are often diaphoretic, pale, and using accessory muscles to breathe. They frequently wheeze on expiration.
21. D. Because cyanosis depends on hemoglobin concentration, patients with anemia do not become cyanotic until they are severely hypoxemic. The opposite is true of polycythemic patients. Patients with low cardiac output have decreased blood volume, and thus, decreased hemoglobin levels.
22. A. In the event that the ET tube slips into the right mainstem bronchus, the left lung will no longer be ventilated, causing atelectasis, NOT pneumothorax.
23. A. Low levels of CO_2 (hypopnea) and a decreased respiratory rate (bradypnea) would characterize hypoventilation, instead of hyperventilation.

Advanced Practitioner Pretest

According to the NBRC, 7% of the questions on the Advanced Practitioner Examination are from the collect and evaluate additional clinical information content category. In addition, the Composite Examination Matrix states that questions in this category assess the advanced practitioner's ability to assess the patient's overall cardiopulmonary status by:

1. Physical examination (including inspection, palpation, percussion, and auscultation)
2. Interview techniques
3. Inspecting of the chest x-ray
4. Inspecting of lateral neck x-rays
5. Performing bedside procedures (including V_D/V_T, transcutaneous O_2/CO_2 monitoring, shunt studies, cardiac output, capnography, pulmonary capillary wedge pressure, mixed venous blood gases, $P(A\text{–}a)O_2$, lung compliance, ECG, and apnea monitoring)
6. Interpreting results of bedside procedures (including pulse oximetry, tidal volume, minute volume, maximum inspiratory and expiratory pressure, tracheal tube cuff pressure, timed forced expiratory volumes, I:E ratio, alveolar ventilation, FVC, peak flow, central venous pressure, pulmonary artery pressures, fluid balance, sleep studies)

The following self-study questions were developed from the NBRC Composite Examination Matrix.

1. Which of the following statements about the technique of palpation are true?

   I. Pneumothorax produces decreased fremitus.
   II. Broken ribs on the left side produces symmetrical expansion of the chest.
   III. Consolidation is associated with decreased fremitus.
   IV. Consolidation is associated with increased fremitus.

   A. II and III
   B. I and IV
   C. II and IV
   D. III and IV

   (9:13)

2. Which of the following statements about the chest roentgenogram is *not* true?

   A. Adult respiratory distress syndrome is associated with ground glass appearance.
   B. Atelectasis appears radiolucent.
   C. Radiolucent structures tend to be black in appearance.
   D. An area of calcification will be white in appearance.

   (9:29–34)

3. The roentgenographic changes most frequently seen in patients with pulmonary emphysema include:

   I. Increased radiolucency
   II. Widened cardiac shadow
   III. Flattened diaphragms
   IV. Decreased anteroposterior diameter

   A. I and IV
   B. I and III
   C. II and IV
   D. III only

   (9:29–34)

4. A neonate exhibits nasal flaring, sternal retractions, HR 40 beats/min, and central cyanosis. Gestational age is estimated at 30 weeks. This patient will most likely require:

   A. No respiratory therapy
   B. Oxygen hood at 30%
   C. Intubation and mechanical ventilation
   D. Nasal CPAP

(14:55–9)

5. Which of the following disorders is known to produce characteristic bronchographic evidence of a lack of the normal tapering of the medium-sized airways?

   A. Bronchiolitis
   B. Cystic fibrosis
   C. Bronchiectasis
   D. Bronchogenic carcinoma

(8: Chap 4)

6. The presence of which of the following when noted on a chest roentgenogram is *most* suggestive of the presence of consolidated lung tissue?

   A. Blunting of the costophrenic angles
   B. Multiple reticulonodular densities that do not coalesce
   C. Areas of increased radiolucency
   D. Areas of increased opacification

(9:29–34)

7. A respiratory therapist is monitoring CO_2 levels in order to determine proper endotracheal tube placement. What would he/she expect to see if the tube is positioned correctly in the trachea?

   A. Very little fluctuation of CO_2 levels
   B. 5% on inspiration, fluctuating to 0% on expiration
   C. 0% on inspiration, fluctuating to 6% on expiration
   D. 10% on inspiration, fluctuating to 30% on expiration

(1:489)

8. Which of the following radiologic findings would *most* likely be seen in a patient who has cor pulmonale?

   I. Left ventricular hypertrophy
   II. Increased pulmonary vascular markings
   III. Right ventricular hypertrophy
   IV. Compensatory hyperinflation

   A. I and III
   B. III and IV
   C. I and II
   D. II and III

(8:67, 94)

9. Which physical findings are characteristic of left lower lobe pneumonia?

   I. Asymmetric chest movement
   II. Venous distention
   III. Productive cough
   IV. Bronchovesicular breath sounds over affected segments

   A. I and III
   B. I, II, and IV
   C. II, III, and IV
   D. I and IV

(9:66–75)

10. Hyperresonance to percussion is *least* likely to indicate which of the following?

    A. Pneumothorax
    B. Asthma
    C. Emphysema
    D. Chronic bronchitis

(13:30–1)

11. The presence of which of the following, when noted on a chest roentgenogram, is *most* suggestive of fluid within the pleural space?

    A. Mediastinal shift to the affected side
    B. Areas of increased radiolucency
    C. Multiple small densities that coalesce into larger densities
    D. Blunting of the costophrenic angles

(9:282–6)

12. On viewing a lateral chest roentgenogram, the respiratory therapy practitioner would most frequently note the presence of pleural fluid in which one of the following locations?

    A. Anterior costophrenic sulcus
    B. Posterior costophrenic sulcus
    C. Mediastinum
    D. Thoracic duct

(9:282–6)

13. Which of the following is *least* likely to be associated with evidence of tracheal deviation on the chest film?

    A. Pleural fluid
    B. Pneumothorax
    C. Pneumonectomy
    D. Lobar atelectasis

(9:29–34)

14. A 12-year-old patient appears cachectic, barrel-chested, with digital clubbing, and cyanosis, and is using accessory muscles. Cough is productive of large amounts of green sputum. These physical findings are typical of which disease?

A. Bronchitis
B. Pneumonia
C. Asthma
D. Cystic fibrosis

(9:168–9)

15. Lateral neck x-ray reveals haziness in the supraglottic area. This is diagnostic of:

A. Croup
B. Laryngotracheobronchitis (LTB)
C. Epiglottitis
D. A and B

(8:255)

16. A patient presents with pulmonary capillary wedge pressure of 30 mm Hg; decreased lung compliance; ventricular hypertrophy and diffuse fluffy opacity on chest x-ray; widened $P(A–a)O_2$; and increased vocal and tactile fremitus. The most likely diagnosis is:

A. Massive atelectasis
B. Noncardiogenic pulmonary edema
C. Cardiogenic pulmonary edema
D. Tension pneumothorax

(8: Chap 7)

17. A patient is being evaluated prior to being enrolled in a pulmonary rehabilitation program. Which of the following should be assessed?

I. Activities of daily living (ADL)
II. Nutrition status
III. Exercise tolerance
IV. Social support systems

A. I and III
B. I, II, and IV
C. I, III, and IV
D. I, II, III, and IV

(20:36)

18. Which is the most accurate measure of left ventricular function?

A. Central venous pressure
B. Pulmonary artery pressure
C. Pulmonary capillary wedge pressure
D. Pulse oximetry

(5:152–6)

19. Which of the following measurements is *least* likely to give an accurate assessment of respiratory muscle strength?

A. Maximum inspiratory pressure
B. Maximum expiratory pressure
C. Vital capacity
D. Maximum voluntary ventilation

(3:693)

20. A patient in the ICU is orally intubated and is being mechanically ventilated. Both delivered volume and peak inspiratory pressures have suddenly decreased. Breath sounds are diminished, and air can be felt at the patient's mouth. The first action of the respiratory therapist should be:

A. Extubate and ventilate with bag/mask.
B. Insert an esophageal obturator until the patient can be reintubated.
C. Attempt to reinflate the cuff.
D. Cut the pilot balloon.

(3:507)

Answer Key

1. B. Air or fluid between the lung and chest wall prevent transmission of sound—fremitus is decreased. Fluid in the lung, however, enhances transmission of sound—fremitus increases. Broken ribs would cause asymetrical chest expansion.
2. B. Adult respiratory distress syndrome is associated with hyaline membrane formation (hazy infiltrates); atelectasis appears as opacification; radiolucent structures tend to be black in appearance; an area of calcification will be white in appearance.
3. B. The CXR of a patient with emphysema will show increased A-P diameter, increased radiolucency (due to air trapping), and flattened hemidiaphragms.
4. C. This patient is in obvious respiratory distress and is approximately 10 weeks premature. Intubation and mechanical ventilation are clearly indicated.
5. C. Bronchiectasis is characterized by abnormal dilatation of the airways.
6. D. Areas of patchy densities (increased opacification) are typical of consolidated lung tissue.
7. C. If the endotracheal tube is properly positioned in the trachea, CO_2 levels will approach 0% on inspiration, fluctuating to 6% on expiration.
8. B. A patient with cor pulmonale (RV failure) would exhibit RV enlargement. Because cor pulmonale is associated with COPD, air trapping would show up as hyperinflation.
9. A. LLL pneumonia would produce decreased expansion on the left, with a productive cough. Bronchial breath sounds would be heard over the affected area.
10. D. Only chronic bronchitis is not characterized by excessive amounts of air caused by air trapping (asthma, emphysema) or air in the pleural space (pneumothorax).
11. D. Blunting of the costophrenic angles is a classic sign of fluid in the pleural space.
12. B. Posterior costophrenic sulcus will be most likely to be blunted on a lateral CXR of a pleural effusion because the posterior lung extends down further than the anterior lung (the effusion is gravity-dependent).
13. A. Pneumothorax, pneumonectomy, and lobar atelectasis all cause tracheal deviation; pleural effusion does not.
14. D. This is the classic presentation of a pediatric patient suffering from cystic fibrosis.

15. C. Haziness in the supraglottic area is typical of epiglottitis; haziness in the subglottic area is typical of croup.
16. C. Cardiogenic pulmonary edema is characterized by increased PWP (PWP is normal in noncardiogenic pulmonary edema). CXR reveals fluffy infiltrates, there is a widened $P(A–a)DO_2$, and increased fremitus due to the presence of fluid.
17. D. It is important to assess all of these aspects of the patient's life prior to their participation in a pulmonary rehabilitation program.
18. C. PWP may be used to evaluate preload, left atrial filling pressure, and LV efficiency in the absence of obstruction.
19. B. Maximum inspiratory pressure, vital capacity, and maximum voluntary ventilation are all used to assess respiratory muscle strength. Maximum expiratory pressure is a reflection of the function of the accessory muscles.
20. D. If the cuff is deflated, this is the easiest problem to remedy, so the RCP should attempt to reinflate the cuff before taking more drastic measures.

C. Perform Procedures and Interpret Results (Entry Level)

Questions in this category are designed to assess the ability of the candidate to recommend and/or obtain additional diagnostic data that may be pertinent in the management of patients requiring respiratory care. It should be pointed out that this category is used to assess the candidate's competency in performing arterial puncture techniques and in handling the sample once it is obtained. Questions on arterial blood gas analysis and arterial blood gas analyzers appear in other categories.

Entry Level Pretest

According to the NBRC, 8.6% of the questions on the Entry Level Examination are from the perform procedures and interpret results category. In addition, the Composite Examination Matrix states that questions in this category assess the ability of the candidate to perform and/or interpret results of procedures to determine:

1. Pulse oximetry
2. Tidal volume
3. Maximum inspiratory and expiratory pressure
4. Minute volume
5. I:E ratio
6. Peak flow
7. Forced vital capacity
8. Timed forced expiratory volumes
9. Tracheal tube cuff pressure
10. Lung mechanics on the intubated patient
11. Alveolar ventilation spirometry before and after bronchodilator
12. Blood gas analysis
13. Co-oximetry results

The following self-study questions were developed from the NBRC Composite Examination Matrix.

1. Which of the following diagnostic procedures would be most valuable in establishing the diagnosis of bronchial asthma?

   A. Simple spirometry
   B. Flow-volume loop analysis
   C. Before and after bronchodilator study
   D. History and physical examination

   (6:190–3)

2. Which of the following conditions is *least* likely to result in erroneous pulse oximetry readings?

   A. Increased carboxyhemoglobin levels
   B. Increased methemoglobin levels
   C. Fetal hemoglobin
   D. External bright lights

   (14:316–20)

3. A patient is intubated and mechanically ventilated. Peak inspiratory pressures increase suddenly, the high-pressure alarm is sounding with each delivered breath, and breath sounds are decreased bilaterally. Which of the following actions should the respiratory care practitioner take at this time?

   A. Extubate the patient.
   B. Attempt to pass a suction catheter through the endotracheal tube.
   C. Call for a stat chest x-ray.
   D. Deflate the cuff.

   (4:156–9)

4. True statements regarding the brachial artery include:

   I. It lies in close proximity to the anterior tibial vein.
   II. Venipuncture cannot occur at this site.
   III. It does not have collateral blood flow.
   IV. It is less superficial than the dorsalis pedis artery.

   A. I and III
   B. III and IV
   C. I and IV
   D. II, III, and IV

   (5:108)

5. When obtaining an arterial sample from a patient who is being treated with sodium warfarin (Coumadin®), the *most* important action for the respiratory therapy practitioner to take is which of the following?

   A. Perform the Allen test
   B. Inform the physician that arterial puncture is contraindicated in this patient

C. Infiltrate the puncture site with 2% lidocaine (Xylocaine®)
D. Take extra precautions to prevent postpuncture bleeding

(5:108–9)

6. Which of the following measurements are useful in evaluating patients with neuromuscular disease?

I. Maximum inspiratory pressure
II. Maximum expiratory pressure
III. Vital capacity
IV. Minute volume

A. I and IV
B. I, II, and III
C. I, III, and IV
D. II and III

(1:910–11)

7. Which of the following determinations would be most beneficial in establishing the presence of respiratory failure?

A. $C(a\text{-}\bar{v})O_2$
B. $P\bar{v}O_2$
C. $PaCO_2$, PaO_2, and pH
D. $P(A\text{–}a)O_2$

(1:846)

8. Which of the following determinations is considered most useful in establishing the presence or absence of tissue hypoxia?

A. PaO_2
B. $S\bar{v}O_2$
C. $C(a\text{-}\bar{v})O_2$
D. Pulse oximetry

(4:116–7)

9. For each 10 mm Hg increase in $PaCO_2$, how much will the HCO_3^- increase?

A. 1 mmol/L
B. 2 mmol/L
C. 5 mmol/L
D. 10 mmo!l/L

(19:61)

10. An unconscious fireman with suspected carbon monoxide poisoning is brought to the emergency department, where he is intubated and placed on a volume-cycled ventilator. Twenty minutes later, arterial blood is analyzed at an FIO_2 of 1.0. This information is presented below:

PaO_2	490 mm Hg
$PaCO_2$	36 mm Hg
pH	7.36
HCO_3^-	18.2 mEq/L
HbCO	32%
Hb	14 g/dL

Which of the following represents the approximate amount of oxygen dissolved in this patient's plasma?

A. 0.4 vol%
B. 0.8 vol%
C. 1.3 vol%
D. 1.5 vol%

(4:116)

11. A 63-year-old patient with a history of bronchiectasis dating to adolescence is admitted to the emergency department with a complaint of dyspnea and excessive sputum production. Arterial blood drawn at that time yields the following data:

FIO_2	0.28
PaO_2	53 mm Hg
$PaCO_2$	62 mm Hg
pH	7.68
HCO_3^-	34 mEq/L
Base excess	+10 mEq/L

The correct interpretation of the above acid-base data would be:

A. Fully compensated respiratory acidosis
B. Fully compensated metabolic alkalosis
C. Partially compensated metabolic alkalosis
D. Laboratory error exists

(19:60–2)

12. A 57-year-old woman is brought to the emergency department after suffering a cerebrovascular accident at home. Results of admission blood gas analysis performed while receiving 4 L oxygen via nasal cannula are revealed below:

PaO_2	182 mm Hg
$PaCO_2$	28 mm Hg
pH	7.63
HCO_3^-	32 mEq/L

Based on the above information, which of the following is the most correct interpretation of the above data?

A. Acute respiratory alkalosis
B. Partially compensated metabolic alkalosis
C. Combined respiratory and metabolic alkalosis
D. Acute metabolic alkalosis

(19: Chap 5)

13. In which of the following conditions would alveolar hyperventilation *without* hypoxemia be a clinical finding?

    I. Carbon monoxide poisoning
    II. Adult respiratory distress syndrome
    III. Cyanide poisoning
    IV. Bacterial pneumonia

    A. I and III
    B. II and III
    C. II and IV
    D. I and IV

(19: Chap 16, 248)

Answer Key

1. C. Before-and-after bronchodilator studies help to establish the diagnosis of asthma (reversible obstructive airways disease).
2. C. Carboxyhemoglobin and methemoglobin are dysfunctional forms of hemoglobin, causing erroneous readings. Bright lights also cause errors in measurement. Fetal hemoglobin has wavelength characteristics within the realm of the pulse oximeter's accuracy.
3. B. In this case, the endotracheal tube may be obstructed. Presence of obstruction may be confirmed by attempting to pass a suction catheter. If this patient had a pneumothorax, breath sounds would be diminished only on one side.
4. B. The brachial artery is large and easy to cannulate, but it has no collateral blood flow, and it lies deeper than the radial or dorsalis pedis arteries.
5. D. If a patient is being treated with an anticoagulant, the RCP needs to take extra precautions to prevent bleeding (applying pressure to the site for a longer period of time, etc.).
6. B. Vital capacity and MIP are useful in assessing diaphragmatic strength, and MEP is helpful in evaluating ability to cough effectively. Minute volume is not useful in the assessment of patients with neuromuscular disease.
7. C. Respiratory failure is defined as $Pa{O_2}$ less than 55 torr on room air, $Pa{CO_2}$ > 50 torr, with the pH showing significant respiratory acidemia.
8. C. Oxygen content is the most significant indicator of tissue oxygenation.
9. A. For each 10 mm Hg increase in $Pa{CO_2}$, the HCO_3^- will increase by 1 mmol/L.
10. D. Oxygen dissolved in the plasma is calculated by multiplying the $P{O_2}$ by 0.003. $490 \times 0.003 = 1.47$.
11. D. The clinical presentation as well as the HCO_3^- and $Pa{CO_2}$ values are inconsistent with a pH of 7.68; a laboratory error exists.
12. C. Both the increased HCO_3^- level and decreased $Pa{CO_2}$ level cause alkalosis; therefore, it is a combined problem.
13. A. In both cyanide and carbon monoxide poisoning, the oxyhemoglobin dissociation curve is shifted to the left, so the available oxyhemoglobin sites hold on to their oxygen more tightly.

D. Perform Diagnostic Procedures, Interpret Results, and Assist in Care Plan (Advanced Level)

Questions in this category are designed to assess the ability of the candidate to recommend and/or obtain additional diagnostic data that may be pertinent in the management of patients requiring respiratory care. Candidates are also expected to assist the physician and other members of the health care team in developing a patient care plan, based on the results of those diagnostic procedures.

Advanced Level Pretest

According to the NBRC, 7% of the questions on the Entry Level Examination are from the above category. Questions in this category assess the ability of the candidate to perform and/or interpret the following:

1. Co-oximetry
2. Pulmonary function tests (including FRC, flow-volume loops, nitrogen washout distribution test, diffusing capacity, TLC, and MVV)
3. V_D/V_T
4. Q_S/Q_T
5. Tests of ventilatory mechanics (including lung compliance, airway resistance, and pressure-volume, flow-volume loops)
6. ECG
7. $P(A\text{–}a)O_2$
8. $C(a\text{-}\bar{v})O_2$

to interpret results of the following:

1. Spirometry before and after bronchodilator
2. Blood gas analysis
3. Pulse oximetry
4. Hemodynamic parameters (including pulmonary artery pressures, pulmonary capillary wedge pressure, and cardiac output)
5. Mixed venous sampling
6. Fluid balance (intake and output)
7. Sleep studies
8. Arterial, umbilical, and/or central venous pressures

and to determine physiologic state, perform quality assurance, and participate in the development of the respiratory care plan. The following self-study questions were developed from the NBRC Composite Examination Matrix (Figure 6).

1. The tracing in Figure 6 was performed on a 53-year-old man. It is most likely that this patient suffers from which of the following disorders?

    A. Pulmonary fibrosis
    B. Severe emphysema
    C. Adult respiratory distress syndrome
    D. Bronchial asthma

(6:43–54)

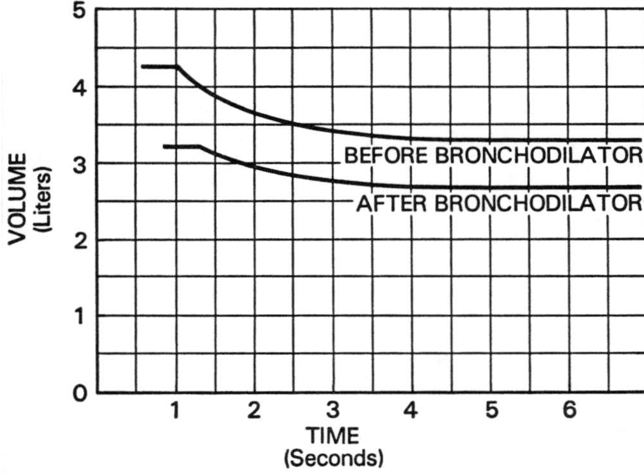

Figure 6.

2. When performing helium dilution and/or nitrogen washout residual volume determinations, the test should begin when the patient is:

   A. At the end of a normal inspiration
   B. At the end of a normal expiration
   C. At the end of a forced expiration
   D. In the middle of a normal tidal volume

   (6:4–8)

3. Pulmonary function tests performed on a patient with chronic obstructive pulmonary emphysema would most likely reveal all of the following *except:*

   A. Decreased FEV_1
   B. Decreased FEF_{25-75}
   C. Increased FEF_{50}
   D. Decreased D_LCO

   (8: Chap 3)

4. Management of the patient in shock generally includes:

   I. Oxygen
   II. Correction of the primary problem
   III. Stabilization of $\dot{V}CO_2$
   IV. Maintenance of fluid balance

   A. I, II, III, and IV
   B. I, II, and III
   C. I, II, and IV
   D. II, III, and IV

   (5:255)

5. Subclavian insertion of a CVP line:

   I. May result in carotid artery puncture
   II. May result in pneumothorax
   III. Is the most commonly used central site
   IV. Is the most commonly used peripheral site

   A. I and III
   B. I and IV
   C. II and III
   D. II and IV

   (5:121–2)

6. The distal lumen of the quadruple-lumen pulmonary artery catheter:

   A. May be used to obtain mixed venous blood
   B. Is located 30 cm from the catheter tip
   C. Is used as the injectate port when measuring C.O.
   D. All of the above

   (5:138–40)

7. You approach Mr. Jones' bedside and observe the following tracing in Figure 7 on his monitor:

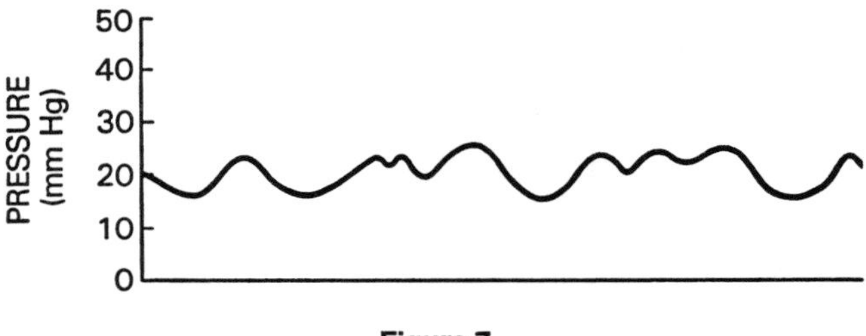

Figure 7.

   You should:

   A. Do nothing—this is an acceptable PA tracing
   B. Advance the catheter with the balloon deflated until you observe a PA tracing
   C. Pull back the catheter with the balloon deflated until you observe a PA tracing
   D. Advance the catheter with the balloon inflated until you observe a PA tracing

   (5:150)

8. If 0.6 cc of air are required to obtain a PCWP, what can you assume?

   A. The catheter tip has slipped into the RV
   B. The catheter tip is too peripheral in the pulmonary circulation
   C. Normal function
   D. The balloon has ruptured

   (5:150)

9. PCWP may be used to estimate the degree of pulmonary edema. A PCWP of 17 mm Hg indicates what level of pulmonary edema?

A. None
B. Mild
C. Moderate
D. Full-blown

(5:313–9)

10. You are performing a fluid challenge for volume replacement on a patient in cardiogenic shock. PCWP = 15 mm Hg. Five minutes into the 10 mL/min infusion, PCWP has increased to 20 mm Hg. What is the appropriate action?

A. Stop immediately
B. Stop at the end of 10 minutes
C. Repeat the challenge using 20 mm Hg as the new baseline
D. Administer a diuretic

(5:257–8)

11. Which of the following disorders are known to frequently result in marked to severe decreases in the diffusion capacity of the lung (D_LCO)?

I. Bronchial asthma
II. Emphysema
III. Idiopathic pulmonary fibrosis
IV. Small airways disease

A. I, III, and IV
B. II, III, and IV
C. I, II, and IV
D. I, II, and III

(6:97–115)

12. 50-kg patient is in the ICU with a diagnosis of sepsis. PCWP = 12 mm Hg; C.O. = 11 L/min; UO is adequate; pH = 7.2; PCO_2 = 57; PO_2 = 41; HCO_3^- = 26. Treatment regimen should include:

A. Antibiotics
B. Volume replacement
C. Intubation/mechanical ventilation
D. A and C

(5:263–70)

13. Which of the following can be determined from a flow-volume loop study?

I. Maximal expiratory flow rate (MEFR)
II. Forced expiratory flow rate at 75% of the vital capacity (FEF_{75})
III. Average flow rate of the middle 50% of the vital capacity
IV. Maximal inspiratory flow rate (MIFR)

A. I, II, and IV
B. II and III
C. I, II, and III
D. II, III, and IV

(6:57–60)

14. RA pressure may be measured using a:

A. Transducer attached to a CVP line
B. HOH manometer attached to a CVP line
C. Proximal lumen of Swan-Ganz
D. Any of the above

(5:118–9, 147)

15. Which of the following pulmonary function determinations is known to yield the largest value for total lung capacity when performed on patients with emphysema?

A. Time-volume studies
B. Flow-volume loop
C. Open analysis circuit nitrogen washout method
D. Full body plethysmography

(6:377–81)

16. Patients exhibiting ventilatory respiratory failure:

I. Have increased RR
II. Have decreased RR
III. Are cyanotic with mild clubbing
IV. Have increased $PaCO_2$

A. I, III, and IV
B. II, III, and IV
C. I and III
D. II and IV

(9:338)

17. Arterial blood pressure is 240/130. What is MAP (mean arterial pressure)?

A. 17 mm Hg
B. 92 mm Hg
C. 167 mm Hg
D. 202 mm Hg

(5:56)

18. You are preparing to insert a radial arterial line. While performing an Allen test, you discover that it takes 4 sec for blood flow to return to the hand. You would now:

A. Proceed with insertion
B. Choose another site
C. Notify the patient's physician
D. None of the above

(5:104)

19. Given the following measurements:

PAP S/D = 40/20 mm Hg

PAP mean = 30 mm Hg

Based on these measurements *alone,* what conclusion can be drawn?

A. Patient requires diuretics
B. Patient requires fluids

C. Patient exhibits PA hypertension
D. Patient exhibits PA hypotension

(5:148–50)

20. CPR has been in progress for 8 min for a 50-kg patient in the coronary care unit. The patient is being ventilated by bag-valve-mask unit. The results of an arterial sample drawn 5 min earlier are Pa_{O_2} 52 mm Hg, Pa_{CO_2} 62 mm Hg, and pH 7.16. Which of the following are indicated?

I. Assure that delivered oxygen is at 100%
II. Increase ventilation rate
III. Maintain ventilation as is
IV. Repeat arterial blood gases

A. I, II, and IV
B. I and III
C. I, III, and IV
D. III and IV

(10:76, 84)

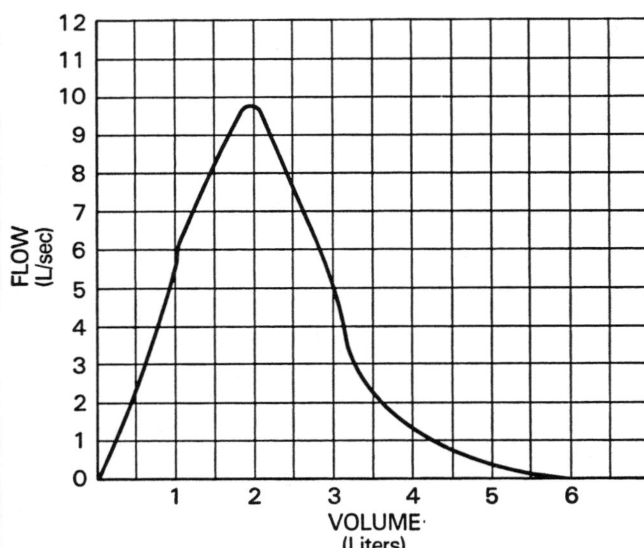

Figure 8.

21. The flow-volume tracing in Figure 8 was obtained from a 56-year-old man. He is 72 inches tall and weighs 195 lb. He has a 20 pack-year history of cigarette smoking. The best interpretation for this loop would be:

A. Small airways disease
B. Early restrictive lung disease
C. Severe combined obstructive and restrictive pulmonary disease
D. Typical Hamman-Rich configuration

(6:57–60)

22. Direct measurement of which of the following types of compliance requires the use of an esophageal balloon?

A. Static effective
B. Static lung (C_L)
C. Static lung-thorax (C_{LT})
D. Static thorax (C_T)

(1:464–5)

23. The spirometric data in Figure 9 were obtained from a 15-year-old, 35-kg girl. Which of the following is the most correct interpret?

A. Obstructive disease
B. Restrictive disease
C. Normal study
D. Mixed obstructive and restrictive disease

(6:44–54)

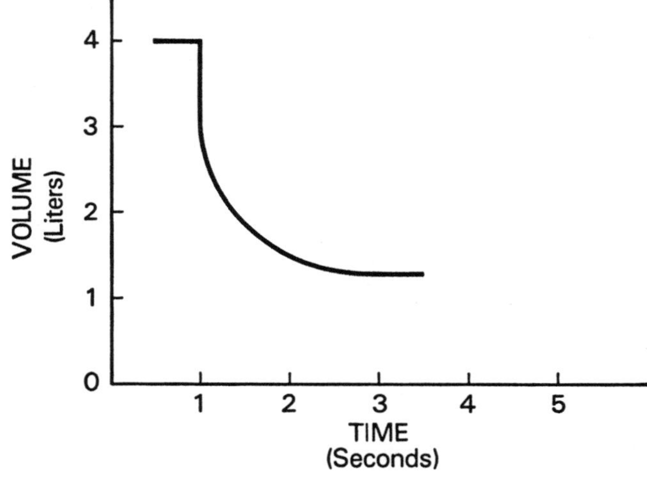

Figure 9.

24. Measurements taken during a sleep study include:

I. EEG
II. ECG
III. Electrodes to detect chest/abdominal movement
IV. CBC

A. I, II, III, and IV
B. I, II, and IV
C. II and III
D. I, II, and III

(9:56–7)

Answer Key

1. B. Because the volume takes a long time to leave the airways/lungs (> 6 sec), we can assume that there is an obstructive process. The tracing worsened after bronchodilator, so we can eliminate asthma, and the other two disorders are restrictive.

2. B. When performing helium dilution and/or nitrogen washout residual volume determinations, the test should begin when the patient is at FRC (the end of a normal expiration).
3. C. Flow rates are decreased (all measures of them) in emphysema, as well as diffusing capacity. RV is increased, sometimes as much as 7 times normal.
4. C. Maintenance of shock generally includes correction of the underlying problem, stabilization of Pa_{O_2}, fluid maintenance, and airway maintenance.
5. C. The subclavian vein is cannulated to provide central access. The only artery in danger of puncture is the subclavian. There is a risk of pneumothorax.
6. A. The distal lumen is used for obtaining mixed venous blood and pulmonary artery pressure monitoring. It is located at the catheter tip. Other statements describe the proximal (RA) lumen.
7. C. Prolonged wedging of the catheter may cause pulmonary infarction. Pull back the catheter, making sure that the balloon is deflated (this avoids valve damage), until you see a PA tracing on the monitor.
8. B. If it only takes 0.6 cc to wedge (normally it takes 1.5 cc), the catheter has probably moved too far into the pulmonary vasculature. It should be pulled back (remember to make sure that the balloon is deflated).
9. A. Pulmonary edema does not become evident until the PWP reaches 18 mm Hg. Varying degrees of pulmonary edema are present at levels greater than this, with "full-blown" pulmonary edema developing with a PWP > 30 mm Hg.
10. B. Performing a fluid challenge using the 3:7 rule requires that you stop at the end of 10 minutes if PWP increases between 3 and 7 mm Hg during fluid administration. If PWP does not increase by at least 3, repeat the challenge; if PWP increases more than 7, stop infusion immediately.
11. B. Because asthma affects the larger airways versus the lung parenchyma and small airways, distribution of ventilation (measured by $D_{L}CO$) is not severely diminished.
12. D. This patient's ABGs indicate that he is in respiratory failure and should be intubated and mechanically ventilated. Antibiotics are indicated to treat the sepsis. Normal PWP suggests that the patient does not require volume replacement.
13. A. Of the choices listed, only the average flow rate of the middle 50% of the vital capacity cannot be determined from a flow-volume tracing.
14. D. RA pressure may be assessed through either the RA (proximal) lumen of the Swan-Ganz, or through the CVP line, using either a transducer or a water column.
15. D. Full body plethysmography yields the greatest value for total lung capacity when performed on patients with emphysema.
16. D. Patients in ventilatory failure are unable to *ventilate;* their respiratory rate is diminished, resulting in increased Pa_{CO_2} levels.
17. C. $MAP = \frac{\text{Systolic pressure + (Diastolic pressure} \times 2)}{3}$

    In this example, [240 + 130(2)]/3 = (240 + 260)/3 = 500/3 = 167.
18. A. If color returns to the hand in less than 7 sec, collateral flow is adequate.
19. C. Systolic, diastolic, and mean PAP are all elevated—characteristic of PA hypertension. Normal values (in mm Hg) are: systolic: 15–25; diastolic: 8–15; mean: 10–20.
20. A. Increased Pa_{CO_2} indicates hypoventilation; it takes only a second to double check that 100% oxygen is being given; ABGs should be repeated after you make these adjustments.
21. A. The tracing indicates small airways disease: PEF is diminished with a slightly concave curve to RV.
22. B. In order to determine static lung compliance, the patient must swallow an esophageal balloon.
23. C. This tracing shows a normal VC.
24. D. Polysomnography monitors EEG, ECG, chest/abdominal movement, pulse oximetry, $P_{ET}CO_2$; generally no blood work is taken.

E. Assess Therapeutic Plan (Entry Level Only)

According to the NBRC, this content category is assessed only on the Entry Level Examination. This category is designed to assess the candidate's ability to determine the appropriateness of the prescribed respiratory care plan and to recommend modifications in this plan where indicated. For example, the respiratory therapy practitioner is asked to perform therapy on a patient with long-standing chronic obstructive lung disease whose baseline arterial carbon dioxide tension is well in excess of 60 mm Hg. In reading this patient's chart, the practitioner notes that part of the physician's care plan involves placing this patient on 6 L oxygen by simple oxygen mask. The respiratory therapy practitioner should be prepared to recommend modifications involving the administration of oxygen to this patient.

In addition, questions in this category deal with the ability of the respiratory therapy practitioner to identify the patient's pathophysiologic state based on available information. For example, a 22-year-old man is admitted to the emergency department in severe hemorrhagic shock following a motorcycle accident. The patient is resuscitated and successfully treated in the emergency department and subsequently transferred to the intensive care unit. Twelve hours later, the patient has tachypnea, tachycardia, and hypertension. Arterial blood gas analysis performed at that time with the patient receiving 8 L oxygen by simple mask revealed an arterial oxygen tension of 40 mm Hg. Based on the foregoing information, the respiratory therapy practitioner should be able to identify that the most likely cause of this patient's symptoms is adult respiratory distress syndrome.

Entry Level Pretest

According to the NBRC, 3.6% of the questions on the Entry Level Examination are from the assess therapeutic plan category. In addition, the Composite Examination Matrix states that questions in this category assess the ability of the candidate to:

1. Review planned therapy to establish therapeutic goals.
2. Determine the appropriateness of prescribed therapy and goals for the patient's physiologic state.
3. Recommend changes in the therapeutic plan as needed.
4. Participate in the development of the respiratory care plan.

The following self-study questions were developed from the NBRC Composite Examination Matrix.

1. The risk of oxygen-induced hypoventilation is apparently minimal in patients with steady-state arterial CO_2 tensions less than:

   A. 50–60
   B. 60–70
   C. 70–80
   D. 80–90

(1:320–1)

2. PEEP therapy is believed to be most effective in the management of which one of the following?

   A. Status asthmaticus
   B. Cardiogenic pulmonary edema
   C. Adult respiratory distress syndrome
   D. Unilateral aspiration pneumonitis

(8: Chap 9)

3. Which of the following statements is (are) true regarding cyanide poisoning?

   I. It is invariably accompanied by arterial hypoxemia.
   II. It is an example of anemic hypoxia.
   III. It is known to result in abnormally high mixed venous oxygen tensions.
   IV. Its primary pathology involves a shift to the right in the oxyhemoglobin dissociation curve.

   A. I and III
   B. II and IV
   C. I and IV
   D. III only

(13:150)

4. The presence of which of the following is believed to be necessary in order for sustained maximal inspiratory maneuvers to be effective in preventing postoperative atelectasis?

   I. Vital capacity less than 15 mL/kg
   II. Patient ability to cooperate
   III. Respiratory rate greater than 25/min
   IV. Effective patient instruction

   A. II and IV
   B. I and IV
   C. III only
   D. II and III

(4:92–4)

5. Continuous positive airway pressure (CPAP) is believed to be of greatest benefit when employed in the treatment of which of the following disorders?

   A. Refractory hypoxemia with hypercarbia
   B. Advanced chronic obstructive pulmonary disease with right ventricular failure
   C. Diffuse microatelectasis with upper airway obstruction
   D. Left lower lobe atelectasis

(4:370)

6. Depression of the peripheral respiratory drive is a known complication when excessive concentrations of oxygen are administered to patients with which of the following pulmonary disorders?

   I. Cystic fibrosis
   II. Pickwickian syndrome
   III. Asphyxia neonatorum
   IV. Infant respiratory distress syndrome

   A. I and II
   B. I and IV
   C. III and IV
   D. II and III

(1:320–1)

7. A tall, thin 20-year-old man presents to the emergency department with a complaint of sharp chest pain and difficulty in breathing. The patient states these symptoms began half an hour previously during a game of racquetball. Chest physical examination reveals a hyperresonant percussion note over the left lung fields and a tracheal shift toward the right thorax. Based on the above information, the most likely cause of this patient's distress is:

   A. Myocardial infarct
   B. Pulmonary embolus
   C. Spontaneous tension pneumothorax
   D. Congenital lobar emphysema

(9:286–9)

8. A 40-year-old man with a history of alcoholism is admitted to the emergency department. He has tachypnea and tachycardia and is febrile. Cough efforts are productive of copious amounts of putrid-smelling sputum. Physical examination also reveals extremely poor dental hygiene. Based on the above information, the most likely cause of this patient's distress is:

   A. Cystic fibrosis
   B. Pulmonary tuberculosis
   C. Anaerobic lung abscess
   D. Chronic bronchitis

(9:75–7)

9. Seventy-two hours after being subjected to an exploratory laparotomy, a 30-year-old man is noted to have both tachypnea and tachycardia. His temperature at this time is 37.5° C. Breath sounds are diminished bibasally, and coughing yields small amounts of mucopurulent sputum. The white blood cell count is noted to be 7000/µL. Based on the above information, the most likely cause of this patient's distress is:

   A. Gram-negative nosocomial pulmonary infection
   B. Pulmonary embolus
   C. Aspiration pneumonia
   D. Postoperative atelectasis

   (9:247, 301)

10. Five days following hip surgery, a 74-year-old woman develops acute dyspnea accompanied by sharp chest pain. Later that afternoon the patient has an episode of hemoptysis. Arterial blood gas analysis at this time reveals arterial hypoxemia with hypocarbia. Which of the following disorders is most likely to be responsible for this patient's distress?

    A. Spontaneous pneumothorax
    B. Pleural effusion
    C. Pulmonary embolus
    D. Massive pulmonary atelectasis

    (9:268–72)

11. A 60-year-old woman is admitted to the hospital after falling at home and fracturing her tibia and femur. Twelve hours later she has tachycardia and tachypnea and is dusky in appearance. Arterial blood is analyzed with the patient receiving 8 L oxygen via simple oxygen mask:

Pa_{O_2}	42 mm Hg
Pa_{CO_2}	32 mm Hg
pH	7.40
HCO_3^-	20 mEq/L

    Based on the above information, the most likely cause of this patient's distress is:

    A. Fat embolus with adult respiratory distress syndrome
    B. Viral pneumonia
    C. Cervical spine transection
    D. Tension pneumothorax

    (9:272–5)

12. Which of the following statements regarding carbon monoxide poisoning is *not* true?

    A. It is considered an indication for the administration of 100% oxygen.
    B. It is associated with smoke inhalation.
    C. It frequently results in a decreased P_{50}.
    D. The rate of carbon monoxide excretion is highest on 21% oxygen.

    (9:210–2)

Answer Key

1. A. The risk of oxygen-induced hypoventilation is minimal in patients with steady-state arterial CO_2 tensions < 50–60 torr.
2. C. ARDS causes severe hypoxemia and is generally managed with PEEP therapy. Obstructive diseases, which already cause increased FRCs, do not respond as dramatically as a restrictive process.
3. D. In cyanide poisoning, the tissues are unable to take up oxygen, so the mixed venous blood will show abnormally high oxygen concentrations. Pa_{O_2} and Sa_{O_2} levels are normal. Anemic hypoxia is caused by low levels of hemoglobin.
4. A. VC < 15 mL/kg is an indication for IPPB. SMI therapy is indicated for cooperative patients with a normal RR and breathing pattern. Patient instruction is always important.
5. D. CPAP works best in a restrictive process, such as atelectasis.
6. A. The first two choices represent obstructive disease processes, where depressed respiratory drive with high FI_{O_2} is a concern.
7. C. This is a classic presentation of spontaneous pneumothorax: thin, white male, hyperresonant percussion note, tracheal shift.
8. C. Poor oral hygiene and copious amounts of putrid sputum are suggestive of anaerobic lung abcess.
9. D. Because there is no indication of infection, choices A and C can be ruled out. Because the patient underwent exploratory surgery, post-op atelectasis is implicated.
10. C. These symptoms are characteristic of pulmonary embolus: sharp chest pain, hypoxemia, hemoptysis. The patient has probably not been ambulatory as well.
11. A. Long bone fracture and dyspnea characterize fat embolism. The ABG values are typical of ARDS.
12. D. The rate of CO removal is highest in HBO, followed by 100% oxygen.

PART 2

Equipment

According to the NBRC, 25% of the Entry Level and 20% of the Advanced Practitioner Examinations are devoted to assessing the candidate's knowledge of respiratory care equipment. Questions in this area are broken down into two entry level and three advanced level subcategories on the examinations:

1. *Select, obtain, and assure cleanliness of equipment.* These questions assess the candidate's knowledge of the classification, principles of operation, and clinically significant design characteristics of all equipment used in respiratory care. The candidate's knowledge of sterilization and disinfection techniques is also evaluated.
2. *Assemble, check, and correct equipment malfunctions.* Questions in this category assess the candidate's ability to ensure the proper operation of all equipment in the performance of respiratory diagnostic and therapeutic procedures.
3. *Perform quality control procedures* (advanced level only). Knowledge of the procedures as applied to blood gas analyzers and co-oximeters, pulmonary function equipment, noninvasive monitors, gas metering devices, and ventilator volume/flow/pressure calibration is assessed in this category.

As stated previously, the major purpose of the NBRC Examination is to determine whether the candidate is competent to perform as a respiratory therapy practitioner. To ensure its validity in this regard, the examination is constructed around the 1992 Respiratory Therapy Job Analysis Survey.

This book is an educational tool. Its goals and ours are twofold. First, we wish to make the candidate familiar with the structure of the examinations; second, we want to help him or her review the fundamental and essential aspects of respiratory therapy that are assessed on these examinations. We believe that classification of respiratory therapy equipment according to *task* (i. e., select, assemble, note operation, correct malfunction) has its greatest validity as a testing tool. A *generic* (i. e., according to name, as in oxygen administration devices) classification system, on the other hand, is appropriate for an instructional guide like this, if for no other reason than its almost universal employment in respiratory therapy textbooks.

In summary, we have "redefined" the following two task-oriented categories:

1. Select and obtain equipment
2. Note operation and correct equipment malfunctions

and incorporated them into the following generic categories:

A. Oxygen administration devices (advanced level assesses 2 only)
B. Humidity and aerosol therapy devices (advanced level assesses 2 only)
C. Ventilators
D. Artificial airways
E. Suctioning devices (entry level only)
F. Gas delivery, metering, and clinical analyzing devices
G. Manometers and gauges
H. Resuscitation devices
I. Incentive breathing devices (entry level only)
J. Patient breathing circuits
K. Percussors and vibrators (entry level only)
L. Environmental devices—Aerosol (mist) tents (advanced level assesses 2 only)
M. Metered dose inhalers (MDI) and spacers (entry level only)
N. Positive expiratory pressure (PEP) mask (advanced level only)
O. Respirometers (advanced level only)
P. Helium/oxygen therapy (advanced level only)
Q. ECG devices (advanced level only)
R. Hemodynamic monitoring devices (advanced level only)
S. Fiberoptic bronchoscopes (advanced level only)
T. Vacuum systems (advanced level only)
U. Ensure the cleanliness of all equipment

We will, because of their specific nature, retain the following two categories as they are reflected in the NBRC Composite Examination Matrix:

1. Ensure the cleanliness of all equipment.
2. Perform quality control procedures.

These categories are further described in the self-study sections that follow.

A. Oxygen Administration Devices

Questions in this category assess the candidate's ability to select and assemble all oxygen administration devices and equipment prior to performing respiratory care procedures. These questions will also test the candidate's understanding of the principles of proper operation and his or her ability to correct all malfunctions of any selected equipment.

Entry Level Pretest

According to the Composite Examination Matrix, questions in this category assess the candidate's understanding of the following types of respiratory therapy equipment:

1. Nasal cannula, mask, reservoir mask (partial rebreathing, nonrebreathing)
2. Tracheostomy collar and T-piece
3. Air entrainment devices
4. CPAP devices (mask and nasal)
5. Oxygen hoods and tents

The following are self-study questions from this category.

1. Which of the following most correctly defines a high flow oxygen delivery system?

   A. One that has a flow rate greater than 30 L/min
   B. One that requires more than one flowmeter to drive the system properly
   C. One whose flow rate is sufficient to meet all patient inspiratory demands
   D. A system that is present only on ventilators that are true constant-flow generators

   (4:125–7)

2. For which of the following reasons should toys with metal gears be kept out of oxygen tents?

   A. The high oxygen contents will make the toys rust.
   B. They are considered a fire hazard.
   C. Children should be resting in the tent, not playing with toys.
   D. The toys can tear the tent canopy, compromising the oxygen-enriched atmosphere.

   (14:234–5)

3. Which of the following statements regarding the nonrebreathing type oxygen mask is (are) true?

   I. It incorporates its own flow-regulating device.
   II. It is believed to be capable of delivering concentrations of oxygen that approach 100%.
   III. It uses a one-way valve between the reservoir bag and the mask.
   IV. It should not be operated with flow rates greater than 8 L/ min.

   A. I and III
   B. II and III
   C. III and IV
   D. I and IV

   (4:125–30)

4. The respiratory therapy practitioner is administering 5 L oxygen via a nasal cannula to a 70-kg patient with a normal ventilatory pattern. Which of the following most closely approximates this patient's FIO_2?

   A. 30%
   B. 35%
   C. 40%
   D. 45%

   (4:129)

5. The most common method of administering oxygen to a newborn is via which of the following?

   A. Nasal cannula
   B. Nasal CPAP prongs
   C. Face tent
   D. Oxygen hood

   (14:231–2)

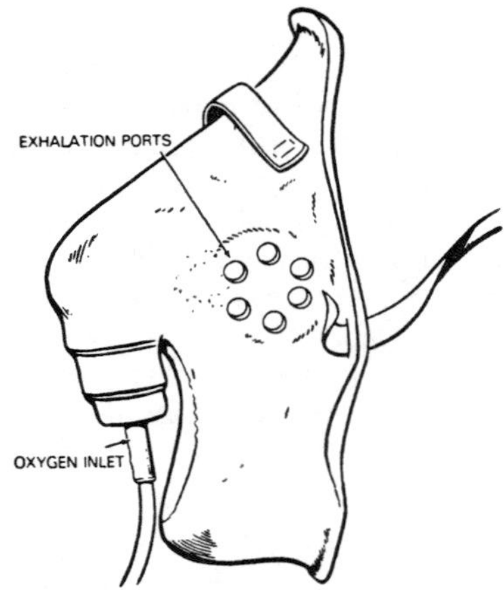

Figure 10.

6. Figure 10 shows a:

   A. Simple oxygen mask
   B. Oxygen-powered breathing device
   C. Anesthesia mask
   D. Nonrebreathing oxygen mask

   (2:60–1)

7. An air entrainment type mask would most likely be used on a patient suffering from which of the following disorders?

   A. Advanced stage emphysema
   B. Silicosis
   C. Carbon monoxide poisoning
   D. Adult respiratory distress syndrome

   (2:64–5)

8. If the air entrainment port of an air entrainment type oxygen mask were to become occluded, which of the following would apply?

    I. The FIO_2 would decrease.
    II. Gas flow to the patient would cease completely.
    III. The FIO_2 would increase.
    IV. Gas flow to the patient would decrease.

    A. I and II
    B. II and III
    C. III and IV
    D. I and IV

(2:64–5)

9. Which of the following statements is (are) true regarding partial rebreathing masks?

    I. There is an air entrainment mechanism built into the reservoir system.
    II. There is a one-way valve between the reservoir system and the mask.
    III. FIO_2s between 60% and 80% are believed to be obtainable.

    A. I only
    B. II only
    C. III only
    D. I and III

(4:125–30)

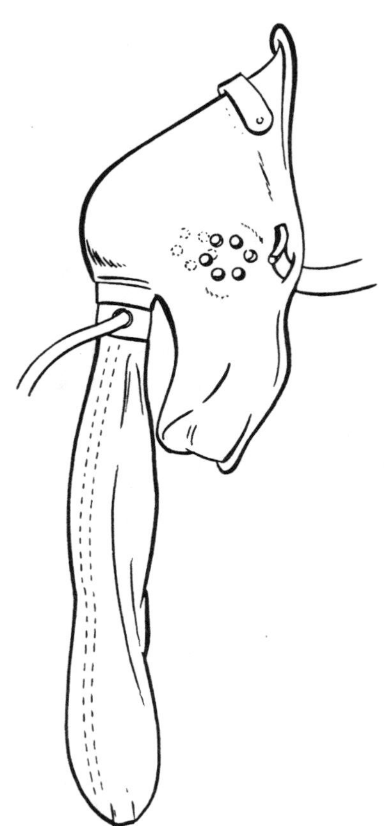

Figure 11.

10. Figure 11 shows which of the following?

    A. Simple mask
    B. Face tent
    C. Partial rebreathing mask
    D. Aerosol mask

(2:63–4)

11. The major disadvantage associated with the use of oxygen hoods is:

    A. The oxygen concentration cannot be controlled.
    B. The temperature inside the hood cannot be controlled.
    C. The absolute humidity within the hood cannot be controlled.
    D. The hood must be removed for feeding.

(14:234–5)

12. Which of the following actions should the respiratory therapy practitioner take to help maintain a constant FIO_2 within an oxygen tent?

    I. Use a canopy that can ensure an enclosed environment.
    II. Avoid opening the canopy unnecessarily.
    III. Use the smallest canopy that is practical.
    IV. Periodically analyze the tent gas at the patient's proximal airway.

    A. I, III, and IV
    B. II, III, and IV
    C. I, II, III and IV
    D. I, II, and III

(14:334–5)

13. Which of the following represents the average volume of an adult patient's anatomic reservoir that must be taken into account when considering low-flow oxygen systems?

    A. 25 cc
    B. 50 cc
    C. 75 cc
    D. 100 cc

(4:128)

14. The partial rebreathing mask is designed to:

    I. Collect the first two thirds of the exhaled gas in the reservoir bag
    II. Allow the patient to draw room air in through the exhalation ports on the side of the mask
    III. *Not* deliver FIO_2s in excess of 0.5

    A. I and II
    B. II only
    C. III only
    D. I and III

(4:125–30)

15. Isolettes (incubators) are designed to allow the operator to provide all of the following *except:*

    A. Control of environmental humidity
    B. Control of environmental temperature
    C. Control of inspired oxygen concentration
    D. Control of alveolar ventilation

(14:234)

16. Which of the following is (are) believed to be an advantage of the nasal cannula as compared with air entrainment mask devices?

    I. The cannula does not have to be removed when the patient is eating.
    II. It may be safely used on patients with irregular ventilatory patterns.
    III. It is generally more comfortable for the patient.
    IV. It eliminates fluctuations in inspired oxygen concentration.

    A. I and III
    B. II and III
    C. II and IV
    D. I, III, and IV

(4:125–30)

17. What is the total flow of a 60% T-piece running at 8 L/min?

    A. 12 L/min
    B. 16 L/min
    C. 19 L/min
    D. 25 L/min

(4:125–30)

18. Which of the following are necessary components of a mask CPAP system?

    I. Soft occlusive mask
    II. Expiratory valve
    III. Continuous flow system
    IV. Oxygen

    A. I, II, III, and IV
    B. II, III, and IV
    C. I and III
    D. I, II, and III

(1:285)

Answer Key

1. D. A high-flow oxygen delivery system provides enough flow to meet all of the patient's inspiratory demands. Examples are the air entrainment and nonrebreathing masks.
2. B. Because oxygen supports combustion, electrical and friction toys are considered fire hazards.
3. B. Nonrebreathing type masks incorporate a one-way valve between the mask and reservoir bag, can deliver nearly 100% oxygen, and should be operated at a flow high enough so that the reservoir bag remains at least one third full on maximal inspiration.
4. C. A nasal cannula running at 5 L will deliver approximately 40% to the patient. To help you remember this, begin with 24% at 1 L/min, and add 4% for each 1-L increase, up to 6 L (44%).
5. D. The most common method of administering oxygen to a newborn is the oxyhood.
6. A. This is a drawing of a simple oxygen mask; it can be identified by the connecting tubing and small exhalation ports arranged in a circle.
7. A. Patients with advanced emphysema would benefit from a high-flow system (able to meet all of the patient's inspiratory demands) that is able to deliver low concentrations of oxygen (24–50%).
8. C. If the air entrainment port were to be occluded, less room air would be drawn in, so both flow and FIO_2 would decrease.
9. C. FIO_2s of 60 to 80% can be delivered with the partial rebreather. There is no valve between the mask and reservoir bag.
10. C. The picture is of a partial rebreathing mask. It can be identified by the reservoir bag and absence of a one-way valve between the mask and bag.
11. D. The oxyhood must be removed in order to feed the infant. All of the parameters listed in the answers *can* be controlled.
12. C. All of those actions listed are important for keeping the FIO_2 constant inside the tent.
13. B. The anatomic reservoir of the nose, nasopharynx, and oropharynx is approximately ⅓ anatomic deadspace (⅓ of 150 cc = 50 cc).
14. B. Patients may draw in room air from the side holes. FIO_2 delivered is 60–80%, and it collects only the first third of exhaled gas in the reservoir bag.
15. D. Alveolar ventilation cannot be controlled in an incubator; it can be controlled, only to an extent, by mechanical ventilation.
16. A. Cannulas can remain on the patient at all times and are generally more comfortable than a mask. They should not be used for patients who have irregular breathing patterns, or when a precise oxygen concentration is desired.
17. B. The following equation can be used to determine the air:oxygen ratio: (100 – concentration)/(concentration – 20) = (100 – 60)/(60 – 20) = 40/40 = 1:1. For every liter of oxygen supplied (8, in this case), there is 1 liter of room air entrained. 8 + 8 = 16
18. A. All of the components are necessary to deliver mask CPAP.

Advanced Level Pretest

According to the Composite Examination Matrix, questions in this category assess the candidate's understanding of the following types of respiratory therapy equipment (assemble, check for proper function):

1. Transtracheal oxygen catheters

Correct malfunctions:

1. Tracheostomy collar and T-piece
2. Air entrainment devices
3. Oxygen hoods and tents
4. CPAP devices
5. Transtracheal oxygen catheters
6. Oxygen conserving devices

The following are self-study questions from this category.

1. A patient has been selected to receive transtracheal oxygen. What benefits can he look forward to?

   A. Improved patient compliance
   B. Using less oxygen
   C. Getting better sleep
   D. All of the above

   (13:408–10)

2. Routine care of the transtracheal oxygen catheter includes all but which of the following?

   A. Cleaning the insertion site
   B. Lavage
   C. Soaking the catheter in a vinegar and water solution
   D. Cleaning the catheter lumen

   (13:410)

3. A patient has been receiving 2 L/min of oxygen delivered via a nasal cannula with a reservoir system for approximately 2 weeks. The patient complains that she feels as if she is not getting enough oxygen. What is the most likely cause of the problem?

   A. Deterioration of the reservoir's plastic
   B. Failure of the reservoir's membrane
   C. Mucous plugging
   D. Failure to properly clean the device

   (1:336–7)

4. If the entrainment port of an air entrainment mask becomes occluded, what will occur?

   A. FIo_2 will increase
   B. FIo_2 will decrease
   C. Patient's respiratory rate will increase
   D. A and C

   (2:64–5)

5. In an oxygen hood, where is the highest concentration of oxygen found?

   A. At the bottom
   B. In the middle
   C. At the top
   D. Oxygen concentration does not vary throughout the hood

   (14:230–1)

6. A neonate is receiving 24% oxygen via hood. One of the infant's inexperienced caregivers decides to tape the holes on top of the hood so that the oxygen does not escape. What will be the likely result?

   A. The FIo_2 will decrease
   B. The Pao_2 will increase
   C. The $Paco_2$ will increase
   D. The pH will increase

   (14:230–1)

7. Which oxygen delivery device is most appropriate for the patient who has just been given a tracheostomy?

   A. T-piece
   B. Transtracheal oxygen catheter
   C. Tracheostomy mask
   D. Face tent

   (4:125–30)

8. A patient is receiving mask CPAP of 10 cm H_2O as part of her home care. She has complained that the system is uncomfortable, and that she experiences difficulty adjusting to the high pressure delivered by the machine. What should the respiratory care practitioner suggest?

   A. Repeat sleep study
   B. BiPAP
   C. Use of ramp function
   D. Partial ventilatory support

   (14:436–7)

Answer Key

1. D. Improved compliance with therapy, better appetite, improved sleep, and less oxygen use are all benefits associated with TTO.
2. C. The TTO catheter should be cleaned along with the site, and lavaged to prevent formation of mucous balls that might occlude the TTO. Soaking in a vinegar solution is not necessary.
3. B. Because the reservoir's membrane fails often (sometimes after only one week), the cost of frequent replacement may be a disadvantage.
4. If the air entrainment port were to be occluded, less room air would be drawn in, so FIo_2 would decrease.
5. C. Higher oxygen levels occur at the top, as the oxygen "layers out."
6. C. The holes at the top are for CO_2 to exit, not for air entrainment. If they are occluded, CO_2 levels inside the hood will increase.
7. C. Tracheostomy masks should be selected over T-pieces for a fresh trach because they put less ten-

sion on the tracheostomy and may be less likely to cause bleeding.

8. C. The ramp function is designed to gradually increase the CPAP over a set period of time, so that the patient is more comfortable and often asleep by the time the desired CPAP level is reached.

B. Humidity and Aerosol Therapy Devices

According to the NBRC, questions in this category are designed to assess the candidate's ability to select and assemble all humidity and aerosol therapy devices prior to performing respiratory care procedures. These questions will also test the candidate's understanding of the principles of proper operation and his or her ability to correct all malfunctions of any selected equipment.

Entry Level Pretest

According to the NBRC Composite Examination Matrix, questions in this category assess the candidate's understanding of the following types of respiratory therapy equipment:

1. Humidifiers (bubble, passover, cascade, wick, and heat moisture exchangers)
2. Aerosol generators (pneumatic and ultrasonic nebulizers)

The following are self-study questions from this category.

1. Which of the following factors will influence the absolute humidity of therapeutic gases that are delivered by a bubble-type humidifier?

   I. The size of the liquid/gas interface
   II. Gas exposure time (unit liter flow)
   III. Type of medical gas administered
   IV. Temperature within the humidifier device

   A. I, II, and IV
   B. III and IV
   C. I, II, and III
   D. II and IV

   (4:57–61)

2. Figure 12 shows a(n):

   A. All-purpose jet nebulizer
   B. Hydronamic nebulizer
   C. Heat moisture exchanger
   D. Ultrasonic nebulizer

   (2:101–3)

3. The device on an ultrasonic nebulizer that converts electrical energy to mechanical/vibrational energy is called a(n):

   A. Electric transducer
   B. Condenser module

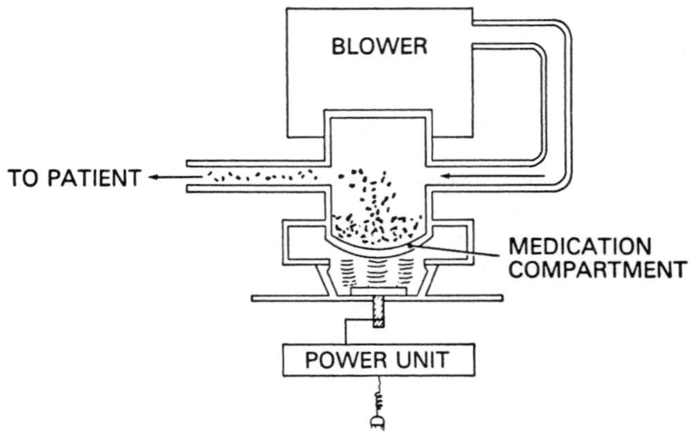

Figure 12.

   C. Piezoelectric transducer
   D. Aerosol generator

   (2:101–3)

4. Which of the following are true statements regarding the cascade humidifier?

   I. It is used to deliver gases at APTD.
   II. It is a type of jet humidifier.
   III. It is not capable of delivering particulate water.
   IV. It can deliver 100% relative humidity

   A. I and II
   B. III and IV
   C. I, III, and IV
   D. II, III, and IV

   (2:85–6)

5. The size of the aerosolized particles that are generated by an ultrasonic nebulizer is believed to be determined by which of the following factors?

   A. Unit ultrasonic frequency
   B. Unit amplitude
   C. Type of solution nebulized
   D. Shape of the ceramic disk

   (2:101–3)

6. The quantity of aerosol produced by an ultrasonic nebulizer is most directly related to:

   A. The type of solution in the nebulizer cup
   B. The shape of the ceramic disk
   C. The setting on unit amplitude control
   D. The device's ultrasonic frequency

   (2:101–3)

7. Figure 13 shows a(n):

   A. Ultrasonic nebulizer
   B. Intermittent sidestream jet nebulizer

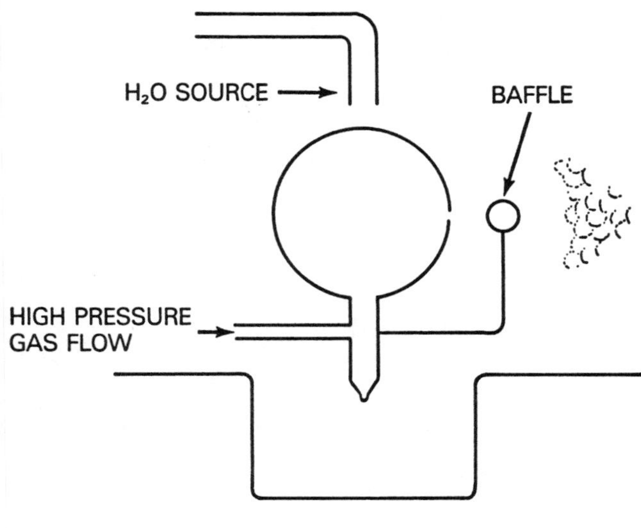

Figure 13.

C. Jet nebulizer
D. Hydronamic nebulizer

(2:102)

8. The majority of particles aerosolized by this device is believed to be in the range of:

A. Less than 10μ
B. 10–20μ
C. 20–30μ
D. 30–40μ

(2:101)

9. The respiratory therapy practitioner would be most concerned about the transmission of nosocomial infection when using which of the following aerosol and/or humidity therapy devices?

A. A jet nebulizer
B. An ultrasonic nebulizer
C. A cascade humidifier
D. A bubble humidifier

(2:101–3)

10. The baffle in a nebulizer serves which of the following purposes?

A. It increases the aerosol output.
B. It decreases the aerosol output.
C. It increases gas density.
D. It breaks up the larger particles into smaller particles.

(2:94)

11. Which of the following is (are) known to occur when water inside a pneumatic nebulizer is heated through the use of an immersion heater?

I. An increased danger of contamination of the liquid
II. An increase in nebulizer flow rate
III. An increase in absolute humidity
IV. An increase in delivered oxygen concentration

A. II and IV
B. III and IV
C. I and III
D. I, II, and III

(2:100–1)

12. Which of the following aerosol therapy devices are reportedly able to deliver aerosols the majority of whose particles are less than 10μ in diameter?

I. Pneumatic jet nebulizers
II. Atomizers
III. Ultrasonic nebulizers
IV. Hydronamic (Babington) nebulizers

A. I and II
B. I and III
C. III and IV
D. I, II, and IV

(2:101–3)

13. Which of the following statements are true regarding heat-moisture exchangers?

I. They are placed between the patient and the tubing circuit.
II. They are also called "artificial noses."
III. Body humidity of 100% can be achieved.
IV. They produce particle sizes of 3–5 μ.

A. I, II, and III
B. II and IV
C. I and II
D. II, III, and IV

(2:88–9)

Answer Key

1. A. All of the responses listed will influence the absolute humidity, with the exception of the type of gas delivered.
2. D. The drawing depicts an ultrasonic nebulizer: the blower, medication cup, and electrical plug identify it.
3. C. The piezoelectric transducer converts electrical energy into mechanical energy.
4. B. The cascade humidifier does not deliver particulate water (this is true only of an aerosol), and it can deliver 100% RH.
5. A. The size of the aerosolized particles that are generated by an ultrasonic nebulizer is believed to be determined by the ultrasonic frequency of the unit.
6. C. The quantity of aerosol produced by an ultrasonic nebulizer is most directly related to the unit's amplitude control setting.
7. D. The illustration shows a hydronamic nebulizer. The water source over the sphere, with a hole directing gas toward a baffle help identify it.

8. A. The hydronamic nebulizer delivers the majority of its aerosol in the range of 3–5 μ.
9. B. Humidifiers do not output particulate water, and the ultrasonic nebulizer produces more particles than a jet nebulizer, increasing the risk of contamination.
10. D. The purpose of a baffle is to break up large particles into smaller ones.
11. C. When an immersion heater is used, the increase in temperature causes an increase in absolute humidity. There is also an increased risk of contamination as the heater is introduced into the liquid.
12. C. Hydronamic and ultrasonic nebulizers both deliver the majority of their aerosol particles in the appropriate particle size range.
13. C. Heat and moisture exchangers are also known as condensing humidifiers or artificial noses, because they perform the functions of the nose (heating and humidifying). They do not produce particulate water, and they can produce a body humidity of only 70–90%.

Advanced Level Pretest

According to the Composite Examination Matrix, questions in this category assess only the candidate's ability to correct malfunctions associated with the following equipment:

1. Aerosol generators (pneumatic and ultrasonic nebulizers)

The following are self-study questions from this category.

1. The respiratory therapy practitioner is operating a jet nebulizer on the 100% oxygen setting using a flow rate of 10 L/min to drive the jet. If he or she were to place this nebulizer on the 40% setting, which of the following would occur?

   I. The aerosol density (mg/L) would increase.
   II. The aerosol output (mL/min) would increase.
   III. The total flow rate delivered by the apparatus would double.
   IV. The total flow rate delivered by the apparatus would quadruple.

   A. I and III
   B. II and III
   C. I and IV
   D. II and IV

   (2:89–93)

2. A patient is receiving ultrasonic nebulizer therapy. The respiratory therapist notes that the aerosol mist has suddenly disappeared. What action should the therapist take?

   A. Replace the piezoelectric disc transducer.
   B. Check the water level in the couplant.
   C. Check the fluid level in the medication cup.
   D. B or C

   (2:101–4)

3. In any given nebulizing device, which of the following may act to baffle the aerosolized particles?

   I. The surface of the water
   II. The sides of the container
   III. A sphere placed in the path of the aerosol's flow
   IV. A bend in the aerosol tubing

   A. I and III
   B. II and III
   C. I, II, III, and IV
   D. I, II, and III

   (2:93–9)

4. The air entrainment port on a pneumatic jet nebulizer serves which of the following purposes?

   I. Increases humidity
   II. Increases total system flow
   III. Decreases the delivered FIO_2
   IV. Provides a larger particle size

   A. II and III
   B. III and IV
   C. I and II
   D. I and IV

   (2:93–9)

Answer Key

1. D. Aerosol output would increase if air were entrained. Total flow would increase from 10 L to 40 L (on 40%, the air:oxygen ratio is 3:1).
2. D. If the water in the couplant is low, or if the medication cup is empty or nearly empty, the aerosol output will decrease.
3. C. Any of the choices may act as a baffle, breaking up large particles into smaller ones.
4. A. The air entrainment ports are designed to decrease the FIO_2 and to increase total flow to the patient.

C. Ventilators

Questions in this category assess the candidate's ability to select continuous mechanical ventilatory equipment prior to performing related respiratory care procedures. These questions also test the candidate's understanding of the principles of operation and his or her ability to correct all malfunctions of any selected equipment.

Entry Level Pretest

According to the NBRC Composite Examination Matrix, questions in this category assess the candidate's understanding of the following types of mechanical ventilators:

1. Pneumatic
2. Electric
3. Microprocessor

The following self-study questions were developed from the NBRC Composite Examination Matrix.

1. If a volume-cycled ventilator has its inspiratory time and inspiratory flow rate held constant, then the respiratory rate becomes a function of which of the following controls?

   A. Tidal volume
   B. Minute volume
   C. Pressure limit
   D. I:E ratio

   (2:163–6)

2. During controlled mechanical ventilation, the inspiratory phase may be initiated by:

   I. An inspiratory timer
   II. An expiratory timer
   III. A pneumatic timer
   IV. An electronic timer

   A. I, III, and IV
   B. I, II, III, and IV
   C. II, III, and IV
   D. I and IV

   (2:163–6)

3. On a volume-cycled ventilator the development of an episode of bronchospasm will most likely result in which of the following occurrences?

   A. A decrease in the delivered tidal volume
   B. An increase in respiratory rate
   C. An increase in the ventilator peak pressure
   D. Altered ventilator sensitivity

   (15:151–2, 181)

4. Which of the following is the most fundamental consideration in determining how a mechanical ventilator is *cycled?*

   A. That which initiates inspiration
   B. That which terminates expiration
   C. That which terminates inspiration
   D. That which initiates apneusis

   (15:128–30)

5. Low-pressure drive pneumatic ventilators generally have which of the following waveforms?

   I. Downward-tapering flow pattern
   II. Upward-tapering flow pattern
   III. Downward-tapering pressure pattern
   IV. Upward-tapering pressure pattern

   A. I and III
   B. II and III
   C. I and IV
   D. II and IV

   (2:158–9)

6. High-pressure drive pneumatic ventilators that generate a constant flow, square-wave pattern are referred to as:

   A. Constant-flow generators
   B. Pneumatic-flow generators
   C. Double-circuit systems
   D. Linear-flow generators

   (2:159)

7. When the gas supply powering a ventilator goes directly to the patient, it is considered to have a:

   A. Double circuit
   B. Single circuit
   C. Fluidic circuit
   D. Bellows system

   (2:158–9)

8. Electrically powered ventilators with rotary-driven pistons produce which type of flow pattern?

   A. Square wave
   B. Sine wave
   C. Decelerating
   D. Accelerating

   (2:160–1)

9. Which of the following is (are) able to be assessed by a ventilator microprocessor during an extended self-test?

   I. Pneumatics
   II. Microprocessor systems
   III. Compressibility factor
   IV. Check for leaks

   A. I, II, III, and IV
   B. I, III, and IV
   C. II and III
   D. I and IV

   (2:360–1)

Answer Key

1. D. As long as the flow rate and inspiratory time are held constant, RR becomes a function of I:E ratio.
2. C. During controlled ventilation, inspiration may be initiated by an expiratory, pneumatic, or electronic timer.
3. C. Bronchospasm (or any type of obstruction) will cause an increase in the peak pressure. Only if this pressure meets the set pressure limit will the delivered tidal volume decrease.
4. B. Whatever terminates expiration is how a ventilator is "cycled." For example, if a expiration ends when a certain tidal volume is delivered, the ventilator is considered to be volume-cycled.
5. C. Low-pressure drive pneumatic ventilators (that use a venturi or fluidic drive) have a downward tapering flow and upward tapering pressure curve.
6. A. High-pressure drive pneumatic ventilators that generate a constant flow, square-wave pattern are referred to as constant-flow generators.
7. B. Single-circuit systems use the same gas to power

the machine and deliver the patient's tidal volume. Double-circuit systems use a separate gas source to power the machine.

8. B. Rotary driven pistons produce a sine-wave flow pattern because they move gradually up, then down.
9. A. All of the mechanisms listed are assessed during an extended self-test.

Advanced Practitioner Pretest

According to the NBRC Composite Examination Matrix, questions in this category assess the candidate's understanding of the following types of ventilators:

1. Pneumatic
2. Electric
3. Fluidic
4. Microprocessor
5. High frequency—jet
6. High frequency—oscillator
7. BiPAP system
8. Transport ventilators
9. Home care ventilators

The following are self-study questions from this category.

1. The phenomenon whereby an airstream passing by a wall will tend to adhere to that wall refers to the:

   A. Schmitt effect
   B. Coanda effect
   C. Flip-flop phenomenon
   D. AND/NAND effect

(2:170)

2. Which of the following correctly describes the fluidic element pictured in Figure 14?

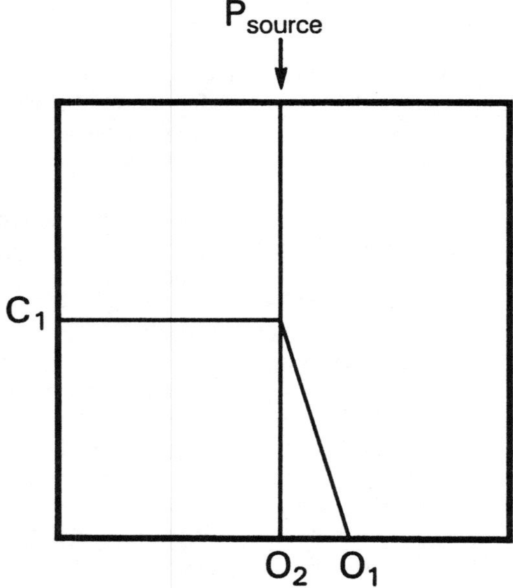

Figure 14.

   A. OR/NOR gate
   B. AND/NAND gate
   C. Flip-flop component
   D. Schmitt trigger

(2:171)

The next two questions refer to Figure 15.

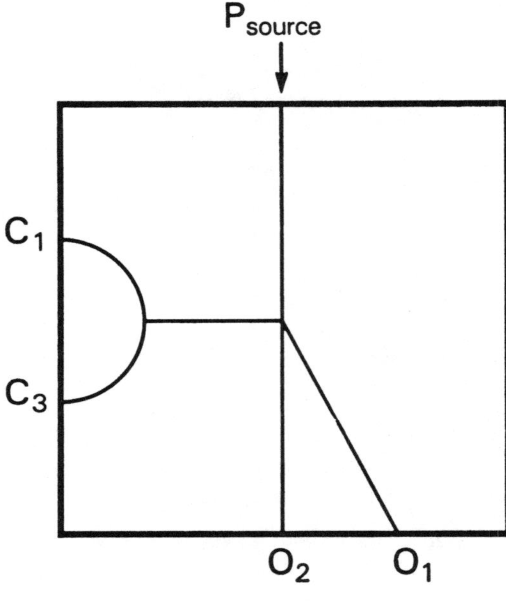

Figure 15.

3. Which of the following best describes the fluidic element pictured above?

   A. OR/NOR gate
   B. Schmitt trigger
   C. AND/NAND gate
   D. Bistable flip-flop element

(2:171)

4. If the previous fluidic element were to have gas under pressure supplied to points P_{source}, C_1, and C_3, gas will exit from tract:

   A. O_2
   B. O_1 and O_2
   C. O_1, O_2, and C_3
   D. O_1

(2:171)

5. A microprocessor ventilator is set to deliver a tidal volume of 700 cc to a patient who is in the early stage of ARDS. The patient's peak inspiratory pressure has increased significantly. Based on this ventilator's closed loop system, what will happen to the delivered tidal volume?

   A. It will decrease.
   B. It will increase.

C. It will remain the same.
D. It will not be delivered at all.

(15:100–1)

6. As you perform a ventilator check, you notice that the peak pressure has increased from 25 cm H_2O to 40 cm H_2O over the last three breaths. The pressure does not return to zero at the end of exhalation, and the patient is not receiving PEEP. What should you do?

A. Increase the pressure limit
B. Increase the tidal volume
C. Increase the flow
D. Decrease the flow

(15:234)

7. Your hospital has just experienced a power outage. Which type of ventilator would be the ideal choice to replace the electrically powered machines?

A. They do not need to be replaced because they all have internal extended battery systems.
B. Pneumatic ventilators
C. Manual resuscitators
D. Microprocessor ventilators

(3:744)

8. Under which of the following situations or conditions are electrically powered ventilators unable to be used?

A. Magnetic resonance imaging
B. Home care
C. CT scan
D. X-ray

(3:744)

9. Which of the following statements are true of high-frequency jet ventilation (HFJV)?

I. Respiratory rates up to 150 breaths/min are utilized.
II. The expiratory phase is passive.
III. It requires the use of a special catheter or endotracheal tube.
IV. Most ventilators can deliver HFJV.

A. I, III, and IV
B. I, II, and III
C. II and IV
D. II and III

(14:332–3)

10. All but which of the following describe high-frequency oscillatory ventilation (HFOV)?

A. Tidal volumes less than dead space are delivered.
B. Respiratory rates as high as 3000 can be delivered.
C. Tracheal tissue damage is a commonly seen side effect.
D. Expiration is active.

(14:332–3)

11. Which of the following statements are true of Bi-PAP?

I. Both IPAP and EPAP are used.
II. It is classified as a form of noninvasive ventilation.
III. It is well tolerated in patients with neuromuscular respiratory insufficiency.
IV. It is well tolerated in children.

A. I, II, III, and IV
B. I, II, and IV
C. II, III, and IV
D. II and III

(14:437)

12. All but which of the following statements are true about transport ventilators?

A. May be volume-limited
B. May be pressure-limited
C. All have the capability of providing PEEP/CPAP
D. Should have a self-contained power supply

(14:389)

13. Positive pressure ventilators used in the home should possess all but which of the following characteristics?

A. Portability
B. Easy to operate
C. Internal battery
D. All of the above

(20:372–3)

14. A patient is receiving mechanical ventilation through a small volume-cycled ventilator in his home. He is in the IMV (SIMV) mode and is unable to generate enough inspiratory effort for spontaneous breathing. Which of the following is the *least* acceptable alternative?

A. Set up an external continuous flow system.
B. Remove the tower of the cascade humidifier.
C. Increase the sensitivity.
D. Switch the patient to assist/control mode.

(20:373)

15. How do HFJV and HFOV effectively accomplish CO_2 removal?

A. Mean airway pressure
B. Tidal volume
C. Flow rate
D. Inspiratory time

(14:333)

16. A patient is receiving noninvasive ventilatory support via the BiPAP® system. Occasionally, this patient has experienced apneic periods during the night. What should the respiratory therapist suggest?

 I. Repeat sleep study
 II. BiPAP® S/T
 III. Iron lung
 IV. Full ventilatory support during the night

 A. I and III
 B. II only
 C. I and II
 D. I and IV

(14:437)

17. A ventilator designed for out-of-hospital transport should possess all but which of the following characteristics?

 A. Operates over extremes of temperature
 B. Uses minimal gas flow above the patient's minute ventilation
 C. Must be able to provide IMV
 D. Consumes minimal power

(13:492)

18. Negative-pressure devices sometimes used in the home include:

 A. Iron lung
 B. Chest cuirass
 C. Pneumosuit
 D. All of the above

(13:360–1)

19. Which of the following statements is true about positive-pressure home care mechanical ventilators?

 A. They are piston driven.
 B. Oxygen is delivered directly from the ventilator.
 C. They are operated by a microprocessor.
 D. Some have negative pressure ventilation capabilities.

(13:358)

20. Which of the following is *not* an advantage of a pneumatically powered mechanical ventilator with fluidic control?

 A. It is safer to operate in the operating room.
 B. Ventilators of this type last longer.
 C. Compressed air consumption is minimal.
 D. It provides a good back-up ventilator source in areas prone to power failures.

(13:251)

Answer Key

1. B. The phenomenon whereby an airstream passing by a wall will tend to adhere to that wall describes the Coanda effect and is the basis for fluidic controls.
2. A. This picture depicts the OR/NOR gate.
3. C. This illustrates the AND/NAND gate.
4. D. If gas under pressure were supplied to point P_{source}, as well as *both* C_1 and C_3, gas will exit from O_1.
5. C. Delivered tidal volume will remain the same; the ventilator compares set and measured variables and will correct delivered volume.
6. C. Risk of auto-PEEP is increased with decreased flow, increased compliance, decreased ET tube size, and increased tidal volume; all of these lead to shorter expiratory times.
7. B. Pneumatic ventilators will allow patients to be ventilated until the power comes back on, without using excessive staff to manually ventilate.
8. A. Electrically powered ventilators cannot be used in MRI procedures. They can be used in the other situations listed.
9. D. HFJV can deliver rates up to 600 and is not available as a mode on most ventilators. Exhalation is passive, and a special catheter or ET tube is necessary in order to deliver HFJV.
10. C. Tracheal tissue damage is not a side effect of HFO. Because it actually produces a positive and negative pressure waveform, expiration is active. RR of 3000 to 4000 have been reported.
11. A. All of the statements are true of BiPAP.
12. C. Not all transport ventilators are capable of providing PEEP.
13. D. Home ventilators should be portable, lightweight, easy to operate, with an internal battery in case of power failure.
14. C. Increasing the sensitivity works only in assist control. The patient on IMV is breathing only through the continuous flow system, which is not regulated by sensitivity.
15. B. These two modes accomplish CO_2 removal primarily through tidal volume control and, to a lesser extent, frequency.
16. B. BiPAP S/T provides a "backup" rate in case of apnea.
17. C. A transport ventilator does not need to be capable of providing IMV; the other characteristics listed, however, are of great importance.
18. D. All of the devices listed are used in the home to provide negative-pressure ventilation.
19. A. Home care positive-pressure ventilators are piston driven. If oxygen is needed, it must be added externally. Only a few are microprocessor vents, and none can also deliver negative pressures.
20. C. Fluidic machines use high amounts of compressed air, and often, small particles of dirt or dust block the small channels. Other answers listed are advantages.

D. Artificial Airways

Questions in this category assess the candidate's ability to select all airway care devices and equipment prior to performing related respiratory care procedures. These questions also test the candidate's understanding of the principles of operation and his or her ability to correct all malfunctions of any selected equipment.

Entry Level Pretest

According to the NBRC Composite Examination Matrix, questions in this category assess the candidate's understanding of the following types of artificial airways:

1. Oropharyngeal and nasopharyngeal airways
2. Endotracheal tubes (oral and nasal)
3. Tracheostomy tubes and buttons
4. Intubation equipment (laryngoscope and blades)

The following self-study questions were developed from the NBRC Composite Examination Matrix.

1. Which of the following statements is (are) true regarding the oropharyngeal airway?

   I. It is well tolerated by all patients.
   II. It is designed to prevent soft tissue upper airway obstruction.
   III. It may be used on semiconscious patients.
   IV. It may induce vomiting.

   A. III and IV
   B. I, II, and III
   C. II, III, and IV
   D. II and IV

   (4:155)

2. Which of the following is the most common material used in the manufacture of endotracheal and tracheostomy tubes?

   A. Natural rubber
   B. Teflon™
   C. Polyvinyl chloride
   D. Polyurethane

   (4:174–6)

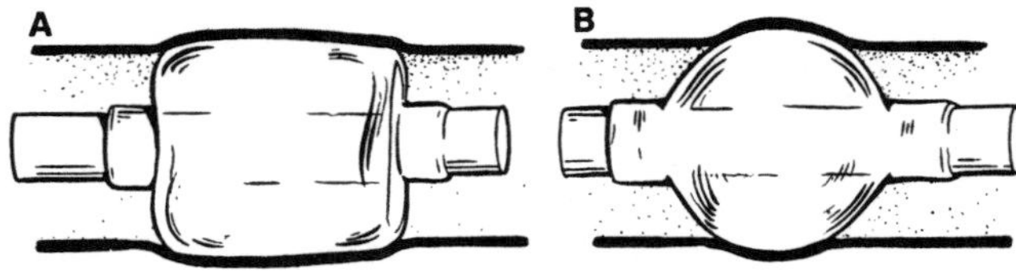

Figure 16.

3. Figure 16 shows:

   I. A high-volume low-pressure cuff and a low-volume, high-pressure cuff
   II. A low-volume high-pressure cuff and a high-volume, high-pressure cuff
   III. A high-volume, high-pressure cuff and a low-volume, low-pressure cuff
   IV. A nasotracheal tube and an anesthesia tube

   A. III and IV
   B. III only
   C. II and IV
   D. I only

   (3:504)

4. Which of the following are true statements regarding the nasopharyngeal airway?

   I. It is indicated to relieve soft tissue obstructions.
   II. It should be used only in comatose patients.
   III. It may be used to facilitate nasotracheal suctioning.
   IV. Epistaxis is a disadvantage.

   A. I and III
   B. II and III
   C. II, III, and IV
   D. I, III, and IV

   (4:155–6)

5. The respiratory therapy practitioner is asked to select an airway care device for a patient with a permanent tracheostomy who is to be discharged. The physician's orders stipulate that the patient's device be able to accomplish all of the following: (a) allow the patient to communicate; (b) provide for administration of IPPB therapy; and (c) provide a patent suction port. Which of the following devices should the practitioner select?

   I. Tracheostomy button
   II. Passy-Muir speaking valve
   III. Tone generator
   IV. Tracheostomy tube with a fenestrated outer cannula

   A. I and III
   B. II and IV
   C. IV only
   D. I, II, and III

   (2:115–19)

6. All but which of the following are advantages of the nasal endotracheal tube over the oral endotracheal tube?

   A. It is easier to pass a suction catheter.
   B. It is more stable to attach respiratory therapy equipment.
   C. It is the endotracheal tube of choice for emergency intubation.
   D. It is more comfortable for the patient.

   (4:169–72)

7. Which of the following statements is (are) true of the laryngoscope?

   A. The handle contains batteries.
   B. Blades come in a variety of sizes, curved or straight.
   C. Handles come in different sizes.
   D. All of the above.

   (13:307)

8. On endotracheal tubes the markings that indicate the tube length from the bevel tip are in which of the following units?

   A. Millimeters
   B. Centimeters
   C. Inches
   D. Angstroms

(2:110–1)

9. Which of the following markings is *least* likely to be found on a standard endotracheal tube?

   A. I.D.
   B. Z-79
   C. I.T.
   D. R.T.

(2:111)

Answer Key

1. D. The oropharyngeal airway can be used only on unconscious patients. Its purpose is relief of upper airway obstruction only (one cannot ventilate through it), and its presence may induce vomiting.
2. C. PVC is the most commonly used tube material because it is compatible with human tissue and flexible to mold at body temperature.
3. D. This drawing depicts a high-volume, low-pressure cuff (A), and a low-volume, high-pressure cuff (B).
4. D. The nasopharyngeal airway is used to relieve soft tissue obstruction, is well tolerated by conscious patients, may cause epistaxis (nosebleed!), and may be used to facilitate nasotracheal suction.
5. D. Only a trach tube with a fenestrated outer cannula can accomplish all of the criteria communicated by the physician. The tone generator and speaking valve can allow communication, but cannot satisfy the other two criteria. Trach buttons must have an adaptor to be able to give IPPB.
6. C. The oral ET tube is the airway of choice for emergency intubation; other statements are true.
7. D. All of these statements about laryngoscopes are true.
8. B. Length of tube is marked in centimeters; I.D. and O.D. are marked in millimeters.
9. D. I.T. = implantation tested; Z-79 is the committee that recommends guidelines for I.T.; I.D. = inside diameter.

Advanced Practitioner Pretest

According to the NBRC Composite Examination Matrix, questions in this category assess the candidate's understanding of the following types of artificial airways:

1. Double-lumen endotracheal tube
2. Exhaled CO_2 detection devices

Candidates are also assessed on their ability to correct malfunctions of the following types of artificial airways:

1. Tracheostomy tubes and buttons
2. Intubation equipment (laryngoscopes and blades)
3. Double-lumen endotracheal tubes
4. Endotracheal tubes (oral and nasal)
5. Exhaled CO_2 detection devices

The following self-study questions were developed from the NBRC Composite Examination Matrix.

1. The most common usage of double-lumen endotracheal tubes is:

   A. In the neonatal ICU
   B. By paramedics in the field
   C. In the emergency room
   D. In the operating room

(16:828–9)

2. Which of the following statements are true about double-lumen endobronchial tubes?

   I. The tracheal lumen has the smaller cuff.
   II. The bronchial lumen has the smaller cuff.
   III. Risk of obstruction is higher than with the single lumen tube.
   IV. They may be used to provide differential levels of PEEP.

   A. I, III, and IV
   B. II, III, and IV
   C. I and IV
   D. II and III

(16:828–9)

3. A patient in respiratory failure has been orally intubated in the emergency room. Exhaled CO_2 measures 0.5%. What should the RCP recommend?

   A. Extubate the patient and reintubate.
   B. Secure the tube as it is.
   C. Obtain a chest x-ray to assure proper placement.
   D. Perform an emergency tracheotomy.

(16:834–5)

4. Measurement of exhaled CO_2 to detect proper endotracheal tube placement may give false negative results under what circumstance(s)?

   A. Central line placement
   B. Cardiopulmonary arrest
   C. Bronchoscopy
   D. All of the above

(13:602–3)

5. Which of the following is *not* true regarding selection of the proper size endotracheal tube for an adult?

   A. Select the largest diameter tube that will fit through the patient's glottis.

B. For nasotracheal intubation, select a tube one half to one size smaller than the oral tube of correct size.
C. Larger diameter tubes require greater work of breathing.
D. Larger tubes require less air for cuff inflation.

(1:469–71)

6. Which of the following statements are true about laryngoscopes?

I. There is less stimulation of the epiglottis with a curved blade.
II. The straight blade allows greater exposure of the glottic opening.
III. Straight blades are preferred for pediatric patients.
IV. The curved blade has a larger blade surface.

A. I, II, and III
B. II, III, and IV
C. I and III
D. I, II, III, and IV

(1:485–6)

7. Which of the following is *not* true about tracheostomy tubes:

A. They come in a variety of sizes.
B. They may be made of synthetics, silver, nylon, or Teflon.
C. They are available in different lengths.
D. They are all equipped with low-pressure, high-volume cuffs.

(1:478)

8. Which of the following statements is (are) true regarding placement of the curved laryngoscope blade during endotracheal intubation of the adult?

A. It is placed under the epiglottis.
B. It is placed above the epiglottis in the vallecula.
C. It is placed between the base of the tongue and the epiglottis.
D. B and C

(1:485–6)

9. A laryngoscope that is used for endotracheal intubation consists of which of the following parts?

I. Blade
II. Handle
III. Light source
IV. Malleable stylet

A. I, II, III, and IV
B. I, II, and III
C. II and III
D. I and II

(1:484–6)

10. When a straight laryngoscope blade is being used to intubate the trachea of an adult patient, which of the following is *not* appropriate?

A. The patient's head and neck should be in the sniffing position.
B. The patient's teeth should not be used as a fulcrum.
C. The tip of the blade should be placed under the epiglottis.
D. The blade should be inserted into the left side of the patient's mouth.

(1:487–9)

Answer Key

1. D. Double-lumen tubes are used in the OR to allow collapse of the operative lung, while ventilating the nonoperative one.
2. B. The bronchial lumen has a smaller cuff because the bronchi is smaller than the trachea. Obstruction is more common because the lumens are smaller than the one in a standard ET tube. The two lumens may also provide different levels of PEEP to each lung.
3. A. $P_{ET}CO_2$ levels should approach 6% on exhalation. The patient is esophageally intubated and should be extubated and reintubated.
4. B. Capnography may give false negative results during cardiac arrest due to decreased blood flow.
5. C. Smaller tubes provide greater airway resistance and increase the patient's work of breathing.
6. D. All of the statement listed are true of laryngoscope blades.
7. D. Some trach tubes are uncuffed.
8. D. The curved blade is placed above the epiglottis (between the base of the tongue and the epiglottis).
9. B. The stylet is an extra piece of equipment designed to give some rigidity to the ET tube so that it is easier to insert.
10. D. The blade should be inserted on the right side of the patient's mouth.

E. Suctioning Devices (Entry Level Only)

Questions in this category assess the candidate's ability to select and assemble all suctioning equipment prior to performing respiratory care procedures. These questions also test the candidate's understanding of the principles of proper operation and his or her ability to correct all malfunctions of selected equipment.

Entry Level Pretest

According to the NBRC Composite Examination Matrix, questions in this category assess the candidate's understanding of the following types of respiratory care equipment:

1. Suction catheters
2. Specimen collectors
3. Oropharyngeal suction devices

The following are self-study questions developed from the NBRC Composite Examination Matrix.

1. Secretions that have accumulated in a patient's oropharynx should be removed by which of the following?

   A. Tonsil tip suction
   B. Standard suction catheter
   C. Murphy suction
   D. Continuous in-line system

   (1:498–9)

2. Wall suction should optimally be set at what pressure?

   A. –50 to –75 mm Hg
   B. –80 to –120 mm Hg
   C. –125 to –150 mm Hg
   D. Research has not determined the optimal pressure setting

   (1:499–500)

3. A tracheostomized patient is suffering from left upper lobe pneumonia, and produces large amounts of sputum. Which suction catheter should you choose to remove his secretions?

   A. Whistle-tip
   B. Open-ended
   C. Aero-Flo
   D. Coude

   (1:500)

4. Which of the following describe the ideal suction catheter?
   I. Has side holes
   II. Has smooth molded ends
   III. Is long enough to pass the tip of the airway
   IV. Is able to withstand negative pressures > 150 cm H_2O

   A. I, II, III, and IV
   B. I, II, and III
   C. II and III
   D. I and II

   (4:183)

5. Continuous-suction catheter systems are advantageous for patients who:

   A. Require high levels of PEEP
   B. Wish to save money
   C. Are on respiratory rates greater than 10
   D. A and C

   (1:500–1)

6. When suctioning, in order to obtain a culture specimen:

   A. Be sure to rinse the suction catheter with sterile water.
   B. Obtain a specimen every 3–5 days.
   C. Place the collection container between the catheter and the suction tubing leading to the wall outlet.
   D. Rinse the catheter with normal saline.

   (4:185)

Answer Key

1. A. Tonsil tip suction is appropriate for removal of oropharyngeal secretions.
2. B. Optimal wall pressure for suction is –80 to –120 cm H_2O.
3. D. The Coude catheter is angled to facilitate suction of the left mainstem bronchus.
4. B. The suction catheter does not need to be able to withstand high negative pressures (–120 cm H_2O is the highest acceptable suction pressure).
5. D. Continuous-suction catheters are good for patients who are on high RR or high PEEP levels, so that they are not completely removed from the ventilator.
6. C. When obtaining a sputum specimen from an intubated patient, if the catheter is rinsed, the specimen can be lost or diluted. Traps are placed between the catheter and suction tubing.

F. Gas Delivery, Metering, and Clinical Analyzing Devices

Questions in this category assess the candidate's ability to select and assemble all medical gas therapy equipment prior to performing respiratory care procedures. These questions also test the candidate's understanding of the principles of proper operation and his or her ability to correct all malfunctions of selected equipment.

Entry Level Pretest

According to the NBRC Composite Examination Matrix, questions in this category assess the candidate's understanding of the following types of respiratory care equipment:

1. Regulators, reducing valves, connectors, and flowmeters
2. Air/oxygen blenders
3. Gas cylinders, bulk systems, and manifolds
4. Oxygen analyzers
5. Air compressors
6. Blood gas analyzers and sampling devices
7. Pulse oximeters

The following are self-study questions developed from the NBRC Composite Examination Matrix.

1. A device that registers flow rate as a result of backpressure created by a fixed orifice is:

   A. A Thorpe tube
   B. A kinetic flowmeter
   C. A rotameter
   D. A Bourdon gauge

   (2:58–9)

2. Which type of O_2 analyzer operates on the fact that oxygen tends to disrupt a magnetic field?

   A. Paramagnetic
   B. Polarographic
   C. Thermoconductive
   D. Electronic

   (13:70–1)

3. When full, cylinders of gaseous oxygen usually contain a pressure of:

   A. 1100 psig
   B. 1000 psig
   C. 2500 psig
   D. 2200 psig

   (2:21–30)

4. The respiratory therapy practitioner can most readily identify the number of stages a given reducing valve has by:

   A. Looking at the pressure gauge
   B. Counting the number of frangible disks
   C. Counting the number of pressure gauges
   D. Counting the number of pop-off valves

   (2:50–3)

5. Which of the following safety systems was designed for use with the connecting valves of large medical gas cylinders (F-H)?

   A. Pin Index Safety System (PISS)
   B. American Standard Safety System (ASSS)
   C. Color Code Safety System
   D. Diameter Index Safety System (DISS)

   (2:26–31)

6. Figure 17 illustrates:
   I. A single-stage reducing valve
   II. The inner mechanism of the Bourdon gauge
   III. A simple example of an oxygen blender
   IV. An adjustable pressure regulator
   V. A DISS wall outlet

   A. I, II, and III
   B. II, III, and IV

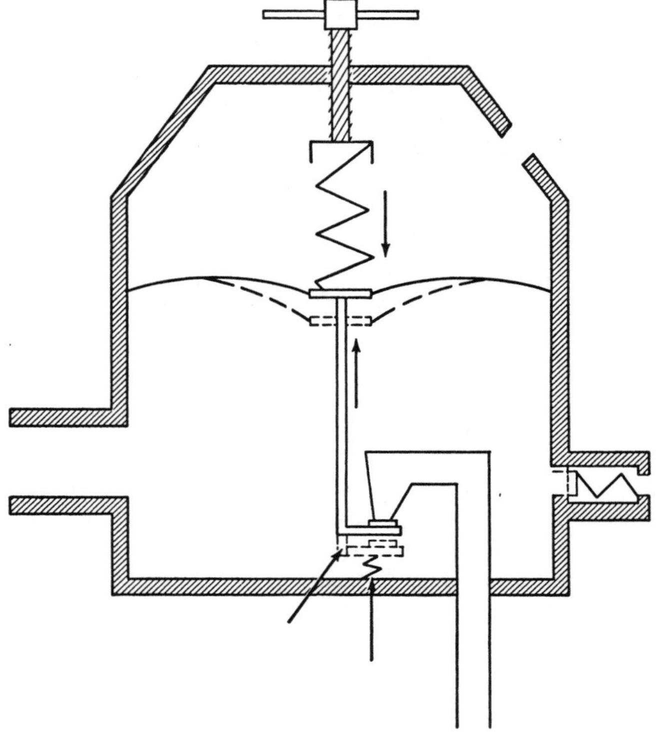

Figure 17.

   C. I and IV
   D. I, III, and IV

   (2:50–3)

7. The diaphragm in Figure 17:
   I. Separates the high-pressure from the low-pressure side of the regulator
   II. Opens the poppet valve when the low-pressure side loses pressure
   III. Closes the poppet valve when the low-pressure side gains pressure
   IV. Allows for the pressure needed to move it to be varied by the user

   A. I, II, and III
   B. III and IV
   C. I, II, III, and IV
   D. I and III

   (2:50–3)

8. Which of the following safety systems was designed for use on small medical gas cylinders (A-E) with post-type valves?

   A. Pin Index Safety System (PISS)
   B. Diameter Index Safety System (DISS)
   C. American Standard Safety System (ASSS)
   D. Color Code Safety System

   (2:26–8)

9. Which of the following organizations is responsible for regulating the purity of compressed medical gases?
   A. Compressed Gas Association
   B. National Formulary
   C. United States Pharmacopeia
   D. Food and Drug Administration

(2:28)

10. When a medical gas cylinder has been designated and stamped with the symbol 3AA, which of the following is true?
    A. It is capable of containing medical quality gases.
    B. It can withstand pressures up to 5000 psig.
    C. It has been produced from heat-treated steel.
    D. It has undergone hydrostatic testing.

(2:24)

11. Which of the following statements regarding the design and construction of medical gas cylinders is *not* true?
    A. Most cylinders must currently undergo hydrostatic testing every 5 or 10 years.
    B. Cylinders must contain a pressure release mechanism to prevent explosion.
    C. The cylinder's marked maximum filling pressure may be exceeded by 50% if needed.
    D. Hydrostatic retesting is performed at $5/3$ of the cylinder service pressure.

(2:23–6)

12. The International Color Code for oxygen is:
    A. White
    B. Green
    C. Brown
    D. Orange

(2:25)

13. Which of the following *most* correctly defines the minimal standard for a bulk oxygen system?
    A. More than 50,000 cubic feet of gaseous oxygen connected and ready for use
    B. More than 480 cylinders of oxygen connected and ready for use
    C. More than 13,000 cubic feet of gaseous oxygen connected and ready for use
    D. More than 4000 cubic feet of liquid oxygen connected and ready for use

(2:32–3)

14. The Food and Drug Administration requires that medical oxygen be at least ___ in purity.
    A. 90%
    B. 99%
    C. 98%
    D. 99.9%

(2:29)

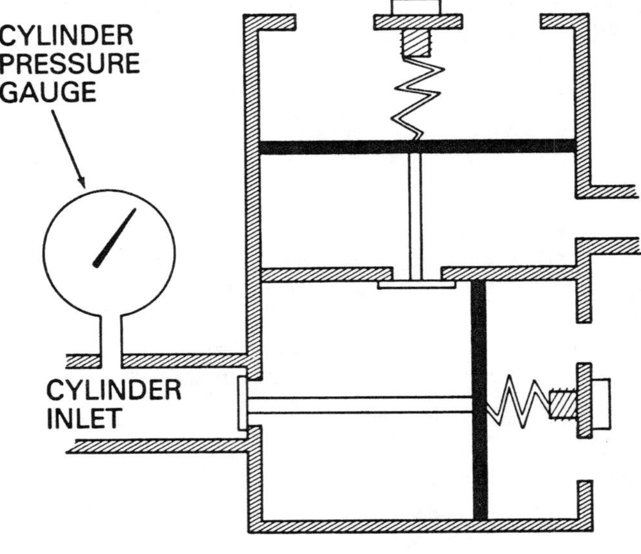

Figure 18.

15. Figure 18 shows:
    I. A triple-stage pressure regulator
    II. Two poppet valves
    III. A double-stage pressure regulator
    IV. Two diaphragms
    V. Five pop-off valves

    A. I, II, and IV
    B. II, III, and IV
    C. I, II, IV, and V
    D. I, III, IV, and V

(2:50–4)

16. Which of the following devices/systems does *not* use a compressor as part of its principle of operation?
    A. Piped vacuum systems
    B. Certain volume ventilators
    C. Molecular sieve type oxygen concentrators
    D. Piped 100% oxygen

(2:33–5)

The next two questions refer to Figure 19.

17. Figure 19 illustrates:
    A. A cylinder valve for sizes A-E cylinders
    B. A single-stage reducing valve
    C. A cylinder valve of cylinder sizes larger then E cylinders
    D. A 50-psi wall outlet

(2:26–8)

18. The number "1" in Figure 19 refers to:
    A. An example of color coding
    B. The outlet of the yoke

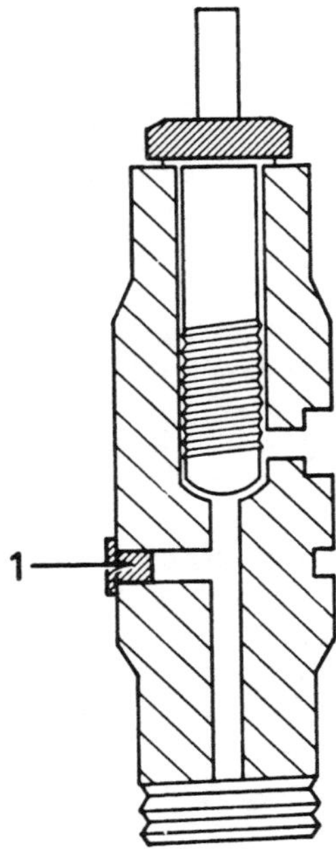

Figure 19.

C. The metal relief valve
D. Female adaptor for PISS system

(2:26–8)

19. Which of the following statements regarding back-pressure-compensated Thorpe tube type flowmeters is *not* true?

A. They are calibrated at 50 psig and 70° F.
B. Their accuracy is not significantly affected by changes in backpressure.
C. Their accuracy is not affected by changes in wall pressure.
D. Their accuracy is affected by changes in position.

(2:54–5)

20. Which of the following is (are) true statements regarding kinetic type flowmeters?

I. Their accuracy is not affected by changes in position.
II. They cannot be backpressure compensated.
III. They use a plunger type device to indicate flow.

A. I and II
B. II only
C. I, II, and III
D. III only

(2:55)

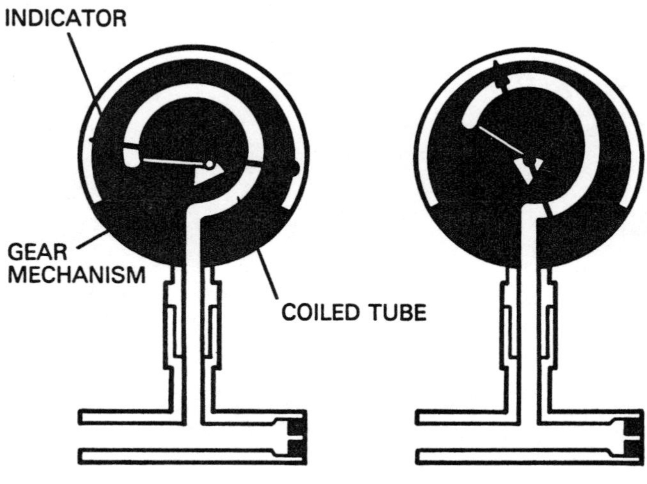

Figure 20.

21. The Diameter Index Safety System would be used on which of the following gas systems?

A. Those with pressures greater than 2200 psig
B. Those with pressures greater than 500 psig
C. Those with pressures greater than 200 psig
D. Those with pressures less than 200 psig

(2:26–8)

22. True statements regarding Figure 20 include:
I. A Thorpe tube is illustrated.
II. A Bourdon gauge is illustrated.
III. A single-stage regulator is shown.
IV. The coiled tube will straighten with increasing pressure.
V. The coiled tube will curl with increasing pressure.

A. I, II, and IV
B. I, II, and III
C. II and IV
D. III, IV, and V

(2:50–1)

23. Which of the following statements regarding the color coding of medical gases are correct?
I. The code for a cylinder containing helium and oxygen is gray and green.
II. The color code for a cylinder containing oxygen and carbon dioxide is brown and green.
III. The color code for a cylinder of compressed air is yellow.
IV. The color code for a cylinder of nitrous oxide is light blue.

A. I and III
B. II and III
C. I and IV
D. III and IV

(2:25)

24. The first stage of a multiple-stage reducing valve will generally lower cylinder pressure to around ___ psig.

    A. 200–1500
    B. 1200–1500
    C. 700–1200
    D. 200–700

    (2:50–3)

25. The most accurate type of oxygen analyzer is:

    A. Physical
    B. Electrical
    C. Mass spectrophotometry
    D. Electrochemical

    (2:143)

26. Oxygen blenders consist of which of the following?

    I. Pressure-regulating valves
    II. Precision-metering device
    III. 30 psig sources of oxygen and compressed air
    IV. Alarm system

    A. I, II, III, and IV
    B. II, III, and IV
    C. I, II, and III
    D. I, II, and IV

    (3:621)

27. Pulse oximeters display:

    A. Oxygen saturation
    B. Partial pressure of oxygen
    C. Oxygen content
    D. Perfusion

    (13:600)

28. The oxygen electrode in a blood gas analyzer is:

    A. Polarographic
    B. Paramagnetic
    C. A Severinghaus electrode
    D. B and C

    (13:78)

29. The CO_2 electrode in a blood gas analyzer:

    A. Is a pH electrode
    B. Is separated from the blood sample by a silica membrane
    C. Measures the change in carbonic acid concentration
    D. A and B

    (13:78)

Answer Key

1. D. A Bourdon gauge registers flow rate as a result of backpressure created by a fixed opening.
2. A. A paramagnetic oxygen analyzer uses a nitrogen-filled glass dumbbell suspended on a filament in a magnetic field. As oxygen is introduced, the dumbbell rotates proportionately.
3. D. When full, cylinders of gaseous oxygen usually contain a pressure of 2200 psig.
4. D. The number of stages in a given reducing valve can be determined by counting the number of pop-offs.
5. B. ASSS was designed for use with the connecting valves of large medical gas cylinders (> F).
6. C. The illustration shows a single-stage reducing valve (one pressure pop-off) with an adjustable regulator (spring that may be adjusted at the top).
7. C. All of the statements describe or are true of the diaphragm in the illustration.
8. A. The PISS was designed for use on small medical gas cylinders (A–E) with post-type valves.
9. D. The FDA regulates gas purity.
10. C. When a medical gas cylinder has been designated and stamped with the symbol 3AA, it means that it is made of heat-treated steel.
11. C. The cylinder's maximum filling pressure may be exceeded by 10%.
12. A. The international color code for oxygen is white.
13. D. Bulk oxygen systems must have more than 20,000 cubic feet of gaseous oxygen connected and ready for use. Other statements are true.
14. B. The FDA requires that medical oxygen be at least 99% pure.
15. B. The illustration is of a double-stage regulator (two pop-offs) with two poppets and two diaphragms.
16. D. Piped oxygen does not utilize a compressor.
17. A. The picture shows a cylinder valve for an A–E size.
18. C. The 1 indicates the relief valve.
19. The backpressure compensated Thorpe tube *is* affected by changes in wall pressure.
20. D. Kinetic flowmeters use a plunger to indicate flow, can be backpressure compensated (they are a type of Thorpe tube), and do not read accurately unless they are vertical.
21. D. DISS is designed for low pressure devices (< 200 psi).
22. C. The picture shows a Bourdon gauge. As the pressure increases, the tube will straighten, indicating a higher pressure reading.
23. D. Compressed air cylinders are yellow; oxygen, green; helium, brown; CO_2 gray; nitrous oxide, light blue.
24. D. The first stage of a multiple-stage reducing valve will generally lower cylinder pressure to around 200–700 psig.
25. C. The most accurate type of oxygen analyzer is mass spectrophotometry; it counts the number of oxygen ions.
26. D. Oxygen blenders consist of pressure-regulating valves, a precision metering device, 50 psig gas sources of oxygen and compressed air, and an alarm system.
27. A. Pulse oximeters display oxygen saturation and, usually, pulse rate.

28. A. The oxygen electrode (Clark) in a blood gas analyzer is polarographic.
29. The CO_2 electrode in a blood gas analyzer is a Severinghaus pH electrode, which is separated from the blood by a silica membrane.

Advanced Level Pretest

According to the NBRC Composite Examination Matrix, questions in this category assess the candidate's understanding of the following types of respiratory care equipment:

1. Oxygen concentrators
2. Portable liquid oxygen systems
3. Capnograph
4. Co-oximeter
5. Transcutaneous O_2/CO_2 monitor

The following are self-study questions developed from the NBRC Composite Examination Matrix.

1. You are taking care of a patient who has end-stage IPF. She requires a nonrebreather continuously, running at 12 L/min. What oxygen system is best for her to have at home?

   A. Conventional cylinders
   B. Liquid oxygen
   C. Concentrator
   D. Oxygen requirements are too high for home use

   (20:340–4)

2. Which of the following is an advantage of oxygen concentrators?

   A. Portability
   B. Lightweight
   C. No need for oxygen resupply
   D. They can also power other respiratory equipment

   (20:340)

3. Which of the following describe liquid oxygen systems (LOX)?

   I. They are unreliable.
   II. They are portable.
   III. No external power source is required.
   IV. LOX is best for homebound patients.

   A. I, II, and III
   B. II and III
   C. III and IV
   D. I, III, and IV

   (20:342–3)

4. One of your home care patients is on a liquid oxygen system. He has not used his oxygen for several days. When he attempts to turn it on, no flow comes out of the system, even though the system has not been used since it was refilled last week. What is the most likely cause of the problem?

   A. The connection has frozen due to the low temperature of liquid O_2.
   B. He accidentally left the flowmeter on at a low flowrate.
   C. The liquid oxygen has evaporated.
   D. He is turning the needle valve the wrong way.

   (20:342–3)

5. Which types of hemoglobin are analyzed by the co-oximeter?

   I. Reduced hemoglobin
   II. Oxyhemoglobin
   III. Carboxyhemoglobin
   IV. Methemoglobin

   A. I, III, and IV
   B. II, III, and IV
   C. I, II, and III
   D. I, II, III, and IV

   (19:334–6)

6. Which of the following is *not* a cause of measurement error(s) associated with co-oximeters?

   A. Lipids in the sample
   B. Cell fragments in the sample
   C. Methylene blue dye
   D. Oxygen saturations below 90%

   (19:336)

7. You have been asked to analyze a sample of fetal blood for carboxyhemoglobin level. If you use adult values for the extinction coefficient, how will your results be affected?

   A. They will be accurate.
   B. They will be in error from 4–7%.
   C. They will be in error by as much as 20%.
   D. You must multiply your result by 1.5.

   (16:492)

8. You are attempting to take a pulse oximetry reading in order to assess oxygen saturation. If no signal can be detected by the oximeter ("insufficient" display), what should the respiratory therapist check?

   A. Presence of digital clubbing
   B. Untrimmed fingernails
   C. Fingernail polish
   D. A and C

   (19:339)

9. All but which of the following is (are) disadvantages associated with transcutaneous monitoring of O_2 and CO_2?

   A. 20–30 min equilibration time
   B. Skin blistering
   C. Skin burning
   D. Unreliable compared to oximetry

   (19:282)

10. Failure of a transcutaneous monitor to accurately reflect Pa_{O_2} and Pa_{CO_2} may be caused by all but which of the following?

    A. Electrode temperature of 37° Celsius
    B. Fetal hemoglobin
    C. Thick skin
    D. Diminished cardiac output

(3:791–2)

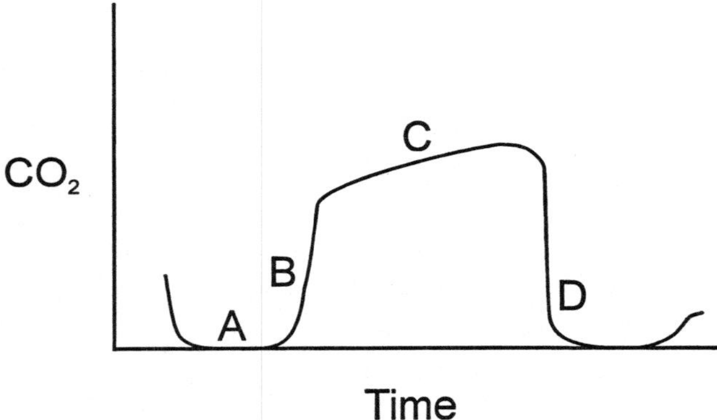

Figure 21. Normal capnogram.

The next two questions are based on Figure 21.

11. Inspiration is represented by:

    A. A
    B. B
    C. C
    D. D

(16:499–500)

12. Gas leaving the alveoli is reflected in:

    A. A
    B. B
    C. C
    D. D

(16:499–500)

13. Under normal circumstances:

    A. $P_{ET}CO_2$ is equal to Pa_{CO_2}.
    B. $P_{ET}CO_2$ is slightly lower than Pa_{CO_2}.
    C. $P_{ET}CO_2$ is slightly higher than Pa_{CO_2}.
    D. $P_{ET}CO_2$ has no correlation with Pa_{CO_2}.

(16:500)

14. What type of condition is indicated by the capnogram in Figure 22?

    A. Restrictive pulmonary disease
    B. Obstructive pulmonary disease

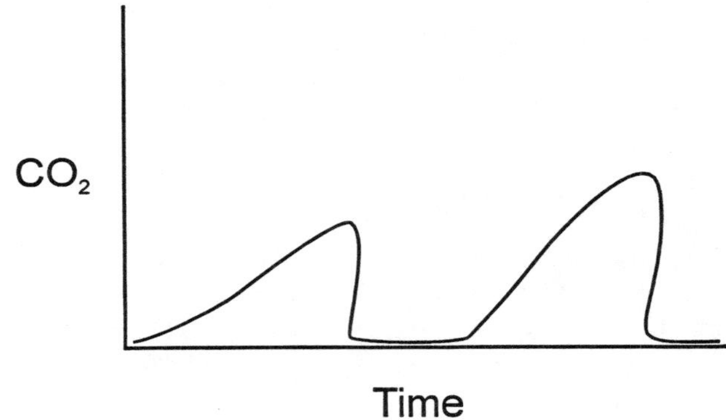

Figure 22.

    C. Hypoventilation
    D. Cardiac compressions

(19:257)

15. Sources of blood gas analyzer calibration errors include all but which of the following?

    A. Inaccurate barometer readings
    B. Insufficient cleaning
    C. Contaminated buffers
    D. All are calibration errors.

(19:321)

16. What is the best way for the respiratory care practitioner to eliminate the "blood gas factor"?

    A. Calibrate with tonometered blood
    B. Calibrate with tonometered gas
    C. Always use referenced buffers
    D. Apply a blood gas factor correction

(13:78–9)

17. Which of the following types of electrodes measure pH?

    I. Clark type
    II. Severinghaus type
    III. Galvanic type
    IV. Sanz type

    A. II and IV
    B. II and III
    C. III and IV
    D. I and IV

(19:288–9)

18. A highly specialized type of glass is used in the pH electrode to separate the known reference buffer from the sample being measured. Which of the following statements about this "pH sensitive glass" is (are) true?

    I. It is permeable to hydrogen ions.
    II. It is permeable to electrons.

III. It is permeable to protons.
IV. It is responsible for the potential difference created between the two solutions.

A. I and III
B. I, III, and IV
C. IV only
D. II and IV

(19:288–90)

19. Which of the following oxygen monitoring devices incorporates modifications of the Clark electrode?

I. Polarographic analyzers
II. Galvanic cell analyzers
III. Transcutaneous devices
IV. Oximeter devices

A. I and III
B. II, III, and IV
C. I and IV
D. I and II

(13:78, 604)

20. The respiratory therapy practitioner is monitoring the transcutaneous oxygen tension of a patient in the intensive care unit. The 70-kg patient's cardiac index is 1.2 L/min/m^2 body surface area. Based on this information, the practitioner would expect which of the following degrees of correlation between $Ptco_2$ and Pao_2?

A. Poor
B. Good
C. Linear
D. Excellent

(13:604)

21. Which of the following types of oxygen analyzers operates by separating gases according to their ionic mass?

A. Paramagnetic
B. Thermal conductivity
C. Modified Clark cell type
D. Mass spectrometer

(13:69)

Answer Key

1. A. Liquid systems cannot provide flow rates > 10 L/min, and concentrators are designed for low-flow use (the higher the flow, the lower the FIo_2). Conventional cylinders is the only option for this patient.
2. C. Although oxygen concentrators are rather cumbersome, they require no resupply of gas and are economical.
3. C. LOX systems are reliable at flow rates up to 10 L/min, have the advantage of portability (best for patients who are mobile), and require no external power source.
4. C. If liquid oxygen is not used for several days, it will evaporate.
5. D. The co-oximeter measures each of the choices listed here.
6. D. Lipids, cell fragments, or dye in the sample will cause measurement error.
7. B. If you use adult values for the extinction coefficient when analyzing fetal hemoglobin for carboxyhemoglobin level, the error will be from 4 to 7%.
8. D. Digital clubbing and fingernail polish interfere with the fiberoptics, and the pulse oximeter cannot pick up any signal.
9. D. Transcutaneous monitoring is reliable, but may cause burning or blistering of the skin if the electrode site is not changed often enough. The 20–30 min equilibration time may be a disadvantage because it is inconvenient.
10. B. Fetal hemoglobin is measured in utero, and is not associated with transcutaneous gas monitoring.
11. A. Inspiration is "A"—CO_2 levels are near 0.
12. C. C represents gas leaving the alveoli; B represents gas leaving the conducting airways (gradual rise).
13. B. Normally, $P_{ET}co_2$ is about 5 mm Hg lower than $Paco_2$.
14. B. This capnogram (characteristic of obstructive disease) delays the upstroke and blurs the distinction between emptying of the conducting airways and emptying of the alveoli.
15. D. All of the choices represent calibration errors.
16. B. Calibrate blood gas electrodes with tonometered gas to eliminate the blood gas factor (when the O_2 electrode forms oxygen gradients around the cathode, which may cause some error in analysis).
17. A. Both Sanz and Severinghaus electrodes measure pH.
18. D. The glass that separates the known reference buffer from the sample being measured in a pH electrode is permeable to electrons and is responsible for the potential difference created between the two solutions.
19. A. Polarographic analyzers and transcutaneous electrodes contain modifications of the Clark electrode.
20. A. Correlation would be poor due to poor perfusion (normal C.I. is 2.5–4.0 L/min/m^2.
21. D. The mass spec separates gases according to mass and counts the number of ions of each gas in the sample.

G. Manometers and Gauges

Questions in this category assess the candidate's ability to select and assemble various manometers and gauges prior to performing respiratory care procedures. These questions also test the candidate's understanding of the principles of operation and his or her ability to correct all malfunctions of any selected equipment.

Entry Level Pretest

According to the Composite Examination Matrix, questions in this category assess the candidate's understanding of the following types of manometers and gauges:

1. Water, mercury, and aneroid manometers
2. Inspiratory and expiratory pressure meters
3. Cuff pressure manometers

The following are self-study questions from this category.

1. Ideally, peak endotracheal intracuff pressures should not exceed:

   A. 15 mm Hg
   B. 25 mm Hg
   C. 40 mm Hg
   D. 50 mm Hg

   (1:472)

2. Hazards of increased intracuff pressures include all but which of the following?

   A. Destruction of ciliated epithelium
   B. Massive atelectasis
   C. Tracheal dilatation
   D. Pressure necrosis of mucosal tissue

   (1:472)

3. Which of the following are true statements about water manometer monitoring technique?

   I. The manometer should be filled to a level slightly less than the estimated pressure reading.
   II. Patients should be removed from mechanical ventilation to obtain readings.
   III. The zero reference point should be placed at the phlebostatic axis.
   IV. Fluctuation of the fluid level with respiration is normal.

   A. I, II, III, and IV
   B. I, II, and III
   C. II and III
   D. III and IV

   (5:126–8)

4. Pressure manometers:

   A. May be evaluated for accuracy by either a water or mercury column
   B. Should be evaluated at zero and at 10 mm Hg
   C. May be evaluated by a supersyringe
   D. A and C

   (1:118–9)

5. An aneroid manometer is attached to the endotracheal or tracheostomy tube. The patient inhales against an occluded airway following maximal exhalation. This describes measurement of:

   A. Negative inspiratory force
   B. Maximal expiratory pressure
   C. Maximal inspiratory pressure
   D. A and C

   (13:593)

6. Normal maximal expiratory pressure is:

   A. 80 to 100 cm H_2O
   B. –80 to –100 cm H_20
   C. 20 to 40 cm H_2O
   D. –20 to –40 cm H_2O

   (6:75)

Answer Key

1. B. Peak endotracheal intracuff pressures should not exceed 25 cm H_2O, so that arterial blood flow to the area is not compromised.
2. B. Atelectasis is not a hazard associated with increased ET tube cuff pressures.
3. D. The water column should be filled with fluid to a level slightly higher than expected; patients should not be removed from mechanical ventilation to take readings; the last two statements are true.
4. A. Pressure manometers should be evaluated for accuracy by either a water or mercury column.
5. D. The maneuver described is NIF or MIP.
6. A. Normal maximal expiratory pressure is 80–100 cm H_2O.

Advanced Practitioner Pretest

According to the NBRC Composite Examination Matrix, questions in this category assess the candidate's understanding of transducers. In addition, the candidate's ability to correct malfunctions associated with transducers will be evaluated on the advanced level examination. The following self-study questions are based on the NBRC Composite Examination Matrix.

1. An intracuff pressure of 60 mm Hg is required in order to maintain a tracheal seal. What might the respiratory therapist conclude from this information?

   A. This is a normal intracuff pressure.
   B. The endotracheal tube may be too small.
   C. The endotracheal tube may be too large.
   D. The patient has developed a tracheoesophageal fistula.

   (1:472–3)

2. Which of the following are true statements about transducers?

   I. They convert mechanical energy to electrical energy.
   II. They convert electrical energy into mechanical energy.
   III. The most common is the strain gauge type.
   IV. Increased flow to the transducer is transmitted as an upward deflection on the monitor.

   A. I, II, III, and IV
   B. I, II, and III
   C. II, III, and IV
   D. I, III, and IV

   (5:86–7)

3. All but which of the following are types of transducers?

   A. Quartz
   B. Strain gauge
   C. Disposable
   D. Amplifier-type

(5:87)

4. What is the purpose of a transducer dome?

   A. Provides a more compressible medium than air for measurement purposes
   B. Separates the transducer from IV fluid
   C. Transmits the electrical signal to the monitor
   D. Electrically damps the system

(5:87)

5. Strain gauges are often used to measure:

   I. Intravascular pressures
   II. Helium concentrations
   III. Intrapulmonary pressures
   IV. Mixed expiratory carbon dioxide concentration

   A. I and III
   B. II and IV
   C. III and IV
   D. II and III

(5:86–7)

6. The term *strain gauge* is most synonymous with:

   A. A pressure transducer
   B. A pressure drop transducer
   C. A thermistor bead transducer
   D. A mercury manometer

(5:86–7)

Answer Key

1. B. If a pressure of 60 cm H_2O must be generated in order to maintain a seal, the endotracheal tube is probably too small.
2. D. Transducers convert mechanical energy into electrical energy. Other statements are correct.
3. D. An amplifier-type is not a type of transducer; all of the others are.
4. B. The transducer dome separates the transducer from IV fluid to prevent electrical shock.
5. A. Strain gauges can measure either intravascular or intrapulmonary pressures.
6. A. Strain gauge is a pressure transducer.

H. Resuscitation Devices

Questions in this category assess the candidate's ability to select and assemble various resuscitation devices prior to performing respiratory care procedures. These questions also test the candidate's understanding of the principles of operation and his or her ability to correct all malfunctions of any selected equipment.

Entry Level Pretest

According to the Composite Examination Matrix, questions in this category assess the candidate's understanding of the following types of resuscitation devices:

1. Manual resuscitators (bag-valve)
2. Mouth-to-valve mask resuscitators

The following are self-study questions from this category.

1. The RCP is asked to select an adult manual resuscitator device for use on the hospital's emergency crash carts. Which of the following features would be *least* advisable for this unit?

   A. A self-expanding bag
   B. A pop-off valve
   C. The ability to deliver at least 85% oxygen with an attached reservoir
   D. A patient ventilating valve that is unaffected by high flow rates

(1:892)

2. Most adult manual resuscitator units have a total volume of which of the following ranges?

   A. 0–500 cc
   B. 500–1000 cc
   C. 1000–1500 cc
   D. 1500–2000 cc

(1:892)

3. Components of a mouth-to-valve device may include all but which of the following?

   A. Nonrebreathing valve
   B. Oxygen supplement inlet
   C. Bacterial barrier
   D. Plastic face shield

(13:294–5)

4. All but which of the following are true of the mouth-to-mask resuscitation unit?

   A. It is not as effective as bag-valve devices.
   B. Breaths should be delivered with an inspiratory time of 1.5–2 sec.
   C. It should contain as small an amount of dead space as possible.
   D. It is more effective than a face shield.

(13:293)

Answer Key

1. B. Because it is sometimes necessary to ventilate very stiff lungs with a manual resuscitator, a pressure pop-off is unnecessary.

2. D. Most adult manual resuscitator units have a total volume of 1500–2000 cc.
3. D. A mouth-to-valve set up requires a mask, not a plastic face shield.
4. A. Mouth-to-valve ventilation is more effective than bag-valve devices; other statements are true.

Advanced Level Pretest

According to the Composite Examination Matrix, questions in this category assess the candidate's understanding of the following types of resuscitation devices:

1. Pneumatic—demand valve
2. Manual resuscitators (bag-valve)
3. Mouth-to-valve mask resuscitators

The following are self-study questions from this category.

1. Which of the following statements regarding pneumatically powered demand valve type resuscitation devices is (are) true?

   I. They are not capable of delivering high concentrations of oxygen to the patient.
   II. Oxygen enters the unit at 200 psi.
   III. They are designed to provide inspiratory flow rates of approximately 100 L/min.
   IV. They are satisfactory only if manual triggering is available.

   A. I and IV
   B. II and III
   C. III and IV
   D. I, II, and III

   (2:137–8)

2. All but which of the following are true about effective use of mouth-to-mask devices?

   A. The rescuer should be positioned at the head of the patient.
   B. The mask is held in place by one hand.
   C. The mandible should be lifted.
   D. The mask should be placed over the patient's nose and mouth.

   (13:293–4)

3. You are performing mouth-to-mask ventilation on an unconscious victim. What can you do to minimize gastric distention?

   A. Deliver low-pressure breaths
   B. Avoid high-volume breaths
   C. Deliver high flows
   D. A and B

   (13:293)

4. All but which of the following are true about resuscitation bag-valve-mask devices?

   A. Flow to the reservoir should be high.
   B. Unidirectional gas flow prevents rebreathing.
   C. Straps to hold the mask on the patient's face should not be used in unconscious patients.
   D. It is physically impossible for the patient to exhaust the gas supply.

   (13:417)

5. You are manually ventilating a patient who has suffered a cardiac arrest. The patient vomits; how do you clear the vomitus from the bag?

   A. Take the bag to the sink and rinse the nonrebreathing valve with tap water.
   B. Get a replacement nonrebreathing valve.
   C. Tap the patient connector on a hard surface while squeezing the bag.
   D. Continue to ventilate.

   (13:304)

6. Which of the following are true regarding flow rates and bag-valve devices?

   I. Optimal flow is 30 L/min for adults.
   II. Optimal flow is 10 L/min for small children and infants.
   III. Smaller tidal volumes result in increased FIO_2 with the next breath.
   IV. High flows may cause certain brands of nonrebreathing valves to jam in the inspiratory position.

   A. I, II, and III
   B. II, III, and IV
   C. I and IV
   D. II and III

   (13:304)

Answer Key

1. C. Pneumatically powered demand valve type resuscitation devices are capable of delivering high concentrations of oxygen to the patient; gas enters the unit at 50 psi; they are designed to provide inspiratory flow rates of approximately 100 L/min; and they are satisfactory only if manual triggering is available.
2. B. The mask should be held in place by two hands.
3. D. To minimize gastric insufflation during mouth-to-mask breathing, deliver breaths of low pressure, flow, and volume.
4. D. If the flow is not high enough, or if the patient's ventilatory requirements suddenly increase, it is possible for the patient to outdraw the system.
5. C. Tap the patient connector on a hard surface while squeezing the bag to remove vomitus quickly.
6. B. Optimal flow for adults is 15 L/min. Other statements are true.

I. Incentive Breathing Devices (Entry Level Only)

Questions in this category assess the candidate's ability to select and assemble various incentive breathing devices prior to performing respiratory care procedures. These questions also test the candidate's understanding of the principles of operation and his or her ability to correct all malfunctions of any selected equipment.

Entry Level Pretest

According to the Composite Examination Matrix, questions in this category assess the candidate's understanding of incentive breathing devices. The following are self-study questions from this category.

1. Which of the following statements are true of volume displacement incentive spirometers?

   I. They quantitatively measure flow generated by the patient.
   II. They measure the actual volume inspired by the patient.
   III. The accuracy of the device is not influenced by inspiratory flow rate.
   IV. They are designed to improve inspiratory muscle strength.

   A. I, III, and IV
   B. II and III
   C. III only
   D. I, II, and IV

   (13:501)

2. All but which of the following are advantages of the incentive spirometer (IS) over IPPB?

   A. IS is a more effective prophylactic technique.
   B. IS is more cost-effective.
   C. With IS, patients potentially receive more frequent therapy.
   D. IS is the treatment of choice for pneumonia accompanied by atelectasis.

   (3:93)

3. Types of "incentive" utilized by incentive breathing devices include which of the following?

   A. Ping-pong balls
   B. Lights
   C. Golf balls
   D. A and B

   (13: Chap 17)

Answer Key

1. B. Volume incentive spirometry devices measure actual volume, as opposed to flow, and are not influenced by inspiratory flow rates.
2. D. IPPB is the treatment of choice for pneumonia accompanied by atelectasis. Other statements are advantages associated with IS.
3. D. Ping-pong balls and lights represent "incentives" utilized by incentive breathing devices.

J. Patient Breathing Circuits

Questions in this category assess the candidate's ability to select and assemble various patient breathing circuits prior to performing respiratory care procedures. These questions also test the candidate's understanding of the principles of operation and his or her ability to correct all malfunctions of any selected equipment.

Entry Level Pretest

According to the Composite Examination Matrix, questions in this category assess the candidate's understanding of the following types of patient breathing circuits:

1. IPPB
2. Continuous mechanical ventilation
3. CPAP
4. PEEP valve assembly

The following are self-study questions from this category.

1. A patient is receiving IPPB therapy with a pressure-cycled machine. The machine does not cycle off when inspiration ends. What is the most likely cause of the problem?

   A. There is a leak in the system.
   B. The pressure setting on the machine is too high.
   C. The circuit's expiratory valve is stuck.
   D. All of the above

   (2:227–35)

2. All but which of the following are acceptable adaptations to the patient connection of an IPPB circuit?

   A. Mouth seal
   B. Tracheostomy tube adaptor
   C. Nose clips
   D. Mask

   (13:224–5)

3. A ventilator breathing circuit must have all but which of the following capabilities?

   A. Flexibility
   B. Presence of ports for monitoring certain variables
   C. Ability to calculate airway resistance
   D. Ability to direct gas flow

   (13:266)

4. Patient circuit compliance accounts for which of the following?

   A. Volume coming out of the ventilator is higher than volume delivered to the patient.
   B. Flow coming out of the ventilator is higher than flow delivered to the patient.
   C. Pressure at the patient's airway opening is higher than pressure measured inside the ventilator.
   D. A and B

   (13:266–7)

5. You have set up a CPAP system for a patient using a variable (adjustable) flow generator. Which of the following is (are) true about this circuit?

 I. Output flow is 100 L/min.
 II. Oxygen concentrations can be varied between 0.30 and 1.0.
 III. A PEEP valve is placed at the mask inlet port.
 IV. A bacterial filter should be placed at the entrainment port.

 A. I, II, and IV
 B. II and III
 C. I, II, III, and IV
 D. III and IV

(13:401)

6. You are asked to set up a mask CPAP system for a patient with atelectasis who is also severely hypoxemic. What equipment do you need?

 I. Variable-flow generator
 II. Fixed-flow generator
 III. PEEP valve
 IV. Pressure manometer

 A. II, III, and IV
 B. II and III
 C. I, III, and IV
 D. I and III

(13:400–1)

7. Which PEEP device is the apparatus of choice in the adult patient?

 A. Opposing flow devices
 B. Orificial resistor
 C. Threshold resistor
 D. Weighted resistor

(17:552)

8. You have been instructed to place a patient on PEEP via a water column. How can you avoid the common problems of noise and altered PEEP levels due to evaporation?

 A. Increase the height of the water column initially.
 B. Put a pressurized balloon valve in-line.
 C. Adjust the immersion depth of the expiratory line.
 D. Divert the patient's exhaled breath to a diaphragm under the water column.

(3:766–7)

Answer Key

1. A. In the event that a pressure-cycled IPPB machine will not cycle off, the RCP should look for a leak in the system.
2. C. Noseclips cannot be added to the patient IPPB circuit.
3. A. A ventilator breathing circuit cannot calculate airway resistance.
4. D. Both flow and volume coming out of the ventilator is higher than volume delivered to the patient due to the effect of compliance on the patient circuit.
5. A. PEEP valve is placed at the outlet port of the mask. Other statements are true.
6. C. A variable-flow generator should be used because fixed-flow generators deliver an FIO_2 of 0.33.
7. C. The threshold resistor is the best choice for PEEP delivery in the adult.
8. D. By diverting the patient's exhaled breath to a diaphragm under the water column, the common problems of noise and altered PEEP levels due to evaporation can be avoided.

Advanced Practitioner Pretest

According to the NBRC Composite Examination Matrix, questions in this category assess the candidate's understanding of the H-valve assembly. In addition, the candidate's ability to correct malfunctions associated with IPPB, CPAP, and continuous mechanical ventilator circuits is evaluated on the advanced level examination. The following self-study questions are based on the NBRC Composite Examination Matrix.

1. High circuit compliance and short expiratory time during mechanical ventilation may lead to which of the following?

 A. Increased delivered tidal volume
 B. Auto-PEEP
 C. Decreased PIP
 D. Increased plateau pressure

(13:267)

2. A patient is receiving IPPB via a pressure-cycled machine with a standard straight mouthpiece. The patient is unable to maintain a seal during inspiration, resulting in volume loss. Which of the following should the RCP do first?

 A. Increase the pressure
 B. Apply noseclips
 C. Apply a mask and headstraps
 D. Apply a mouth seal

(13:224–5)

3. A fixed-flow generator is being used to deliver 20 cm H_2O PEEP via mask to a patient in the ICU. This patient had previously been receiving 5 cm H_2O PEEP. Which of the following statements is (are) true of this setup?

 A. Total output will increase with the increased pressure.
 B. Flow and FIO_2 will remain unchanged.
 C. FIO_2 will increase with the increased pressure.
 D. A and B

(13:400–1)

4. Which of the following equipment is required for an H-valve IMV system?

   I. One-way valve
   II. Reservoir tubing
   III. Flowmeter separate from the ventilator system
   IV. Oxygen source

   A. I, II, and III
   B. I, III, and IV
   C. II, III, and IV
   D. I, II, III, and IV

(3:762–3)

5. Which of the following statements are true about ambient reservoir (H-valve) IMV?

   I. It is equivalent to SIMV.
   II. It can be used only in control mode.
   III. Breath stacking may occur.
   IV. It is incompatible with the use of PEEP.

   A. I, II, III, and IV
   B. I, II, and III
   C. II and III
   D. I and II

(3:762–3)

Answer Key

1. B. High circuit compliance and short expiratory time during mechanical ventilation may lead to auto-PEEP (air is trapped because there is not enough time to exhale fully).
2. B. Applying noseclips is the easiest and least traumatic solution for the patient; try this first.
3. C. With downstream pressure at or > 15 cm H_2O, output decreases, and FIO_2 increases to about 0.37.
4. D. All of the selections are necessary for H-valve setup.
5. C. Because IMV is not synchronous with ventilator breaths, breath stacking may occur. PEEP may be used in conjunction with IMV.

K. Percussors and Vibrators (Entry Level Only)

Questions in this category assess the candidate's ability to select and assemble various types of percussors and vibrators prior to performing respiratory care procedures. These questions also test the candidate's understanding of the principles of operation and his or her ability to correct all malfunctions of any selected equipment.

Entry Level Pretest

According to the Composite Examination Matrix, questions in this category assess the candidate's understanding of percussors and vibrators. The following are self-study questions from this category

1. Which of the following are true about mechanical percussors?

   I. They may be electric.
   II. They may be pneumatic.
   III. They are more effective than manual percussion.
   IV. Most devices control both intensity and frequency of percussion.

   A. I, II, III, and IV
   B. I, II, and III
   C. I, II, and IV
   D. II, III, and IV

(13:507–8)

2. How long should mechanical percussors be applied to any one location on the patient's thorax?

   A. 30 to 60 sec
   B. 1 to 2 min
   C. 2 to 5 min
   D. At least 5 min

(13:507–8)

3. What action should the RCP take in the event that a mechanical percussor overheats?

   A. Leave the patient in drainage position and wait until the unit cools down.
   B. Discontinue therapy and allow the unit to cool down.
   C. Discontinue therapy and return for the next scheduled treatment.
   D. Continue with therapy.

(13:510)

Answer Key

1. C. Mechanical percussors have not been shown to be more or less effective than manual percussion. The choice is the RCP's and/or patient's preference.
2. A. The mechanical percussors should be applied to any one location on the patient's thorax for no longer than 30 to 60 sec.
3. B. If a unit overheats, discontinue therapy and allow it to cool down. Therapy may be resumed after the unit has sufficiently cooled, or the RCP may complete treatment manually.

L. Environmental Devices—Aerosol (Mist) Tents

Questions in this category assess the candidate's ability to select and assemble aerosol tents prior to performing respiratory care procedures. These questions also test the candidate's understanding of the principles of operation and his or her ability to correct all malfunctions of any selected equipment.

Entry Level Pretest

According to the Composite Examination Matrix, questions in this category assess the candidate's understanding of aerosol (mist) tents. The following are self-study questions from this category:

1. Which of the following statements about mist tents are true?

   I. Electrical toys may not be used inside the tent.
   II. High concentrations of oxygen (> .50) can be provided.
   III. Flow rates must be at least 30 L/min to flush the tent of CO_2.
   IV. Mist tents are indicated for the treatment of bronchiolitis.

   A. I, II, III, and IV
   B. I and IV
   C. II, III, and IV
   D. II and III

   (14:233–4)

2. All but which of the following are limitations to the use of aerosol tents?

   A. They are poorly tolerated by patients.
   B. They are difficult to maintain.
   C. They are cumbersome.
   D. Patients who need oxygen must wear a hood inside the tent.

   (14:233–4)

Answer Key

1. B. Only low to moderate (< 0.50) concentrations of oxygen can be provided with a mist tent. A minimum flow rate of 10–15 L/min is necessary to prevent CO_2 build-up. Other statements are true.
2. D. The mist tent may not be the optimal choice for patients who require high concentrations of oxygen.

Advanced Practitioner Pretest

According to the NBRC Composite Examination Matrix, questions in this category assess the candidate's ability to correct malfunctions associated with aerosol (mist) tents. The following self-study questions are based on the NBRC Composite Examination Matrix.

1. A patient is resting comfortably in an aerosol tent. The RCP is asked to analyze the oxygen concentration in the tent, and finds that it is approximately 10% lower than the FIO_2 setting on the nebulizer. What is the most likely cause of the problem?

   A. The cooling unit is not operating properly.
   B. Total gas flow is decreased.
   C. There is not a tight seal around the canopy.
   D. Nebulizer entrainment ports are obstructed.

   (14:233–4)

2. All but which of the following types of pediatric patient diseases/disorders may benefit from an aerosol tent?

   A. Cystic fibrosis
   B. Croup
   C. Epiglottitis
   D. Foreign body aspiration

   (3:622)

Answer Key

1. C. It is difficult to keep a tight seal around the canopy due to patient care demands. Each time the tent is opened, room air is drawn in, decreasing the FIO_2.
2. D. Foreign body aspiration is not an indication for a mist tent.

M. Metered Dose Inhalers (MDI) and Spacers (Entry Level Only)

Questions in this category assess the candidate's ability to select and assemble a metered dose inhaler prior to performing respiratory care procedures. These questions also test the candidate's understanding of the principles of operation and his or her ability to correct all malfunctions of any selected equipment.

Entry Level Pretest

According to the Composite Examination Matrix, questions in this category assess the candidate's understanding of metered dose inhalers and spacers. The following are self-study questions from this category.

1. The propellant gas used in MDIs is which of the following?

   A. Hydrocarbons
   B. Lecithin
   C. Sorbitan trioleate
   D. Chlorofluorocarbons

   (7:47)

2. The MDI consists of which of the following components?

   I. Propellant
   II. Canister
   III. Drug
   IV. Metering valve

   A. I, II, III, and IV
   B. I, II, and III
   C. II, III, and IV
   D. I, III, and IV

   (7:47)

3. Spacers are designed to have all but which of the following effects?

   A. Decreased size of aerosol particles
   B. Decreased deposition of drug in the oropharynx
   C. Diminished side effects
   D. All of the above

(7:51–2)

4. How should the RCP instruct a patient to care for his or her MDI?

   I. Rinse the mouthpiece daily.
   II. Clean the mouthpiece with ethyl alcohol daily.
   III. Float canister in water to determine content level.
   IV. Dispose of after 150 puffs.

   A. I, II, and IV
   B. I and IV
   C. I and III
   D. II and III

(7:51)

Answer Key

1. D. The propellant gas used in MDIs is chlorofluorocarbons.
2. A. All of the following are components of the MDI.
3. D. All of the choices represent positive effects associated with spacer use.
4. C. MDI mouthpiece should be rinsed daily. The canister can be floated in a basin of water to determine the content level. Each canister contains about 200 puffs.

N. Positive Expiratory Pressure (PEP) Mask (Advanced Level Only)

Questions in this category assess the candidate's ability to select and assemble a positive expiratory pressure mask prior to performing respiratory care procedures. These questions also test the candidate's understanding of the principles of operation and his or her ability to correct all malfunctions of any selected equipment.

Advanced Level Pretest

According to the Composite Examination Matrix, questions in this category assess the candidate's understanding of PEP masks. The following are self-study questions from this category.

1. Components of a PEP mask include which of the following?

   I. Pressure manometer
   II. One-way valve
   III. Mask, or mouthpiece and noseclips
   IV. Expiratory resistance

   A. I, II, and IV
   B. II, III, and IV
   C. I, II, and III
   D. I, II, III, and IV

(1:641)

2. You have been asked to set up a PEP system for a cystic fibrosis patient. How much expiratory resistance should you select?

   A. One that provides a PEP of 5–10 cm H_2O at end exhalation
   B. One that provides a PEP of 10–15 cm H_2O at end exhalation
   C. One that provides a PEP of 5–10 cm H_2O in midexhalation
   D. One that provides a PEP of 10–15 cm H_2O in midexhalation

(1:641)

3. Which of the following are true statements about PEP therapy?

   I. It is well established that PEP therapy is more effective than chest PT.
   II. It allows independent treatment by patients.
   III. The PEP technique should be employed for 5–15 min.
   IV. Another name for PEP is FET.

   A. I, II, and III
   B. II and III
   C. II, III, and IV
   D. II and IV

(1:643)

Answer Key

1. D. All of the components listed are necessary for proper setup of PEP therapy.
2. D. Select resistance that provides a PEP of 10–15 cm H_2O in midexhalation.
3. B. PEP therapy has not been shown to be more effective than chest PT, but it can be done independently by the patient. The technique should be done for 5–15 min, and may be repeated over 10–30 min. FET = forced expiratory technique, and is another name for huff coughing.

O. Respirometers (Advanced Level Only)

Questions in this category assess the candidate's ability to select and assemble various respirometers prior to performing respiratory care procedures. These questions also test the candidate's understanding of the principles of operation and his or her ability to correct all malfunctions of any selected equipment.

Advanced Level Pretest

According to the Composite Examination Matrix, questions in this category assess the candidate's understanding of the following respirometers:

1. Flow-sensing devices (pneumotachometer)
2. Positive displacement

The following are self-study questions from this category.

1. A differential pressure pneumotachograph uses which of the following principles of operation to sense flow?

   A. Measures a change in electric current created by a change in temperature
   B. Measures a drop in pressure across a fixed flow-resistant element
   C. Measures a change in pressure across a variable orifice
   D. Measures a change in gas flow turbulence

   (13:34–5)

2. A hot-wire anemometer pneumotachograph uses which of the following principles of operation to measure flow?

   A. Measures a change in electrode current created by a change in temperature
   B. Measures the drop in pressure across a fixed flow-resistant element
   C. Measures a change in pressure across a variable-orifice mechanism
   D. Measures a change in an ultrasonic signal

   (13:34–5)

3. A Tissot spirometer serves which of the following purposes?

   A. Acts as a reservoir for inspired gases
   B. Collects expired gases
   C. Measures the volume of the expired gases
   D. B and C

   (13:71–2)

4. Which of the following are spirometers that employ positive displacement to measure volume?

   A. Turbine spirometer
   B. Dry rolling-seal spirometer
   C. Water-seal spirometer
   D. B and C

   (13:33–4)

Answer Key

1. B. A differential pressure pneumotachograph measures a drop in pressure across a fixed flow-resistant element.
2. A. A heated-wire anemometer measures a change in electrode current created by a change in temperature.
3. D. A Tissot spirometer collects expired gases and measures the volume of that gas.
4. D. Both water-seal and dry rolling-seal spirometers use positive displacement to measure volume.

P. Helium/Oxygen Therapy (Advanced Level Only)

Questions in this category assess the candidate's ability to select and assemble equipment to deliver helium/oxygen therapy prior to performing respiratory care procedures. These questions also test the candidate's understanding of the principles of operation and his or her ability to correct all malfunctions of any selected equipment.

Advanced Level Pretest

According to the Composite Examination Matrix, questions in this category assess the candidate's understanding of helium/oxygen therapy. The following are self-study questions from this category.

1. Helium/oxygen therapy may be beneficial in treating which of the following diseases?

   A. Fibrosis
   B. COPD
   C. Atelectasis
   D. B and C

   (1:628–9)

2. Which of the following are true about helium/oxygen therapy?

   I. Helium/oxygen mixtures lower the work of breathing.
   II. Helium/oxygen mixtures cannot be delivered through a nasal cannula.
   III. Special flowmeters must be used when administering helium/oxygen mixtures.
   IV. Helium is generally mixed with 70% or 80% oxygen.

   A. I, II, and IV
   B. II, III, and IV
   C. I, II, and III
   D. I, II, III, and IV

   (1:628–9)

3. What effect does helium/oxygen therapy have on the cough mechanism?

   A. Enhances it
   B. Makes it less effective
   C. Has no effect
   D. Is only a concern in the intubated patient

   (1:628–9)

Answer Key

1. B. Helium/oxygen therapy is used in obstructive disease processes where breathing a less dense gas mixture makes it easier to ventilate.
2. A. Helium/oxygen mixtures may be delivered using a standard flowmeter as long as the appropriate correction factor is used.
3. B. Helium encourages laminar flow; because coughing depends on the ability to create turbulent flow, the cough mechanism may be impaired.

Q. ECG Devices (Advanced Level Only)

Questions in this category assess the candidate's ability to select and assemble equipment to perform ECGs. These questions also test the candidate's understanding of the principles of operation and his or her ability to correct all malfunctions of any selected equipment.

Advanced Level Pretest

According to the Composite Examination Matrix, questions in this category assess the candidate's understanding of the following ECG devices:

1. ECG machines (12-lead)
2. Cardiac leads

The following are self-study questions from this category:

1. A negative electrode placed on the right arm and a positive electrode placed on the left arm most correctly describes which of the following standard, electrocardiographic leads?

   A. Lead I
   B. Lead II
   C. Lead III
   D. aVR

(18:212–3)

2. Which of the following correctly describes precordial leads?

   I. They represent a vertical view of the heart.
   II. They represent a horizontal view of the heart.
   III. They are bipolar.
   IV. They are unipolar.

   A. I and III
   B. I and IV
   C. II and III
   D. II and IV

(18:213)

3. Which of the following techniques may improve electrical contact when performing an ECG?

   A. Cleaning the patient's skin with betadine
   B. Cleaning the electrode connections
   C. Applying only a thin layer of electrode cream
   D. All of the above

(18:216)

4. Which of the following statements is (are) true of the 12-lead ECG machine?

   I. A small square on ECG paper represents one millivolt.
   II. A large square on ECG paper represents 0.20 sec.
   III. The machine is actually a voltmeter.
   IV. Artifact may ruin a good ECG tracing.

   A. I, II, and III
   B. I, III, and IV
   C. II, III, and IV
   D. II and IV

(18:218)

Answer Key

1. A. This describes Lead I.
2. D. Precordial leads are unipolar and provide a horizontal view of the heart.
3. B. Cleaning the patient's skin with isopropyl alcohol, cleaning the electrode contacts and connections, and applying more electrode cream all improve electrical contact.
4. C. A small square = 0.04 sec (there are five small squares in a large square).

R. Hemodynamic Monitoring Devices (Advanced Level Only)

Questions in this category assess the candidate's ability to select and assemble hemodynamic monitoring equipment. These questions also test the candidate's understanding of the principles of operation and his or her ability to correct all malfunctions of any selected equipment.

Advanced Level Pretest

According to the Composite Examination Matrix, questions in this category assess the candidate's understanding of the following hemodynamic monitoring devices:

1. Arterial catheters
2. Pulmonary artery catheters (Swan-Ganz)
3. Cardiac output

The following are self-study questions from this category.

1. Use of a properly functioning quadruple lumen Swan-Ganz pulmonary artery catheter gives the respiratory therapy practitioner the ability to monitor all of the following *except:*

   A. Pulmonary artery systolic pressure
   B. Central venous pressure
   C. Cardiac output
   D. Arterial blood pressure

(5: Chap 9)

2. A properly functioning indwelling *peripheral* arterial catheter gives the respiratory therapy practitioner the ability to monitor which of the following parameters?

   I. Mean arterial pressure
   II. Systolic arterial pressure
   III. Central venous pressure
   IV. Diastolic arterial pressure

   A. I, II, and IV
   B. I, II, III, and IV
   C. II, III, and IV
   D. I, II, and III

   (5: Chap 7)

3. Indwelling peripheral arterial catheters are known to use which of the following devices to measure pressure?

   A. Water column manometers
   B. Pressure drop transducers
   C. Heat transfer transducers
   D. Strain gauges

   (5: Chap 7)

4. Which of the following is actually measured by indwelling pulmonary artery oximeters?

   A. The tension of oxygen dissolved in arterial blood
   B. The oxyhemoglobin concentration of mixed venous blood
   C. The tension of oxygen dissolved in mixed venous blood
   D. The oxyhemoglobin saturation of arterial blood

   (5:201)

5. You approach a patient's bedside and observe an RV tracing on the monitor. How should you proceed?

   A. Do nothing; this is an acceptable PA tracing.
   B. Advance the catheter with the balloon deflated until you observe a PA tracing.
   C. Advance the catheter with the balloon inflated until you observe a PA tracing.
   D. Pull back the catheter with the balloon deflated until you observe a PA tracing.

   (5: Chap 9)

6. Which of the following factors affect cardiac output?

   I. Preload
   II. Afterload
   III. Myocardial contractility
   IV. Coordinated contraction of myocardial muscle fibers

   A. I, II, and III
   B. II, III, and IV
   C. I, II, and IV
   D. I, II, III, and IV

   (5: Chap 10)

7. Which of the following is (are) indication(s) for insertion of a CVP line?

   I. Assess volume status.
   II. Estimate cardiac function.
   III. Measure preload.
   IV. Measure C.O.

   A. I and II
   B. I, II, and III
   C. II, III, and IV
   D. I, II, III, and IV

   (5: Chap 8)

8. Which of the following is true about the distal lumen of the Swan-Ganz catheter?

   A. It may be used to obtain mixed venous blood.
   B. It is located 30 cm from the catheter tip.
   C. It is used as the injectate port when measuring C.O.
   D. All of the above

   (5: Chap 9)

9. Prior to Swan-Ganz catheter insertion, the RCP should perform which of the following?

   A. Set up a He/O_2 tank for balloon inflation.
   B. Test balloon integrity.
   C. Wet the catheter with hypotonic saline.
   D. All of the above

   (5: Chap 9)

10. If 4 cc of air are inserted into the balloon port of the Swan-Ganz catheter, and you still see a PA tracing on the monitor, what can you assume?

    A. The catheter tip has slipped into the RV.
    B. The catheter tip is too peripheral in the pulmonary circulation.
    C. Function is normal.
    D. The balloon has ruptured.

    (5: Chap 9)

11. When obtaining PCWP with the Swan-Ganz catheter, for how long should the balloon be inflated?

    A. 15 sec
    B. 30 sec
    C. 45 sec
    D. 60 sec

    (5: Chap 9)

12. *Optimally,* what position would the patient assume when hemodynamic data is being collected?

    A. Prone
    B. Supine
    C. Semi-Fowler's
    D. Full sitting

    (5: Chap 9)

13. You are preparing to insert a radial arterial line. While performing an Allen test, you discover that it takes 20 sec for blood flow to return to the hand. How should you proceed?

    A. Proceed with insertion.
    B. Choose another site.
    C. Notify the patient's physician.
    D. None of the above.

(5: Chap 7)

Answer Key

1. D. Arterial blood pressure cannot be measured with a pulmonary artery catheter; the PA catheter measures pulmonary artery pressures rather than arterial pressures.
2. A. Arterial catheters can measure all arterial pressures. Central venous pressure may be assessed with a CVP line.
3. D. Strain gauges measure arterial pressures.
4. B. The oxyhemoglobin concentration of mixed venous blood is the actual measurement taken by a PA oximeter.
5. C. If an RV tracing is observed (the PA catheter has slipped back into the RV), inflate the balloon and advance until a PA tracing is observed.
6. D. All of those factors listed affect cardiac output.
7. A. The CVP catheter is capable of assessing volume status and/or cardiac function. The other two choices would be appropriate indications for Swan-Ganz catheter insertion.
8. A. The distal (PA) lumen may be used to obtain mixed venous blood; other functions listed are accomplished through the RA port.
9. B. Test balloon integrity prior to insertion. CO_2 is the inflation medium of choice for the balloon.
10. D. If more than 1.5 cc of air is injected into the balloon port, and a PWP cannot be obtained, the RCP should assume that the balloon is ruptured.
11. A. Inflate the balloon for a maximum of 15 sec to minimize the risk of infarction.
12. B. The patient should be supine with the transducer at heart level during hemodynamic data collection.
13. C. If blanching persists longer than 15 sec, select another site; collateral circulation is inadequate.

S. Fiberoptic Bronchoscopes (Advanced Level Only)

Questions in this category assess the candidate's ability to select and assemble bronchoscopy equipment. These questions also test the candidate's understanding of the principles of operation and his or her ability to correct all malfunctions of any selected equipment.

Advanced Level Pretest

According to the Composite Examination Matrix, questions in this category assess the candidate's understanding of fiberoptic bronchoscopes. The following are self-study questions from this category.

1. In what position should the fiberoptic bronchoscope optimally be stored?

    A. Coiled loosely
    B. Lying straight on a vertical surface
    C. Hanging straight
    D. In a drawer

(1:696)

2. Which of the following statements are true regarding fiberoptic bronchoscopy?

    I. Brushings are performed for obtaining biopsies.
    II. The naris, hypopharynx, and larynx of patients are anesthetized.
    III. Biopsy forceps should be tested prior to the procedure.
    IV. Oxygen should be available.

    A. I, II, III, and IV
    B. I, II, and III
    C. II, III, and IV
    D. III and IV

(1:696–9)

3. Which of the following can be performed with the fiberoptic bronchoscope?

    A. Cytologic specimen collection
    B. Bronchoalveolar lavage
    C. Biopsy
    D. All of the above

(1:696–702)

Answer Key

1. C. The bronchoscope should be stored hanging straight.
2. C. Brushings obtain cytologic specimens. Other statements are true.
3. D. All of the choices are possible functions of the fiberoptic bronchoscope.

T. Vacuum Systems (Advanced Level Only)

Questions in this category assess the candidate's ability to select and assemble a vacuum system. These questions also test the candidate's understanding of the principles of operation and his or her ability to correct all malfunctions of any selected equipment.

Advanced Level Pretest

According to the Composite Examination Matrix, questions in this category assess the candidate's understanding of the following vacuum systems:

1. Regulators
2. Pleural drainage devices

The following are self-study questions from this category.

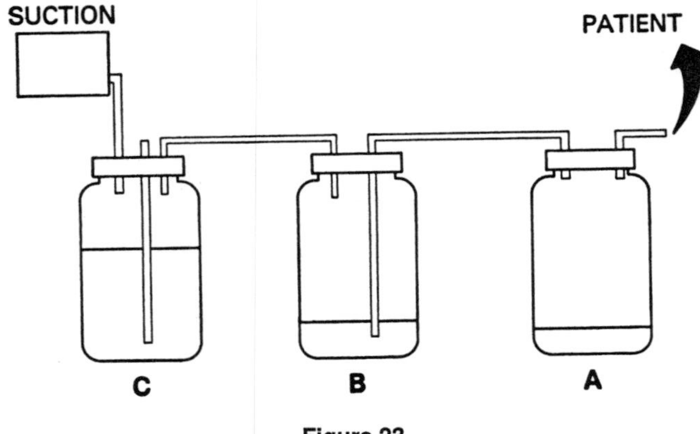

Figure 23.

1. Which of the following statements regarding three-chamber chest suction systems such as that pictured in Figure 23 is (are) true?

   I. Constant bubbling in the suction control bottle indicates evacuation of air from the pleural space.
   II. The tube should be placed 15–20 cm below the surface in the water-seal chamber.
   III. The tube in the suction control bottle should be placed approximately 2 cm below the surface of the water.
   IV. Bottle B is the water-seal chamber.

   A. I only
   B. II and IV
   C. IV only
   D. III and IV

   (4:372–5)

2. While caring for a patient with a commercial three-compartment pleural evacuation system, the respiratory therapy practitioner notes that bubbling has stopped in the pressure control chamber. Which of the following may be responsible for this?

   I. Excessive levels of wall suction
   II. Absence of a lung leak
   III. Leak somewhere in the system
   IV. Inadequate levels of suction

   A. II and IV
   B. III and IV
   C. I and II
   D. II, III, and IV

   (4:372–5)

3. True statements regarding chest tube removal include:

   I. The procedure should be performed during a forced inspiratory maneuver.
   II. It must be preceded by clinical and radiologic evidence of lung reexpansion.
   III. It is usually not performed during administration of continuous ventilatory support.

   A. I and III
   B. II and III
   C. II only
   D. I, II, and III

   (4:372–5)

4. Which of the following statements regarding chest tube placement is (are) true?

   I. It may be indicated in the treatment of open pneumothorax.
   II. A thoracotomy is performed between the sixth and eighth ribs when air removal is desired.
   III. It should not be performed on an elective basis.

   A. I only
   B. II and III
   C. I and III
   D. II only

   (4:372–5)

5. While caring for a patient who has a triple-bottle chest drainage system, the respiratory therapy practitioner notes intermittent bubbling in the underwater seal compartment. Which of the following is most likely responsible for this?

   A. Excessive suction
   B. Leak in the system
   C. Wide fluctuations in intrapleural pressure
   D. Evacuation of pleural gas

   (4:372–5)

6. Which of the following statements regarding triple-bottle chest drainage systems is (are) true?

   I. They can be used for fluid evacuation.
   II. They include a suction control compartment.
   III. They may be used in the treatment of tension pneumothorax.

   A. I and II
   B. II only
   C. I, II, and III
   D. II and III

   (4:372–5)

Answer Key

1. C. Because this bottle determines the level of suction, the tube in the suction control bottle should be placed at least 15 cm below the surface of the water.

The tube should be placed 2 cm below the surface in the water-seal chamber. Constant bubbling in the suction control bottle indicates that the suction source is more than the level of immersion of the tube.
2. B. A leak somewhere in the system or inadequate levels of suction could account for absence of bubbling in the suction control chamber.
3. C. Removal of the chest tube(s) can occur as long as the lung has reexpanded (whether the patient is on mechanical ventilation or not). Chest tubes are removed on exhalation.
4. A. Insertion is between the fourth and fifth intercostal spaces; insertion should not be limited to elective cases.
5. A. If the water-seal chamber bubbles, suction is too high.
6. C. Each statement is true.

U. Ensure the Cleanliness of All Equipment

According to the NBRC, questions in this category assess the candidate' s ability to ensure that all respiratory care equipment has been properly decontaminated, disinfected, and/or sterilized prior to being used in patient care procedures.

Entry Level Pretest

According to the NBRC's Composite Examination Matrix, questions in this category assess the candidate's understanding of equipment cleanliness as follows:

1. Select the appropriate agent and disinfection/sterilization technique.
2. Perform disinfection and/or sterilization procedures.
3. Monitor the effectiveness of sterilization procedures.

The following self-study questions were developed from the NBRC Composite Examination Matrix.

1. Which of the following methods can be used to sterilize the widest variety of respiratory therapy equipment?

A. Acid glutaraldehyde
B. Steam autoclaving
C. Gas sterilization
D. Alkaline glutaraldehyde

(17: Chap 42)

2. Which of the following agents or methods of disinfection/sterilization is *not* considered tuberculocidal?

A. Ethylene oxide
B. Pasteurization
C. 90% isopropyl alcohol
D. All are tuberculoidal

(17: Chap 42)

3. How long must a piece of equipment be soaked in alkaline glutaraldehyde for complete sterilization to occur?

A. 1–2 hr
B. 6–8 hr
C. 10–24 hr
D. 48–72 hr
E. Sterilization cannot be achieved with this agent.

(17: Chap 42)

4. Which of the following agents or methods are considered sporicidal when used properly?

I. Alkaline glutaraldehyde
II. Gamma radiation
III. Pasteurization
IV. Acid glutaraldehyde
V. 90% isopropyl alcohol

A. I, II, and IV
B. II, IV, and V
C. II and V
D. I and II

(17: Chap 42)

5. True statements about ethylene oxide include:

I. It is considered tuberculocidal.
II. It must be used in conjunction with heat and humidity.
III. It is considered a means of sterilization.
IV. It can be employed on most types of equipment.

A. II, III, and IV
B. I, II, III, and IV
C. II and IV
D. I, III, and IV

(17: Chap 42)

6. Which of the following statements regarding the disadvantages or hazards of the ethylene oxide sterilization process is (are) true?

I. It is expensive.
II. Ethylene oxide is flammable.
III. It cannot be used to sterilize electrical equipment.
IV. It is toxic to human tissues.

A. I and II
B. II and IV
C. I, II, and IV
D. I and IV

(17: Chap 42)

Answer Key

1. C. Gas sterilization sterilizes the widest variety of respiratory therapy equipment.
2. D. Each method listed is tuberculoidal.
3. C. A piece of equipment must be soaked in alkaline glutaraldehyde for 10–12 hr in order for complete sterilization to occur.
4. A. All but 90% isopropyl alcohol and pasteurization are sporicidal.
5. B. All are true of ethylene oxide.
6. C. Ethylene oxide can be used to sterilize electrical equipment; other statements are true.

Advanced Practitioner Pretest

According to the NBRC Composite Examination Matrix, questions in this category assess the candidate's ability to monitor the effectiveness of sterilization procedures and perform quality control procedures for the following types of respiratory therapy equipment:

1. Pulmonary function equipment
2. Gas metering devices
3. Blood gas analyzers and sampling devices
4. Noninvasive monitors
5. Co-oximeters
6. Ventilator volume/flow/pressure calibration

The following self-study questions were developed from the NBRC Composite Examination Matrix.

1. The use of spore-containing culture strips has been recommended to monitor the effectiveness of which of the following means of sterilization?

   I. Ethylene oxide
   II. Acid glutaraldehyde
   III. Autoclaving
   IV. Alkaline glutaraldehyde

   A. I and III
   B. II and IV
   C. III and IV
   D. II only

   (17: Chap 42)

2. Which of the following statements regarding ethylene oxide indicator tape is (are) true?

   I. A change in color indicates exposure to 50% relative humidity at a temperature of 30°C or greater.
   II. A change in color indicates exposure to ethylene oxide gas only.
   III. A change in color indicates that complete sterilization has been achieved.

   A. I only
   B. II only
   C. III only
   D. I and II

   (17: Chap 42)

3. Which of the following statements about the care of home respiratory therapy equipment is (are) true?

   I. Equipment should not be allowed to air dry.
   II. All equipment should be sterilized every 24 hr.
   III. All water must be drained from tubing.
   IV. Thorough cleaning and disinfection is a reasonable goal.

   A. I, II, and III
   B. I and III
   C. III and IV
   D. II and IV

   (17: Chap 42)

4. Which of the following methods has *not* been recommended to monitor the effectiveness of a respiratory therapy department's sterilization/disinfection processes?

   A. Random culturing of equipment during its shelf life
   B. Random culturing of equipment after physical washing
   C. Random culturing of equipment while in patient use
   D. Random culturing of equipment after undergoing a sterilization process

   (17: Chap 17)

5. The respiratory therapy practitioner is asked to calibrate a given spirometer to ensure that volume measurements are accurate. In order to do so the practitioner should select:

   A. A rotameter device
   B. A Bourns LS-75 spirometer
   C. A calibrated "super" syringe
   D. A biologic control subject

   (6: Chap 11)

6. The technique of tonometry may be used to establish quality control for which of the following devices?

   I. pH electrodes
   II. Clark electrodes
   III. Severinghaus electrodes
   IV. Helium meters

   A. I and III
   B. II and III
   C. I, III, and IV
   D. I, II, and III

   (1:949)

7. Which of the following methods of calibration should be performed most frequently on blood gas analyzers?

   A. 1 point
   B. 2 point

C. 3 point
D. 3 point double blind

(1:949)

8. Highly accurate samples of known calibrated gases are used to ensure the accuracy of which of the following devices?

I. Clark electrode
II. Galvanic cell devices
III. Sanz electrode
IV. Severinghaus electrode

A. I and IV
B. II and IV
C. I and III
D. III and IV

(1:947–8)

9. The periodic analysis of solutions or gases whose predetermined Po_2, Pco_2, and pH are not known to the respiratory therapy practitioner best describes:

A. 1-point calibration
B. 2-point calibration
C. Tonometry
D. External quality assurance

(1:947–9)

10. Which of the following statements regarding volume/flow/pressure output waveforms (for calibration) of a mechanical ventilator is (are) true?

I. Negative values correspond to inspiration.
II. These are affected by resistance and compliance.
III. Waveforms often contain "noise."
IV. Waveforms do not show the effects of resistance on the expiratory side of the patient circuit.

A. I and IV
B. I, II, and III
C. II and IV
D. I and III

(13:263–5)

11. Which of the following represent methods of quality control utilized in the pulmonary function laboratory?

I. Automated syringes
II. Simple large-volume syringe
III. Sine-wave rotary pumps
IV. Explosive decompression devices

A. I, II, and III
B. I and II
C. II and III
D. I, II, III, and IV

(6:348–51)

Answer Key

1. A. The use of spore-containing culture strips has been recommended to monitor the effectiveness of ethylene oxide and autoclaving.
2. B. A change in the color of the tape indicates exposure to ethylene oxide.
3. C. Equipment must be allowed to air dry in the patient's home; sterilization every 24 hr is impractical and unnecessary.
4. B. Culturing after physical washing has not been recommended.
5. C. A calibrated super syringe should be used for spirometer calibration.
6. B. Tonometry is used to calibrate Clark and Severinghaus electrodes (O_2 and CO_2).
7. A. One-point calibration is performed most often.
8. A. Highly accurate gas samples are used for calibration of the Clark and Severinghaus electrodes.
9. D. Quality assurance is described here.
10. C. Positive values correspond to inspiration; "noise" is not present as it is during normal use.
11. D. All of the choices represent methods of quality control in the PFT lab.

PART 3

Therapeutic Procedures

From the standpoint of number of questions, the therapeutic procedures content category is the most important of the three major examination sections. Fifty percent of the questions on the Entry Level Examination are drawn from this area. On the Advanced Practitioner Examination this category comprises 60% of the total questions.

A convincing case can also be built that, on the whole, these questions are the most difficult on the examination. As was pointed out at the beginning of this book, NBRC examination questions as well as the ones in this book are designed to assess three levels of complexity: recall, application, and analysis. These three levels represent the hierarchy of cognitive or intellectual skills. Questions that assess analytical skills are the most difficult because they frequently require the candidate to use both abstract thinking and good judgment in their solution. The therapeutic procedures category is comprised of approximately 50% application-type questions on the entry level examination, while approximately half of the items on the advanced level exam are analysis-type questions.

In general, questions in the therapeutic procedures content category assess the candidate's ability to perform those tasks that the 1992 Job Survey identified as being essential to the practice of respiratory therapy procedures. This survey is divided into 12 competencies as follows:

A. Educate patients (entry level only)
B. Control infection (entry level only)
C. Maintain airway
D. Mobilize and remove secretions (entry level only)
E. Ensure ventilation
F. Ensure oxygenation
G. Assess patient response to therapy (evaluate, monitor, and record patient's response to respiratory care)
H. Modify therapy/make recommendations based on patient's response
I. Perform cardiopulmonary resuscitation (entry level only)
J. Perform emergency procedures (advanced level only)
K. Maintain records and communication
L. Assist physician with special procedures and conduct pulmonary rehabilitation and home care (advanced level only)

A. Educate Patients (Entry Level Only)

According to the NBRC, the content category "educate patients" is assessed only on the Entry Level Examination. Questions in this category are designed to assess the candidate's ability to explain to the patient the proper procedure for performing therapy that the physician has ordered and the specific therapeutic goals involved. These should be presented to the patient in the simplest and most easily understandable terms possible to achieve an optimal therapeutic outcome.

Entry Level Pretest

According to the NBRC, 5.7% of the questions on the Entry Level Examination are from the educate patients content category. The following self-study questions were developed from the NBRC Composite Examination Matrix.

1. The respiratory therapy practitioner is asked to instruct a 61-year-old patient with advanced pulmonary emphysema in breathing retraining exercises. In interviewing the patient, the chief complaint was his inability to exhale completely. In which of the following exercises should the therapist instruct this patient?

   A. Segmental breathing exercises
   B. Diaphragmatic breathing
   C. Pursed lip breathing
   D. Cough instruction

   (12:219–20)

2. The respiratory therapy practitioner is asked to instruct a patient who has chronic obstructive pulmonary emphysema in breathing retraining exercises. In so doing the patient should be taught to breathe:

   I. Using pursed lip techniques
   II. Slowly and deeply
   III. With abdominal muscles contracted during inspiration
   IV. With use of the diaphragm

   A. I, II, and IV
   B. II, III, and IV

C. I, III, and IV
D. I, II, III, and IV

(12:219–22)

3. Which of the following factors can act to improve the effectiveness of a patient's cough?

I. Placing the patient in a high Fowler's position
II. Supporting the patient's incision during efforts
III. Having the therapist demonstrate effective techniques
IV. Extending the trunk slightly backward while patient is coughing

A. II, III, and IV
B. I, II, and III
C. I and III
D. I, II, III, and IV

(20:57–7, 238–9)

4. The respiratory therapy practitioner is asked to write an instructional pamphlet to be distributed to outpatients enrolled in a large pulmonary rehabilitation program. Which of the following would be the *least* appropriate topic for this paper?

A. Diet and fluid intake
B. Reconditioning exercises
C. Acid-base and electrolyte disturbances
D. Proper use and hazards of prescribed drugs

(12:207–8)

5. The respiratory therapy practitioner is asked to teach a patient methods of caring for his home respiratory therapy equipment. Recommended instructions would include:

I. Culturing techniques
II. Proper assembly of all equipment
III. Proper use of aldehyde sterilization agents
IV. Thorough washing, rinsing, and drying techniques

A. I and IV
B. I, II, and III
C. II, III, and IV
D. II and IV

(20:339–58)

Answer Key

1. C. PLB allows the patient to prevent premature airways collapse by exerting backpressure on the airways to hold them open by exhaling through pursed lips.
2. A. COPD patients may benefit from breathing through pursed lips, using their diaphragms (this muscle uses less oxygen), and breathing slowly and deeply. Abdominal muscles should be contracted during expiration.
3. B. Extending the trunk back while coughing is uncomfortable and serves no purpose. The other three choices, however, are helpful and useful suggestions.
4. C. All of the suggestions but this one potentially offer the patient practical information that can be applied to daily life.
5. D. Patients receiving respiratory care at home need to know how to put their equipment together and how to clean it; other choices are inappropriate.

B. Control Infection (Entry Level Only)

According to the NBRC, the control infection content category is assessed only on the Entry Level Examination. The questions in this category are designed to assess the candidate's ability to protect the patient from nosocomial infection through adherence to generally accepted infection control policies and procedures. For instance, if the respiratory therapist notes that a patient on whom he or she is going to perform respiratory care procedures is in strict isolation, the practitioner should be aware that before entering the patient's room, he or she must implement universal precautions.

Entry Level Pretest

According to the NBRC, 5.7% of the questions on the Entry Level Examination are from the control infection content category. The following self-study questions were developed from the NBRC Composite Examination Matrix.

1. Which of the following most correctly describes the term *nosocomial infection?*

A. A non-hospital-acquired gram-negative infection
B. One that results from treatment by medical or surgical personnel
C. One that occurs while the patient is in the hospital
D. A gram-negative infection that results from cross-contamination

(9:406)

2. Which of the following microorganisms is most likely to contaminate the water reservoirs of respiratory therapy equipment?

A. *Escherichia coli*
B. *Proteus* species
C. Beta-hemolytic *Streptococcus*
D. *Pseudomonas aeruginosa*

(1:397–410)

3. All of the following types of respiratory therapy equipment have been associated with nosocomial pulmonary infections. Which of the following has been implicated as having the potential to cause the greatest damage?

   A. Ultrasonic nebulizers
   B. Heated pneumatic jet type nebulizers
   C. Hydronamic type nebulizers
   D. Cold bubble humidifiers

   (1:397–410)

4. All of the following methods of transmitting disease have been associated with the development of nosocomial infections. Which is believed to be the single major cause?

   A. Droplet contamination by coughing and sneezing
   B. Use of respiratory therapy devices
   C. Increased resistance and virulence of hospital flora
   D. Poor handwashing technique

   (1:397–410)

5. Following placement of an endotracheal or tracheostomy tube, contamination of the tracheobronchial tree can be prevented by which of the following techniques?

   A. Proper handwashing technique
   B. Sterile suctioning technique
   C. Changing all related respiratory therapy equipment at least every 8 hr
   D. None of the above

   (4:177–80)

6. All of the following organisms are frequently implicated in the development of nosocomial respiratory tract infection. The presence of which one of the following is *most* suggestive of contamination by aerosol therapy equipment?

   A. *Staphylococcus aureus*
   B. *Hemophilus influenzae*
   C. *Serratia* species
   D. Pneumococcus

   (1:397–410)

7. Which of the following is *not* part of the normal or resident flora of the upper respiratory tract?

   A. *Candida albicans*
   B. *Hemophilus* species
   C. *Staphylococcus* species
   D. *Klebsiella* species

   (1:397–410)

8. Which of the following are most frequently implicated in the development of nosocomial pulmonary infections?

   A. Viruses
   B. Gram-positive bacteria
   C. Fungi
   D. Gram-negative bacteria

   (1:397–410)

9. Patients with which of the following disorders/conditions should be placed in reverse (protective) isolation?

   A. Small for gestational age newborns
   B. *Pseudomonas* pulmonary infections
   C. Extensive burns
   D. Tuberculosis

   (1:406–8)

10. The respiratory therapy practitioner should be aware that *Mycobacterium* tuberculosis is transmitted to the host primarily by:

    A. Fomite contamination
    B. Direct skin-to-skin contact
    C. Inhalation of contaminated droplets
    D. Handling of infected sputum

    (9:85–6)

Answer Key

1. C. A nosocomial infection is one that occurs while the patient is in the hospital.
2. D. *Pseudomonas aeruginosa* is most likely to contaminate water reservoirs in RT equipment.
3. A. Because of the density and amount of output of particulate water by these devices, they are most likely to cause contamination.
4. D. Poor handwashing technique by hospital personnel is the major cause of nosocomial infection.
5. D. All of the choices can prevent infection, but the patient's airway is contaminated soon after he is intubated.
6. C. *Serratia* is the most likely organism to contaminate aerosol therapy equipment.
7. D. Only *Klebsiella* species does not grow in the upper airway under normal circumstances.
8. D. Gram-negative bacteria are responsible for causing most hospital-caused infections.
9. C. Patients with severe and/or extensive burns must be protected from the organisms that may be carried by hospital personnel; their immune system is impaired and they have lost the protective barrier of their skin.
10. C. TB is transmitted by inhaled droplets through a laugh, cough, sneeze, etc.

C. Maintain Airway

According to the NBRC, questions in this category are designed to assess the candidate's ability to conduct therapeutic procedures to achieve maintenance of a patent airway. Also assessed is the candidate's knowledge of the care and placement of the various types of artificial airways. *It should be pointed out at this time that humidity therapy is assessed only on the Entry Level Examination and that the technique of endotracheal intubation is assessed only on the Advanced Practitioner Examination.*

Entry Level Pretest

According to the NBRC, 5.7% of the questions on the Entry Level Examination are from the maintain airway content category. In addition, the Composite Examination Matrix states that questions in this category assess the candidate's ability to perform the following related tasks:

1. Maintain adequate humidification (humidity therapy).
2. Position patient properly to maintain airway patency.
3. Insert oropharyngeal and nasopharyngeal airways.
4. Maintain proper cuff inflation and proper position of endotracheal and tracheostomy tubes within the patient's airway.

The following self-study questions were developed from the NBRC Composite Examination Matrix.

1. Which of the following statements regarding the reported advantages of nasal over orotracheal tubes is (are) true?

    I. Less skill is required in placement.
    II. They are preferred whenever long-term intubation is anticipated.
    III. A larger caliber tube may be used.
    IV. They are generally tolerated better by the patient.

    A. I, III, and IV
    B. I, II, and IV
    C. II only
    D. II and IV

    (4:169–72)

2. Which of the following is the correct progression of the anatomic structures of the upper airway?

    I. Vocal cords
    II. Arytenoid cartilage
    III. Oropharynx
    IV. Epiglottis
    V. Uvula

    A. III, I, IV, II, and V
    B. IV, III, II, V, and I
    C. IV, III, II, I, and V
    D. III, V, IV, II, and I

    (17:36–43)

3. Which of the following would be the preferred method of maintaining airway patency in an unconscious patient who is not in respiratory distress?

    A. Nasopharyngeal airway
    B. Oropharyngeal airway
    C. Orotracheal intubation
    D. Nasotracheal intubation

    (17:422)

4. Postextubation complications of tracheal intubation include(s):

    I. Tracheomalacia
    II. Tracheoesophageal fistula
    III. Glottic and subglottic edema
    IV. Mucosal ischemia
    V. Tracheal stenosis

    A. I, III, and V
    B. II, III, and V
    C. I, IV, and V
    D. V only

    (4:195–205)

5. Methods of reducing the incidence of tracheal tube cuff-related side effects include:

    I. Use of pressure-limited cuffs
    II. Use of high residual volume type cuffs
    III. Use of Fome type cuffs
    IV. Monitoring of intracuff pressures

    A. I, II, III, and IV
    B. I and III
    C. II, III, and IV
    D. II and IV

    (17:428–8)

6. Which of the following statements regarding tracheal dilatation is (are) true?

    I. It will not occur if low intracuff pressures are used.
    II. It is not associated with positive pressure ventilation.
    III. It may result in leakage of tidal gases.
    IV. It may lead to esophageal compression.

    A. I and III
    B. III only
    C. III and IV
    D. II and IV

    (17:428–9)

7. The respiratory therapy practitioner is called to the recovery room. The patient in question is in a deep coma and, according to the anesthesiologist, has no upper airway reflexes. As this patient regains consciousness, which of the following reflexes will return first?

    A. Gag
    B. Tracheal
    C. Carinal
    D. Swallowing

    (4:156)

8. The trachea of the average adult is approximately ___ cm in length.

   A. 7–9
   B. 8–10
   C. 12–14
   D. 14–16

   (4:3–7)

9. Which of the following is generally considered the route of *first* choice in establishing the emergency airway?

   A. Orotracheal intubation
   B. Nasotracheal intubation
   C. Tracheotomy
   D. Cricothyroidotomy

   (4:166–8)

10. When using a nasopharyngeal airway, the distal end should:

    A. Be level with the uvula
    B. Be level with the tip of the tongue
    C. Displace the tongue forward, preventing obstruction
    D. Partially open the epiglottis

    (4:155–6)

11. In general, use of high-pressure tracheal tube cuffs is *least* likely to result in which of the following?

    A. Tracheal aspiration
    B. Tracheal necrosis
    C. Tracheal malacia
    D. Tracheal stenosis

    (4:157–8)

12. Which of the following actions would *not* be performed as part of the procedure of tracheal tube cuff care?

    A. Suctioning below the cuff
    B. Suctioning above the cuff
    C. Deflating the cuff prior to suctioning the upper airways
    D. Hyperoxygenating before and after the procedure

    (4:186–7)

Answer Key

1. D. Nasotracheal ET tubes are more difficult to insert, more comfortable for the patient, preferred for extended intubation, and require a slightly smaller tube (one to half size smaller).
2. D. This sequence represents the progression of anatomic airway structures.
3. B. Oropharyngeal airways are designed to relieve soft tissue obstruction in the unconscious patient.
4. A. TE fistula and mucosal necrosis are not complications of tracheal intubation; the other choices are.
5. A. All of these can and should be used to reduce the incidence of side effects.
6. C. Tracheal dilatation may result in loss of tidal volume around the affected area, and may eventually cause esophageal compression.
7. C. Reflexes are lost from the top, down, and regained from the bottom, up. The carinal reflex is the "bottom" airway reflex.
8. C. The adult trachea is about 12–14 cm long.
9. A. Oral ET intubation is the emergency airway of choice.
10. C. The nasopharyngeal airway should be inserted so that it displaces the tongue forward, preventing obstruction.
11. A. High-pressure tracheal tubes are rarely seen because of these complications; tracheal aspirations is not a hazard.
12. C. If the cuff were to be deflated prior to upper airway suctioning, the secretions above the cuff would move into the lung.

Advanced Practitioner Pretest

According to the NBRC, 1–2% of the questions on the Advanced Practitioner Examination are from the maintain airway and remove secretions content category. In addition, the Composite Examination Matrix states that questions in this category assess the candidate's ability to perform the following related tasks:

1. Select appropriate endotracheal tubes.
2. Perform endotracheal intubation and extubation.
3. Change tracheostomy tubes.
4. Perform extubation.
5. Initiate positive expiratory pressure (PEP) mask.
6. Select closed system suction catheter.

The following self-study questions were developed from the NBRC Composite Examination Matrix.

1. Immediate complications of endotracheal intubation may include:

   I. Laryngeal trauma
   II. Iatrogenic hypoxia
   III. Tracheal stenosis
   IV. Endobronchial intubation

   A. I, II, and IV
   B. I, II, and III
   C. I, II, III, and IV
   D. I and III

   (4:195–8)

2. Endotracheal intubation may facilitate the administration of emergency life support in which of the following ways?

   I. Metabolic acidosis can be successfully treated.
   II. Aspiration pneumonitis may be prevented.

III. A possible route for sodium bicarbonate administration is assured.
IV. Ventilation with 100% oxygen may be assured.

A. I and III
B. II, III, and IV
C. II and III
D. II and IV

(4:152–75)

3. In patients with cervical spine trauma, visualization of the larynx during nasotracheal intubation may be aided by:

I. Flexion of the head and neck
II. Modified jaw thrust maneuvers
III. Use of the fiberoptic laryngoscope
IV. Hyperextension of the head and neck

A. III only
B. II only
C. II and III
D. I and III

(1:484–5)

4. Which of the following statements about neonatal intubation is (are) true?

I. It should not be used when CPAP therapy is ordered.
II. The expiratory grunt mechanism may be abolished.
III. Cuffed tubes are not employed.
IV. The tip of the tube should be placed approximately 2 cm from the carina.

A. I and IV
B. II only
C. II and III
D. II, III, and IV

(14:289–92)

5. Successful orotracheal intubation in the average adult patient is indicated by which of the following?

I. Bilateral chest wall movement during inspiration
II. The endotracheal tube's 13-cm mark at the patient's gum line
III. Equal and bilateral breath sounds

A. I and III
B. II and III
C. III only
D. II only

(4:164)

6. Which of the following statements is (are) true regarding endotracheal intubation as a means of establishing the airway during cardiopulmonary resuscitation?

I. It should not be attempted by untrained personnel.
II. Preoxygenation is not essential if personnel and equipment are immediately available.
III. It should be performed prior to removal of an esophageal obturator airway.

A. I only
B. I and III
C. II and III
D. I, II, and III

(4:162)

7. True statements regarding tracheal intubation using the straight laryngoscope blade include:

I. With adults, it is used to lift the epiglottis.
II. With newborns, placement in the vallecula is frequently recommended.
III. Its use is contraindicated in the emergency setting.
IV. It is preferred for use on stout, short-necked patients.

A. I and III
B. II and III
C. I, II, and IV
D. I and II

(13:307–8; 14:289–92)

8. Prompt neonatal intubation and supportive ventilation is indicated by which of the following?

I. Presence of unilateral choanal atresia
II. Apgar score of 0–3
III. Prolonged periods of apnea

A. II only
B. III only
C. I and II
D. II and III

(14:289–92)

9. Which of the following size (I.D.) endotracheal tubes should the respiratory therapy practitioner select for an average-size, 7-year-old child?

A. 3.5–4.0 mm
B. 4.5–5.0 mm
C. 5.5–6.0 mm
D. 6.5–7.0 mm

(14:287)

10. Which of the following statements regarding the anatomy and physiology of the neonatal upper airway as compared with that of the adult is (are) true?

I. The tongue is proportionately larger.
II. The newborn is a nose breather.
III. The cricoid is the most narrow portion.

A. II only
B. I, II, and III
C. I and II
D. II and III

(14:289–92)

11. Immediately before performing endotracheal tube extubation, which task would the RCP be *least* likely to perform?

    A. Deflation of the cuff
    B. Hyperoxygenation
    C. Suction
    D. Hyperventilation

(4:191)

12. Closed system suction catheters are *least* appropriate for which type of patient?

    A. Patients receiving high levels of PEEP
    B. Patients receiving high levels of oxygen
    C. Patients receiving high doses of corticosteroids
    D. Patients who are hemodynamically compromised

(4:184)

13. Which of the following is the most common indication for use of the PEP mask?

    A. Asthma
    B. Bronchiolitis
    C. Cystic fibrosis
    D. Idiopathic pulmonary fibrosis

(1:644–5)

Answer Key

1. A. All but tracheal stenosis are complications of intubation that are relatively immediate.
2. D. Metabolic problems should not be treated with respiratory manipulations; aspiration may be prevented because the patient no longer has to protect his airway. Ventilation with FIO_2 of 100% is easier to do if the patient is intubated!
3. C. Modified jaw thrust and use of the fiberoptic laryngoscope make nasotracheal intubation easier in the cervical-spine injury patient.
4. D. Because of the child's natural airway narrowing, cuffed tubes are not used for intubation; intubation may establish the expiratory grunt meachanism; tip of the tube should sit about 2 cm from the carina.
5. A. Proper tube placement can be assessed by presence of equal, bilateral breath sounds and bilateral chest excursion.
6. B. Preoxygenation before an intubation attempt is always indicated; other statements are true.
7. D. With adults, the straight blade is used to lift the epiglottis. In newborns, placement in the vallecula is frequently recommended.
8. D. Intubation is indicated for prolonged apneic periods and for a poor APGAR (0–3).
9. C. A 7-year-old should be intubated with a size 5.5 or 6.0 mm ET tube.
10. B. All of these are true statements about the neonate's airway.
11. D. It is not necessary to hyperventilate the patient prior to extubation. The other steps, however, are important.
12. C. Patients who are on high FIO_2s or PEEP, or who are unstable hemodynamically may benefit from closed system catheters.
13. C. PEP therapy is most commonly used on CF patients.

D. Mobilize and Remove Secretions (Entry Level Only)

According to the NBRC, the mobilize and remove secretions category is assessed only on the Entry Level Examination. Questions in this category are designed to assess the candidate's ability to conduct therapeutic procedures to achieve removal of bronchopulmonary secretions. *It must be pointed out at this time that this content category is meant to include not only the more traditional aspects of bronchial hygiene therapy, such as suctioning, aerosol therapy, postural drainage, and percussion, but is also meant to include the administration of pharmacologic agents via the aerosol route.*

Entry Level Pretest

According to the NBRC, 3% of the questions on the Entry Level Examination are from the mobilize and remove secretions content category. In addition, the Composite Examination Matrix states that questions in this category assess the candidate's ability to perform the following related tasks:

1. Administer prescribed pharmacologic agents (bronchodilators, mucolytics, saline, etc.).
2. Perform postural drainage.
3. Perform percussion and vibration.
4. Suction endotracheal and tracheostomy tubes.
5. Perform nasotracheal and orotracheal suctioning.
6. Instruct and encourage proper coughing techniques.
7. Administer aerosol therapy.

The following self-study questions were developed from the NBRC Composite Examination Matrix.

1. Improving tracheobronchial hygiene is an established clinical goal of which of the following respiratory care modalities?

    I. Aerosol therapy
    II. IPPB therapy
    III. Sustained maximal inflation therapy (incentive spirometry)

    A. I and III
    B. II and III
    C. I only
    D. I, II, and III

(4:103–8)

2. The strong β_2 activity of isoproterenol has been shown to directly result in which of the following unwanted actions?

   I. Increased airway smooth muscle tone
   II. Dilatation of the pulmonary vasculature
   III. Systemic arterial hypertension
   IV. Bradyarrhythmias

   A. I and III
   B. II only
   C. II and III
   D. III and IV

   (7:146)

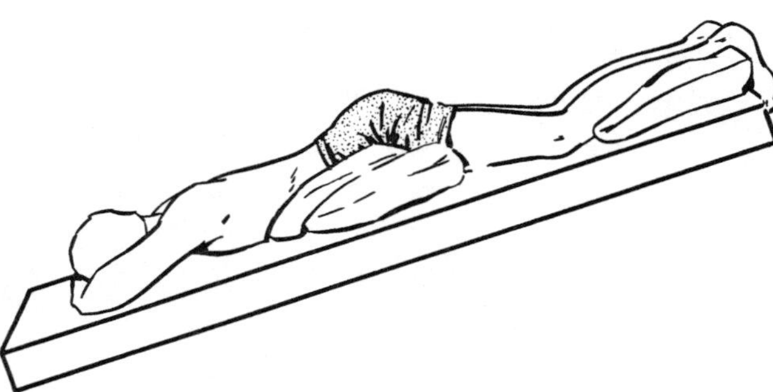

Figure 24.

3. Figure 24 shows the patient in the prone Trendelenburg's position. In this position, which segment will drain?

   A. Lower lobe, apical basal segment, bilaterally
   B. Lower lobe, medial basal segment, bilaterally
   C. Lower lobe, posterior basal segment, bilaterally
   D. Lower lobe, anterior basal segment, bilaterally

   (4:94–103)

4. In general, the minimum vital capacity necessary to provide an effective cough is believed to be:

   A. 15 mL/kg
   B. 25 mL/kg
   C. 40 mL/kg
   D. 15 mL/lb

   (4:89)

5. Which of the following have been described as complications of airway suctioning?

   I. Tracheitis
   II. Decreased intracranial pressure
   III. Atelectasis
   IV. Cor pulmonale

   A. I and III
   B. II and III
   C. II, III, and IV
   D. I, II, and III

   (4:180–4)

6. Which two of the following lung segments are the most common sites of retained secretions among hospitalized patients?

   I. Superior basal
   II. Anterior basal
   III. Lateral basal
   IV. Posterior basal
   V. Medial basal

   A. I and III
   B. I and IV
   C. II and III
   D. III and IV

   (4:94–103)

7. Which of the following are unwanted effects of metaproterenol therapy that the respiratory therapy practitioner should be aware of?

   I. Short duration of action
   II. Tachyarrhythmias
   III. Slowness to peak
   IV. Excessive vasopressor activity

   A. II and III
   B. I and III
   C. II, III, and IV
   D. I, II, III, and IV

   (7:146–7)

8. Which of the following may be considered contraindications to postural drainage techniques?

   I. Recent food consumption
   II. Putrid lung abscess
   III. Undrained empyema
   IV. Intracranial hypertension
   V. Mucosal edema

   A. I and III
   B. II, III, and IV
   C. I, III, and IV
   D. I and V

   (4:94–103)

9. Prone, a pillow under the patient's abdomen, and the bed flat describes the position for draining:

   A. Basal lobes, apical segment
   B. Basal lobes, posterior segment
   C. Basal lobes, lateral segment
   D. Basal lobes, anterior segments

   (4:94–103)

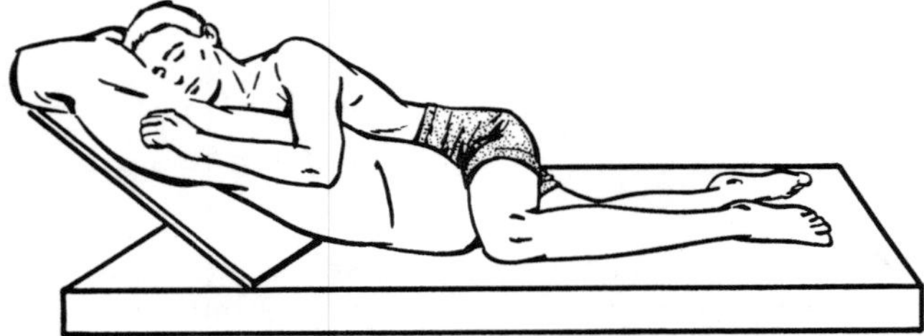

Figure 25.

10. Figure 25 shows a patient lying on his right side with head at a 30° angle and chest and abdomen at a 45° angle. In this position, which segment will drain?

    A. Upper lobe, posterior segment on the left
    B. Upper lobe, apical segment on the right
    C. Upper lobe, anterior segment on the left
    D. Upper lobe, posterior segment on the right

(4:94–103)

11. In patients with extrinsic asthma, cromolyn sodium has been shown to:

    I. Reduce the frequency of allergic asthmatic episodes
    II. Reduce the need for systemic corticosteroids
    III. Treat acute bronchospasm

    A. I and III
    B. II and III
    C. I and II
    D. II only

(7:267–82)

12. Which of the following bronchodilators might the respiratory therapy practitioner recommend for use by asthmatics because of a long duration of action?

    I. Albuterol
    II. Metaproterenol
    III. Terbutaline
    IV. Isoetharine

    A. I, II, and III
    B. II and III
    C. II, III, and IV
    D. I and II

(7: Chap 5 and 7)

13. Which of the following statements regarding the bronchospasm that may accompany administration of acetylcysteine is (are) true?

    I. It may be preventable through concurrent administration of a bronchodilator.
    II. It is the least important of acetylcysteine's side effects.
    III. It is caused by its sympatholytic activity.

    A. I only
    B. II and III
    C. I, II, and III
    D. I and II

(7:212)

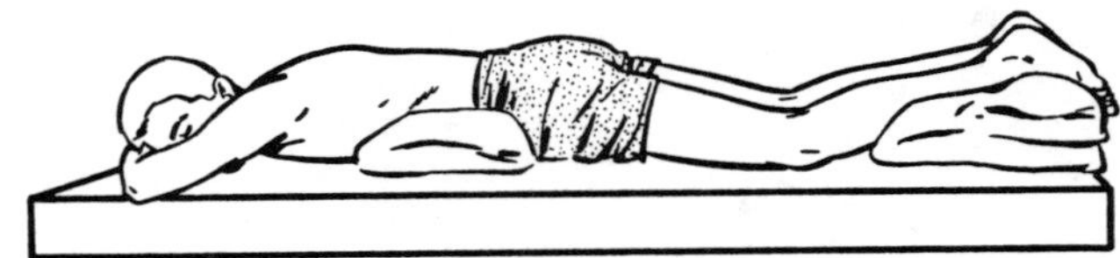

Figure 26.

14. Figure 26 shows the patient in a prone position with a pillow under the abdomen and ankles. In this position, what segment will drain?

    A. Upper lobe, apical segments bilaterally
    B. Upper lobe, anterior segments bilaterally
    C. Lingula, superior lobe, on the left
    D. Lower lobe, apical segment bilaterally

(4:94–103)

15. Which of the following are recommended methods for determining the location of pulmonary infiltrates for purposes of drainage?

    I. Patient historical data
    II. Bedside physical examination
    III. Analysis of pulmonary angiography
    IV. Chest roentgenograms
    V. Arterial blood gas analysis

    A. I and III
    B. II and IV
    C. III and V
    D. II and V

(4:94–103)

16. The respiratory therapy practitioner is asked to perform chest physical therapy on a patient with multiple lung abscesses. On reviewing chest films and other pertinent data, the practitioner notes the presence of consolidation throughout both lung fields apically and basally. The practitioner should drain these segments in which order?

    A. Basal segments first, then middle segments, and apical segments last
    B. Right lung field first, left lung field last
    C. Apical segments first, then middle segments, and basal segments last
    D. Apical segments first, then basal segments, and middle segments last

(13:204–6)

17. In which of the following conditions is chest physical therapy usually considered an essential part of the therapeutic regimen?

I. Cystic fibrosis
II. Adult respiratory distress syndrome
III. Myasthenia gravis
IV. Lung abscess
V. Bronchiolitis

A. II and IV
B. I and IV
C. III and IV
D. I and II

(4:94–5)

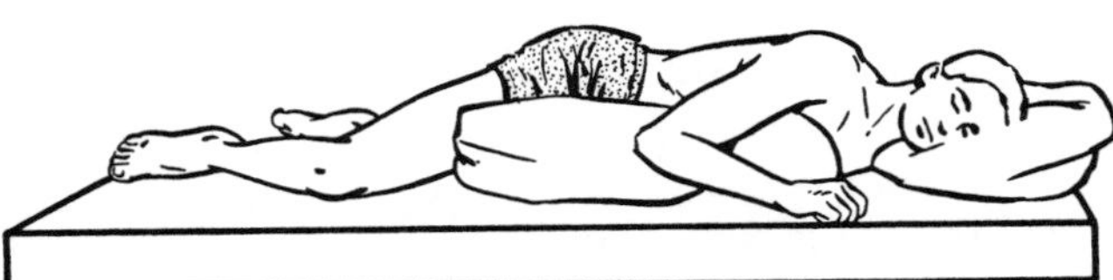

Figure 27.

18. Figure 27 shows the patient lying on his left side with the right leg ahead of the left. In this position, which segment will drain?

A. Upper lobe, anterior segment on the right
B. Lower lobe, posterior-basal segment on the right
C. Upper lobe, apical-posterior segment on the left
D. Upper lobe, posterior segment on the right

(13:204–6)

19. Recommended levels of subatmospheric suctioning pressure in adult and pediatric populations include:

I. Adult: 100–180 mm Hg
II. Pediatric: 60–80 mm Hg
III. Adult: 80–160 mm Hg
IV. Pediatric: 60–120 mm Hg
V. Adult: 80–120 mm Hg
VI. Pediatric: 40–120 mm Hg

A. II and III
B. I and II
C. II and V
D. I and VI

(4:180–4; 14:286–9)

20. Which of the following statements regarding racemic epinephrine is (are) true?

I. It may be indicated in the treatment of croup.
II. It may be indicated in the treatment of adult respiratory distress syndrome.
III. It possesses a strong decongestant action.
IV. It is a more potent bronchodilator than isoproterenol.

A. II and III
B. I and III
C. I and IV
D. III and IV

(7:145–7)

21. Select the false statement about metaproterenol.

A. Central nervous system side effects may be noted.
B. It is completely free of β_1 side effects.
C. Duration of action is relatively long.
D. Oral preparations are available.

(7:146–7)

Answer Key

1. D. All of the above therapies are techniques to improve bronchial hygiene.
2. B. Dilatation of the pulmonary vasculature is an unwanted side effect of isoproterenol.
3. C. This illustration shows the proper position for draining the lower lobe, posterior basal segment, bilaterally.
4. A. The minimum vital capacity necessary to provide an effective cough is 15 mL/kg.
5. A. Tracheitis and atelectasis have been reported as complications of suctioning, along with hypoxemia and dysrhythmias. They can be avoided by using the proper size catheter and the correct pressure range, and limiting the procedure to 15 sec.
6. B. The superior and posterior basal segments are the most common sites of retained secretions in the hospitalized patient due to their positioning.
7. A. Tachyarrhythmias and a slowness to peak (30–60 min) are associated with metaproterenol use.
8. C. Patients with undrained empyema, with high ICP, or those who have just eaten all possess relative contraindications to chest PT.
9. A. The description is correct for drainage of the basal lobe, apical segment.
10. A. This patient is positioned to drain the upper lobe, posterior segment on the left side.
11. C. Cromolyn sodium may decrease the frequency of allergic asthma attacks, and may decrease the need for systemic corticosteroid treatment. It is contraindicated in patients who are in the midst of an attack; the histamine has already been released in this case, which is what this drug is designed to prevent.
12. A. All of the choices except isoetharine have a long duration of action.
13. A. The bronchospasm that some patients experience with acetylcysteine administration may be minimized by giving it with a bronchodilator.
14. D. This position will drain the lower lobe, apical segment bilaterally.
15. B. CXR and chest physical exam (inspection, palpation, percussion, and auscultation) help the RCP determine appropriate lung segments to drain.
16. C. Apical segments should be drained first, then middle segments, and basal segments last.
17. B. Patients with lung abcess and cystic fibrosis patients typically have excessive fluid or secretions that

need to be drained; this is not true of the other entities.

18. D. This positions the patient to drain the upper lobe, posterior segment on the right.
19. C. Pediatric patients should be suctioned using negative pressures of 60–80 mm Hg; adults, 80 to 120 mmHg.
20. B. Racemic epinephrine is often used to treat croup. It provides a decongestant and bronchodilator effect.
21. B. Metaproterenol has minimal beta-one side effects; other statements are descriptive.

E. Ensure Ventilation

Questions in this category are designed to assess the candidate's ability to conduct therapeutic procedures that will help the patient achieve adequate, spontaneous, and artificial ventilation. A major goal of this content category is to assess the candidate's understanding of the physiologic basis, indications, contraindications, and hazards of intermittent positive pressure breathing (IPPB) therapy and continuous mechanical ventilatory therapy.

Entry Level Pretest

According to the NBRC, 7.1% of the questions on the Entry Level Examination are from the ensure ventilation content category. In addition, the Composite Examination Matrix states that questions in this category assess the candidate's ability to perform the following related tasks on an entry level:

1. Instruct in proper breathing techniques.
2. Encourage deep breathing.
3. Instruct and monitor techniques of incentive spirometry.
4. Administer prescribed bronchodilators.
5. Initiate and adjust IPPB therapy.
6. Select appropriate ventilator.
7. Select appropriate ventilator settings.
8. Institute and modify weaning procedures.
9. Initiate and adjust continuous mechanical ventilation when settings are specified.
10. Initiate and adjust IMV, SIMV, and pressure support ventilation (PSV) to maintain adequate alveolar ventilation.

The following self-study questions were developed from the NBRC Composite Examination Matrix.

1. The respiratory therapy practitioner is asked to initiate mechanical ventilation on a woman who is 5 ft, 3 in. tall and weighs 220 lb. Select the appropriate delivered tidal volume for this patient.

   A. 300 mL
   B. 400 mL
   C. 600 mL
   D. 1000 mL

   (15:181–3)

2. Which of the following are true regarding the hyperventilation that can complicate IPPB therapy?

   I. Symptoms include dizziness and tingling of extremities.
   II. It is a rare side effect.
   III. It can usually be prevented through proper patient instruction.
   IV. It is never a serious hazard.

   A. I, III, and IV
   B. II and IV
   C. I, II, and III
   D. I and III

   (4:90–2)

3. The physician's order for IPPB should *not* specify which one of the following?

   A. FIO_2
   B. Ventilator flow rate
   C. Ventilator sensitivity
   D. B and C

   (4:85–92)

4. Which of the following is invariably considered to be an absolute contraindication for IPPB therapy?

   A. Active tuberculosis
   B. Hemoptysis
   C. Untreated tension pneumothorax
   D. Pulmonary emphysema

   (4:90)

5. The primary use of sustained maximal inspiratory therapy (incentive spirometry) is to:

   A. Treat atelectasis
   B. Mobilize secretions
   C. Decrease the work of breathing
   D. Prevent atelectasis

   (4:93–4)

6. When used for the administration of continuous ventilatory support, pressure-cycled ventilators may have which of the following disadvantages?

   I. Volume delivery may be unreliable.
   II. Precise FIO_2 administration may require equipment modification.
   III. They are generally more expensive than volume-cycled ventilators.
   IV. They cannot be adapted to include exhaled tidal volume monitors.

   A. I and II
   B. I and IV
   C. II, III, and IV
   D. I, II, and IV

   (2:217, 241)

7. Hand-held, unpressurized nebulizers are an effective means of administrating adrenergic bronchodilators. Their use over that of positive pressure devices (IPPB) may be encouraged in all but which one of the following cases?

   A. Patients with intrinsic asthma
   B. Patients with abdominal distention
   C. Patients with severely diminished pulmonary reserves
   D. Patients who have had thoracic surgery

   (4:89)

8. The volume of anatomic deadspace in a healthy 100-kg adult is believed to be:

   A. 100 mL
   B. 220 mL
   C. 150 mL
   D. 250 mL

   (1:763)

9. Which of the following is *not* an example of pulmonary barotrauma that may result from the administration of continuous ventilatory support?

   A. Subcutaneous emphysema
   B. Tension pneumothorax
   C. Pulmonary interstitial edema
   D. Cardiovascular depression

   (15:241–4)

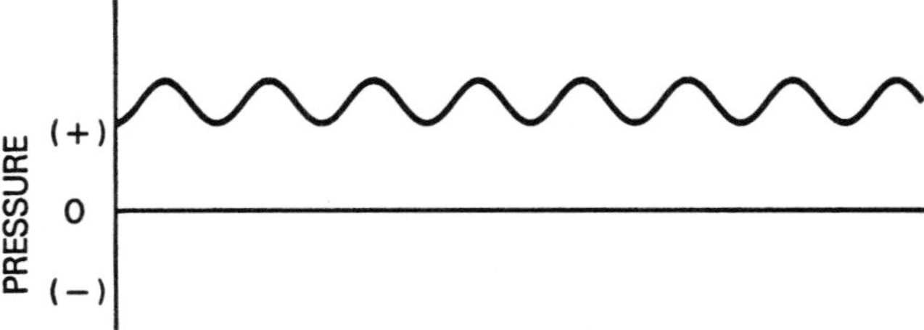

Figure 28.

10. The pressure waveform shown in Figure 28 is most accurately described by which of the following terms?

    A. NEEP
    B. ZEEP
    C. PEEP
    D. CPAP

    (15:366–70)

11. When instructing a patient on proper breathing technique during administration of an aerosolized bronchodilator, which of the following would be *least* likely to be included in the instructions?

    A. Inspiratory hold
    B. Slow breaths
    C. Deep breaths
    D. Inspire through the nose

    (4:64)

12. Which of the following modes of continuous mechanical ventilation would be appropriate for the patient who is being weaned from mechanical ventilation?

    I. SIMV
    II. HFJV
    III. PSV
    IV. Inverse ratio ventilation

    A. I, II, III, and IV
    B. I, II, and III
    C. I and III
    D. II and IV

    (15:496–503)

Answer Key

1. C. Ideal body weight for this patient is approximately 115 lb, or 52 kg. Using 12 cc/kg, V_T would be 625 cc.
2. D. Proper patient instruction can generally prevent the dizziness that may occur with hyperventilation during IPPB.
3. D. The order for IPPB need not specify machine flow rate or sensitivity; these are manipulated as needed by the RCP.
4. C. Untreated tension pneumothorax is the only absolute contraindication to IPPB.
5. D. The main goal of IS is prevention of atelectasis.
6. A. Pressure-cycled ventilators may deliver varied tidal volumes; precise FIO_2 delivery requires modification (beyond air mix).
7. C. Patients with severely diminished pulmonary reserves (inadequate $V_C < 15$ cc/kg), cannot breathe deeply enough on their own to receive maximum benefit from the bronchodilator therapy.
8. C. The volume of anatomic deadspace in a healthy 100-kg adult is 150 cc.
9. D. Cardiovascular depression may be a complication of PPV, but it is not barotrauma.
10. D. CPAP is depicted here.
11. D. Patients should be instructed to take slow deep breaths with an inspiratory hold through their *mouth.*
12. A. SIMV and pressure support are appropriate for the patient who is being weaned from mechanical ventilation.

Advanced Practitioner Pretest

According to the NBRC, 1–2% of the questions on the Advanced Practitioner Examination are from the ensure ventilation category. In addition, the Composite Examination Matrix states that questions in this category assess the candidate's ability to perform the following related tasks on an advanced practitioner level:

1. Instruct in inspiratory muscle training techniques.
2. Initiate and adjust continuous mechanical ventilation when settings are specified and when they are not specified.
3. Initiate and adjust inverse ratio ventilation (IRV).
4. Initiate and adjust airway pressure release ventilation (APRV).
5. Initiate and adjust pressure control ventilation.
6. Initiate nasal/mask ventilation.
7. Initiate and adjust external negative pressure ventilation.

The following self-study questions were developed from the NBRC Composite Examination Matrix.

1. Mechanical hyperventilation may be used therapeutically to:

   I. Decrease intracranial pressure
   II. Prevent patient "fighting" of the ventilator
   III. Aid the management of respiratory acidosis
   IV. Reduce the urine output

   A. I, III, and IV
   B. I and IV
   C. II and IV
   D. I, II, and III

   (15:229–30)

2. Which of the following would generally be considered indications for continuous mechanical ventilation of the newborn?

   I. Prolonged apnea
   II. Pa_{O_2} of 40 mm Hg on 50% oxygen
   III. Pa_{O_2} of 40 mm Hg on 12 cm H_2O CPAP and 80% oxygen
   IV. Pa_{CO_2} of 60 mm Hg on 30% oxygen

   A. I, II, III, and IV
   B. I and IV
   C. I, III, and IV
   D. I, II, and III

   (14:326–31)

3. Widely accepted physiologic indications for continuous mechanical ventilation include:

   I. Vital capacity less than 10 mL/kg
   II. Negative inspiratory force less than 50 cm H_2O
   III. V_D/V_T greater than 0.6
   IV. $P(A\text{–}a)_{O_2}$ greater than 200 mm Hg (on 100% O_2)
   V. Pa_{CO_2} greater than 60 mm Hg in patients with chronic obstructive pulmonary disease

   A. I and III
   B. II and III
   C. I, III, and IV
   D. II, IV, and V

   (15:75–91)

4. Controlling mechanical ventilation through the use of skeletal muscle paralysis is an accepted part of the management of respiratory failure secondary to which of the following disorders?

   A. Drug overdose
   B. Myasthenia gravis
   C. Flail chest
   D. Cardiogenic pulmonary edema

   (9:294–7)

5. Instructions for inspiratory muscle training (IMT) include all but which of the following?

   A. Train at 40–50% of maximum inspiratory pressure.
   B. Perform IMT 4–5 days per week.
   C. Perform two IMT sessions daily.
   D. Training sessions should last about 15 min each.

   (20:504–5)

6. Which of the following statements are true of the chest cuirass?

   I. It must be custom made for each patient.
   II. It is inappropriate for patients who have no repiratory drive.
   III. It is difficult to regulate I:E ratios.
   IV. It has not been associated with the hazard of abdominal pooling of blood.

   A. I, II, III, and IV
   B. I, III, and IV
   C. II, III, and IV
   D. I, II, and III

   (2:168–9)

7. Nasal/mask ventilation is most appropriate for which of the following types of disorders?

   A. Bronchiectasis
   B. Obstructive sleep apnea
   C. Central sleep apnea
   D. Cystic fibrosis

   (2:188)

8. Which of the following describes airway pressure release ventilation?

   A. Assisted ventilation with intermittent levels of CPAP
   B. Inverse ratio ventilation with IPAP
   C. IPAP and EPAP
   D. Spontaneous ventilation with intermittent levels of CPAP

   (15:124)

9. The RCP should be familiar with the risks associated with inverse ratio ventilation. Which of the following is the *least* harmful of those risks?

   A. Pneumothorax
   B. Diminished cardiac output
   C. Patient may require sedation and paralysis
   D. Elevated peak inspiratory pressure and airway pressure

(15:414–15)

10. Which of the following types of patients would be most likely to benefit from pressure controlled ventilation?

   A. Patients with absent respiratory drive
   B. Patients with impaired neuromuscular respiratory function
   C. Patients with decreased lung compliance and increased airway resistance
   D. Patients with increased lung compliance

(15:175–7)

Answer Key

1. D. Mechanical hyperventilation is appropriate for decreasing intracranial pressure, preventing the patient from "fighting" the ventilator, and to treat respiratory acidosis.
2. A. Neonates should be mechanically ventilated if the $PaO_2 < 50$ torr; $PaCO_2 > 55$ torr; and for apnea.
3. A. Inadequate VC and $V_D/V_T > 60\%$ are physiologic indications for mechanical ventilation.
4. C. Paralysis and sedation are sometimes necessary to minimize paradoxical chest movement in the patient with flail chest until the flail segment can heal.
5. A. Patients should train at 25–35% of PI_{max}, measured at FRC.
6. C. The chest cuirass comes in a variety of sizes, and does not usually have to be custom fit for the patient (patients with severe kyphoscoliosis are an exception). Other statements are true of the chest cuirass.
7. B. Nasal mask ventilation is most appropriate for the treatment of obstructive sleep apnea.
8. D. APRV may be defined as spontaneous breathing at an elevated baseline pressure (CPAP).
9. C. The least harmful risk associated with IRV is that the patient may require sedation and paralysis. With VCIRV, increasing the RR may lead to dangerously high peak and mean airway pressures.
10. C. Patients with decreased lung compliance (stiff lungs) and increased airway resistance would benefit most from PCV; these patients are difficult to ventilate.

F. Ensure Oxygenation

Questions in this category are designed to assess the candidate's ability to conduct therapeutic procedures necessary to achieve adequate arterial and tissue oxygenation. It must be pointed out that the questions on the Advanced Practitioner Examination are concerned with ensuring adequate oxygenation through the use of respiratory waveform manipulation maneuvers such as PEEP and CPAP.

Entry Level Pretest

According to the NBRC, 5.7% of the questions on the Entry Level Examination are from the ensure oxygenation category. In addition, the Composite Examination Matrix states that questions in this category assess the candidate's ability to perform the following related tasks on an entry level:

1. Administer oxygen (on or off the ventilator).
2. Administer PEEP therapy.
3. Administer CPAP therapy.
4. Prevent iatrogenic hypoxemia (oxygenate before and after suctioning and equipment changes).
5. Position the patient to prevent hypoxemia.

The following self-study questions were developed from the NBRC Composite Examination Matrix.

1. In a healthy, resting, adult subject at sea level, the content of oxygen in the arterial blood (CaO_2) is approximately:

   A. 5 vol%
   B. 10 vol%
   C. 15 vol%
   D. 20 vol%

(4:115–16)

2. The respiratory therapy practitioner is caring for a patient who has a severe left-sided infiltrate. Positioning the patient on the unaffected side would most likely lead to which of the following?

   I. Drainage of involved segment
   II. Worsening PaO_2
   III. Improvement of V/Q relationships
   IV. Increasing PaO_2

   A. I and II
   B. II only
   C. IV only
   D. I, III, and IV

(8:122–33)

3. Which of the following is the primary physiologic effect of PEEP and CPAP therapy?

   A. Increase in cardiac output
   B. Decrease in $PaCO_2$
   C. Increase in anatomic deadspace
   D. Increase in functional residual capacity

(4:337–9)

4. Which of the following neonatal disorders are believed to be the result of the toxic effects of oxygen?

   I. Bronchopulmonary dysplasia
   II. Infant respiratory distress syndrome
   III. Retrolental fibroplasia
   IV. Asphyxia neonatorum

   A. II and IV
   B. I and III
   C. I, III, and IV
   D. I, II, and III

(14:235–9)

5. Which of the following conditions is (are) known to cause intrapulmonary (right-to-left) shunting?

   I. Sarcoidosis
   II. Left ventricular failure
   III. Ventricular septal defects
   IV. Adult respiratory distress syndrome

   A. I, III, and IV
   B. II and IV
   C. II only
   D. III and IV

(4:236–9)

6. Which of the following statements regarding the administration of helium and oxygen mixtures is (are) true?

   I. It is usually indicated in the management of acute restrictive disorders.
   II. Low gas density may decrease the work of breathing.
   III. It should not be used on patients prone to air-trapping.
   IV. It is of particular benefit when used as a vehicle for medical aerosols.

   A. I and IV
   B. III and IV
   C. I, II, and IV
   D. II only

(13:171)

7. In which of the following conditions may the administration of hyperbaric oxygen be indicated?

   I. Carbon monoxide poisoning
   II. Diaphragmatic hernia
   III. Gas gangrene infections

   A. I and III
   B. I only
   C. III only
   D. I and II

(13:165–7)

8. Figure 29 shows:

   A. A shunt unit
   B. A deadspace unit
   C. A normal unit
   D. A silent unit

(4:236–7)

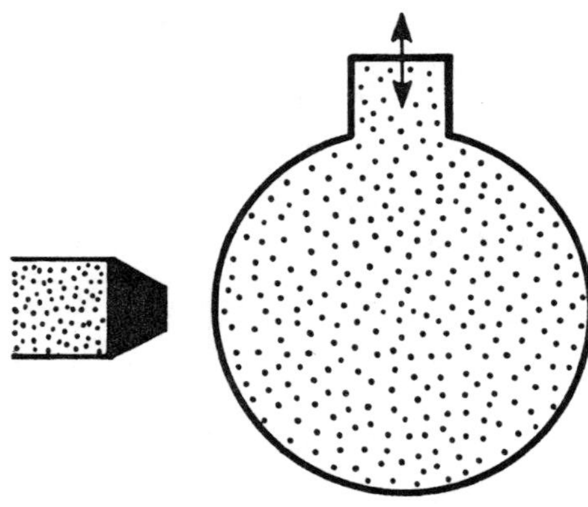

Figure 29.

9. The most efficient mechanism the body has to compensate for arterial hypoxemia is:

   A. Pulmonary vasoconstriction
   B. Increased peripheral vascular resistance
   C. Increased cardiac output
   D. Cerebral vasodilation

(5:203–5)

10. The environmental temperature range in which the newborn's oxygen consumption is lowest refers to which of the following?

   A. Thermal neutral zone
   B. Homeothermic zone
   C. Thermoregulatory zone
   D. Hypothermic zone

(17:361)

11. Which of the following are common clinical goals of oxygen therapy?

   I. To improve alveolar ventilation
   II. To reduce pulmonary workloads
   III. To reduce myocardial workloads
   IV. To increase urine output

   A. II and IV
   B. I and III
   C. II and III
   D. IV only

(4:122–3)

12. Which position is associated with the highest PaO_2 among individuals with normal lungs?

   A. Supine
   B. Upright (erect)
   C. Low Fowler's
   D. High Fowler's

(3:146–50)

13. Which of the following will enhance the tendency of oxygen to dissociate from the hemoglobin molecule at the tissue level?

I. Acidosis
II. Hypocarbia
III. Hyperthermia

A. II and III
B. I only
C. I and II
D. I and III

(4:113, 115)

14. Tissue hypoxia will most frequently lead to which one of the following disorders?

A. Cardiogenic shock
B. Lactic acidosis
C. Hypercapnia
D. Cor pulmonale

(19:238)

15. The primary therapeutic goal of PEEP therapy is to:

A. Improve pulmonary compliance
B. Decrease pulmonary extravascular water
C. Increase the oxygen tension of the arterial blood
D. Improve $Paco_2$

(4:368)

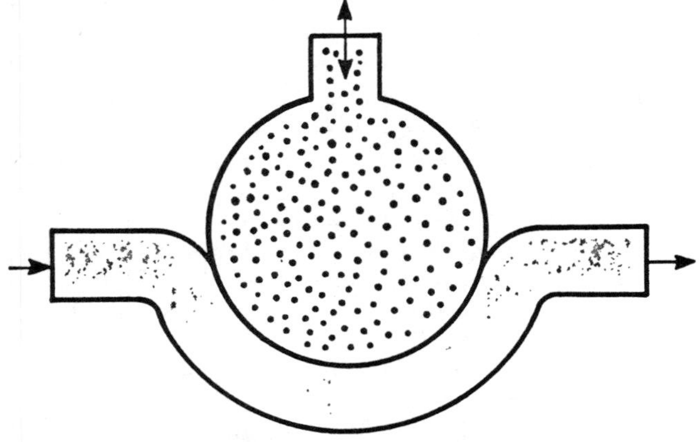

Figure 30.

16. Figure 30 shows:

A. A shunt unit
B. A deadspace unit
C. A silent unit
D. A normal unit

(4:238)

17. Hypoxemia due to diffusion defects is associated with which of the following conditions?

A. Chronic bronchitis
B. Bronchial asthma
C. Sarcoidosis
D. Barbiturate overdose

(1:189–91)

The next two questions refer to the following illustration:

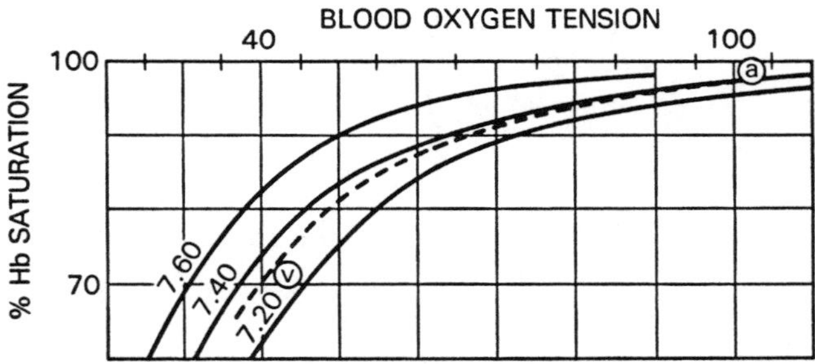

Figure 31.

18. In Figure 31 a dashed line is used to represent the change in blood pH that accompanies tissue oxygenation. Which of the following statements regarding this physiologic shift in the oxyhemoglobin dissociation curve is (are) true?

I. It is known as the Haldane effect.
II. It is known to enhance the unloading of oxygen at the tissue level.
III. It is associated with a decrease in blood P_{50}.
IV. It represents a decrease in the affinity of hemoglobin for oxygen.

A. I and III
B. I, III, and IV
C. III only
D. II and IV

(4:113–17)

19. Which of the following is *least* likely to cause the oxyhemoglobin dissociation curve to shift to the right?

A. Hyperthermia
B. Acidosis
C. Decreased red blood cell 2-3 diphosphoglycerate
D. Hypercarbia

(4:113–17)

20. Recognized hazards of PEEP therapy include which of the following?

I. Cardiovascular embarrassment
II. Microatelectasis
III. Pulmonary barotrauma
IV. Arterial hypertension

A. I and III
B. II and IV
C. IV only
D. II and III

(4:344, 380)

21. Which of the following statements regarding pulmonary oxygen toxicity is *not* true?

A. It is the PIO_2, not the FIO_2, that is causative.
B. The duration of exposure is a critical factor.
C. Prevention usually consists of lowering FIO_2 to 0.4 as rapidly as possible.
D. One may safely administer 100% oxygen for up to 96 hrs.

(4:147–8)

22. Which of the following statements represent(s) indications for PEEP therapy?

I. Treat refractory hypoxemia.
II. Enhance ventilator weaning.
III. Allow reductions of FIO_2 to nontoxic levels.

A. I only
B. II and III
C. I and III
D. I, II, and III

(4:368–9)

23. Which of the following statements is (are) true regarding indications for CPAP therapy?

I. Enhance ventilator weaning.
II. Treat refractory hypoxemia.
III. Provide more effective alveolar ventilation.
IV. Allow for administration of nontoxic levels of oxygen.

A. I and II
B. I, II, and IV
C. II and III
D. III and IV

(4:368–9)

24. Patients who have longstanding chronic obstructive pulmonary disease are sometimes placed on continuous home oxygen therapy. Which of the following should be present for the patient to derive substantial benefit from this expensive mode of therapy?

A. Ventilation-perfusion mismatch
B. Severe pulmonary hypertension
C. A 40 packs/year smoking history
D. Hypercarbia

(5:292)

25. Which of the following should be monitored immediately after placing a patient on PEEP therapy?

A. PaO_2
B. FEV_1
C. Effective static compliance
D. Arterial blood pressure

(13:282)

Answer Key

1. D. Normal oxygen content of arterial blood (CaO_2) is approximately 20 vol%.
2. D. Positioning the patient on the unaffected side would most likely lead to drainage of the affected segment, increased PaO_2 and better V/Q.
3. D. The primary function of PEEP is to increase FRC.
4. B. BPD and RLF are results of toxic effects of oxygen on neonates.
5. B. LV failure and ARDS are two causes of intrapulmonary shunting.
6. D. Helium/oxygen therapy lowers the work of breathing and is used in the treatment of obstructive lung diseases.
7. A. HBO is indicated for treatment of CO poisoning and gas gangrene, the bends, cyanide poisoning, and skin grafts.
8. B. This shows a deadspace unit (ventilation without perfusion).
9. C. Increasing C.O. is the body's most efficient means of correcting for arterial hypoxemia.
10. A. Thermal neutral zone is the environmental temperature range in which the newborn's oxygen consumption is lowest.
11. C. Clinical goals of oxygen therapy include decreased work of breathing and myocardial work.
12. B. The upright position is associated with the highest PaO_2 in those with normal lungs.
13. A. The curve is shifted to the right due to an increase in H^+ ion concentration, $PaCO_2$, 2-3 DPG, and temperature. Decreases in any of these shift the curve to the left, and oxygen is not given up as readily to the tissues.
14. B. Tissue hypoxia will lead to lactic acidosis.
15. C. The primary goal of PEEP therapy is to increase the oxygen tension of the arterial blood. While lung compliance may also improve, this is not the *primary* goal.
16. B. This depicts a normal V/Q relationship.
17. C. In sarcoidosis, fibrin is laid down in the a/c membrane, making it difficult for gas to diffuse across the membrane.
18. D. The shift represents a decrease in the affinity of hemoglobin for oxygen, which enhances the unloading of oxygen at the tissue level.
19. C. See explanation for question 13 above.
20. A. PEEP does not directly lead to atelectasis or arterial hypertension.
21. D. 100% oxygen may safely be administered for only 24 hours.

22. C. PEEP may allow the reduction of FIO_2 to safe levels (< 50%), and treat hypoxemia that had previously been unresponsive to oxygen therapy.
23. B. The above benefits listed for PEEP (question 22), as well as an aid to ventilator weaning, are benefits of CPAP.
24. B. Pulmonary hypertension is caused by longstanding hypoxemia (vasoconstriction). Oxygen may reduce the patient's PA HTN.
25. D. Arterial blood pressure should be monitored in order to determine if cardiac compromise has occurred (stroke volume will be diminished in one cardiac cycle).

Advanced Practitioner Pretest

According to the NBRC, 1–2% of the questions on the Advanced Practitioner Examination are from the ensure oxygenation category. In addition, the Composite Matrix states that questions in this category assess the candidate's ability to perform the following related tasks on an advanced practitioner level:

1. Initiate and adjust BiPAP therapy to treat hypoxia.
2. Initiate and adjust combinations of IMV, SIMV, PEEP therapy, pressure support, and pressure control ventilation to treat hypoxia.

The following self-study questions were developed from the NBRC Composite Examination Matrix.

1. Which of the following statements regarding BiPAP therapy are true?

   I. Therapy is similar to pressure support ventilation and CPAP.
   II. It is a noninvasive mode of ventilation.
   III. Elevated $Paco_2$ is a contraindication.
   IV. Cardiovascular embarrassment is not a hazard.

   A. II and IV
   B. I and IV
   C. III and IV
   D. I and II

   (13:359)

2. Indications for continuous positive airway pressure (CPAP) therapy in the newborn would include which of the following?

   I. Pao_2 of 40 mm Hg on 35% oxygen
   II. $Paco_2$ of 80 mm Hg on 21% oxygen
   III. Pao_2 of 40 mm Hg and $Paco_2$ of 50 mm Hg on 80% oxygen
   IV. Pao_2 of 40 mm Hg on 70% oxygen

   A. I, II, and III
   B. III and IV
   C. IV only
   D. II and IV

   (14:266)

3. Methods of treating hypoxemia that is unresponsive to oxygen administration include which of the following?

   I. PEEP
   II. Use of large mechanical tidal volumes
   III. NEEP
   IV. Supine positioning

   A. I and III
   B. I and II
   C. II, III, and IV
   D. II and IV

   (4:135–40)

4. Which of the following is *least* likely to be a clinical goal of the administration of PEEP therapy?

   A. Improve CO_2 homeostasis
   B. Treat refractory oxygenation failure
   C. Allow administration of nontoxic levels of oxygen
   D. Improve existing pulmonary pathology

   (4:368–9)

5. The most acceptable method of reducing the incidence of pulmonary oxygen toxicity is to:

   A. Administer He/O_2 mixtures instead
   B. Administer megadoses of vitamin E
   C. Administer PEEP and reduce the FIO_2 to 40% as rapidly as possible
   D. Place patient on 21% oxygen for 1 hr each shift

   (4:347–51)

6. The respiratory therapy practitioner is monitoring a 15-year-old patient who is receiving an FIO_2 of 0.6 via a T tube setup. The following data are noted at this time:

Respiratory rate	32
Pao_2	40 mm Hg
$Paco_2$	36 mm Hg
pH	7.38
Base excess	–3.8 mEq/L

   Historical data: Patient is seen 3 days post admission for acute viral pneumonia and has been on continuous mechanical ventilation for 24 hr.

   True statements regarding this situation include:

   I. Refractory oxygenation failure exists.
   II. PEEP would be detrimental.
   III. An FIO_2 of 1.0 would increase the Pao_2 dramatically.
   IV. CPAP may be beneficial.

   A. I, II, and IV
   B. I and IV
   C. II, III, and IV
   D. I and III

   (4:356–61)

7. Acute decreases in venous return seen following administration of PEEP or CPAP therapy may result in which of the following?

   I. Decreased cardiac output
   II. Depression of the systolic blood pressure
   III. Decreased urine output
   IV. Increased $P\bar{v}O_2$

   A. I, II, and III
   B. II and III
   C. I, III, and IV
   D. I only

   (4:344–5)

8. Among patients who are not being monitored with a pulmonary artery (Swan-Ganz) catheter, which of the following would provide the most accurate information regarding the proper level of positive end-expiratory pressure (PEEP)?

   A. Arterial blood pressure
   B. Effective static compliance
   C. $\dot{Q}_S/\dot{Q}_T$
   D. $PaCO_2$

   (13:592)

9. The respiratory therapist is administering continuous ventilatory support to a 60-year-old patient 48 hr post emergency laparotomy. The patient is on a volume ventilator with an FIO_2 of 0.7, 5 cm H_2O PEEP, a tidal volume of 12 cc/kg, and a rate of 15 in the assist mode. The following arterial blood gases are obtained on these settings:

PaO_2	39 mm Hg
$PaCO_2$	42 mm Hg
pH	7.33
HCO_3^-	18 mEq/L
Base excess	–4.6 mEq/L

   Based on the above information, the therapist should recommend which of the following?

   A. Increase FIO_2
   B. Increase respiratory rate
   C. Increase FIO_2 and decrease tidal volume
   D. Increase PEEP

   (4:347–51)

10. Which of the following type of neonatal patient would be *least* likely to be ventilated with pressure control mode?

    A. IRDS
    B. PaO_2/FIO_2 ratio below 100
    C. Bronchopulmonary dysplasia
    D. Peak airway pressure > 35 cm H_2O

    (15:556–7)

11. A patient in the ICU is being mechanically ventilated on an SIMV 4 with a spontaneous respiratory rate of 24 breaths/min. Attempts to wean the patient further have been unsuccessful. The spontaneous RR increases further, and the patient becomes fatigued quickly. What could the RCP recommend?

    A. Pressure control ventilation
    B. Pressure support ventilation
    C. Inverse ratio ventilation
    D. BiPAP

    (15:174–6)

Answer Key

1. D. BiPAP is a noninvasive ventilation mode that uses IPAP and EPAP; it is similar to pressure support ventilation and CPAP. Often used for the treatment of obstructive sleep apnea; patients with increased CO_2 levels are commonly seen. Cardiovascular compromise is a hazard, as with any form of PEEP.
2. B. Ability to maintain $PaCO_2$ at or below 50 to 55 torr, and/or $PaO_2 < 50$ to 60 torr with an $FIO_2 > 50\%$.
3. B. Use of large tidal volumes and PEEP are methods used to treat refractory hypoxemia.
4. A. PEEP is not indicated for improving CO_2 levels. All of the others are clinical indications.
5. C. Application of PEEP with reduction of FIO_2 is an effective method of treating oxygen toxicity.
6. B. Refractory hypoxemia is evidenced by the severe hypoxemia on an FIO_2 of .60. CPAP would be the therapy indicated.
7. A. Physical evidence of decreased venous return includes diminished cardiac output, decreased urine output (caused by decreased perfusion), and decreased arterial systolic pressure.
8. B. Effective static compliance can give the best clue to best PEEP level in the patient who is not being monitored with a pulmonary artery catheter.
9. D. Because the patient's hypoxemia is severe in spite of a delivered FIO_2 of .70, the PEEP level should be increased.
10. C. A patient with BPD would be least likely to be ventilated with PCV; all of the other answers are criteria for pressure controlled ventilation.
11. B. This patient needs assistance in overcoming the resistance of the breathing circuit and ET tube —pressure support is able to overcome these, decreasing the patient's work of breathing.

G. Assess Patient Response to Therapy (Evaluate, Monitor, and Record Patient's Response to Respiratory Care)

Questions in this category are designed to assess the candidate's ability to evaluate and monitor the patient's response to respiratory care techniques. This is one of the most important and difficult content categories on the NBRC examinations—13% of the questions on the Advanced Practitioner Examination are drawn from this area. Questions in this category share a similar scenario: a patient is receiving respiratory care. During that therapy, various bedside and/or laboratory diagnostic data are made available to the respiratory therapy practitioner. Based on that data, the practitioner must make an assessment. That is, the practitioner must evaluate the patient's response to the respiratory therapy techniques in question. Typical questions involve the practitioner noting that a hazardous reaction to therapy is taking place. Other questions may involve determining whether hypoxemia is due to low V/Q or shunting.

Entry Level Pretest

According to the NBRC, 7.1% of the questions on the Entry Level Examination are from this content category. In addition, the Composite Examination Matrix states that questions in this area are designed to test the candidate's ability to evaluate and/or obtain bedside and laboratory data to assess patient response to respiratory care procedures by monitoring the following:

1. Vital signs
2. Cardiac arrhythmias
3. Pulse oximetry
4. Auscultation
5. Subjective response to therapy
6. Cough and sputum evaluation
7. FIO_2 and oxygen liter flow
8. Basic spirometry
9. Arterial blood gas and acid-base data
10. Subjective and objective response to continuous ventilatory support (take and assess ventilator parameters)
11. Alarm systems
12. Endotracheal or tracheostomy tube cuff pressure
13. Ventilatory parameters (tidal volume, respiratory rate, airway pressures, I:E ratios, and maximum inspiratory pressures)

The following are self-study questions from this category.

1. A satisfactory definition of respiratory insufficiency is:

   A. Inability to maintain normal arterial blood gases
   B. Ability to maintain normal arterial blood gases only by increasing cardiopulmonary workloads
   C. $Paco_2$ less than 30 mm Hg with a Pao_2 less than 50 mm Hg
   D. Inability to maintain normal venous blood gases

   (9:337)

2. Which of the following statements regarding cyanosis is *least* true?

   A. Patients may be cyanotic but not significantly hypoxic.
   B. Cyanosis is not usually considered a reliable clinical sign.
   C. Hypoxia may exist without the presence of cyanosis.
   D. In general, central cyanosis is considered a sign of hypoxia.

   (9:20–22)

3. The presence of which of the following may be used to assess that a 70-kg patient is capable of being weaned from continuous ventilatory support?

   I. $P(A–a)o_2$ less than 600 mm Hg
   II. Vital capacity less than 10–15 mL/kg
   III. V_D/V_T less than 0.8
   IV. Resting spontaneous minute volume greater than 15 L/min
   V. Pao_2 greater than 70 mm Hg on 40% oxygen
   VI. Negative inspiratory force greater than 20–30 cm H_2O

   A. I, II, V, and VI
   B. V and VI
   C. III, IV, and V
   D. I, III, and V

   (15:496–7)

4. The decision to initiate continuous ventilatory support in patients with myasthenia gravis is most frequently made by assessment of which of the following parameters?

   A. $Paco_2$
   B. FEV_1
   C. Vital capacity
   D. $\dot{Q}_S/\dot{Q}_T$

   (9:313)

5. The single most important therapeutic effect resulting from the administration of oxygen to a patient with chronic obstructive pulmonary disease who has developed cor pulmonale is:

   A. Decreased right ventricular workloads
   B. Decreased left ventricular workloads
   C. Decreased work of breathing
   D. Improved renal function

   (4:122–3)

6. Which of the following clinical signs does *not* indicate the presence of respiratory distress in the newborn?

   A. Nasal flaring
   B. Expiratory grunting
   C. Tachypnea
   D. Loud crying

   (14:55–9)

7. The clinical diagnosis of ventilatory failure is best assessed by noting which of the following laboratory measurements?

   A. $Pa{O_2}$
   B. $C(a\text{-}\bar{v})O_2$
   C. $Pa{CO_2}$
   D. Maximal voluntary ventilation maneuvers

(15:227–30)

8. For which of the following should the respiratory care practitioner allow one point when using the APGAR scoring system?

   I. Absent reflex irritability
   II. Weak respiratory effort
   III. Pulse rates less than 100
   IV. Central or generalized cyanosis
   V. Some flexion of extremities

   A. II, III, and V
   B. I, III, and IV
   C. II and III
   D. II, III, IV, and V

(14:37)

9. The respiratory therapy practitioner is assessing a patient who has become distressed while receiving continuous ventilatory support. Bedside examination performed while the patient is being ventilated with a bag-valve unit reveals a dull percussion note on the left side. Further physical examination reveals a hyperresonant percussion note on the right side. Under these circumstances, the cause of this patient's distress may be assessed most rapidly by:

   A. Obtaining stat arterial blood gases
   B. Obtaining a portable chest roentgenogram
   C. Retracting the endotracheal tube slightly
   D. Paging the physician

(15:254–6)

10. The respiratory therapy practitioner is monitoring a patient in the intensive care unit who is being ventilated with a volume ventilator. Suddenly the high-pressure alarm begins sounding regularly. Possible causes include:

   I. Patient fighting the ventilator
   II. Mobilization of a large mucus plug
   III. Tension pneumothorax
   IV. Kinking of endotracheal tube

   A. I, II, and III
   B. II and IV
   C. I, III, and IV
   D. I, II, III, and IV

(15:254–6)

11. The respiratory therapy practitioner is performing a physical examination on a patient who has become distressed during continuous ventilatory support. Auscultation reveals absent breath sounds over the right basal lung field. Percussion yields a flat note over the right basal and middle lobes. There is also a noticeable tracheal shift to the left. Based on the above information, the most probable cause of the patient's distress is:

   A. Left-sided pneumothorax
   B. Right-sided hemothorax
   C. Right mainstem intubation
   D. Herniation of endotracheal tube cuff

(9:298)

12. Which of the following are findings that would indicate slippage of an endotracheal tube into the right mainstem bronchus during continuous mechanical ventilation?

   I. Musical inspiratory note
   II. Hyperresonant percussion note on the right side
   III. Decrease in effective static compliance
   IV. Decreased aeration on the left side

   A. I, II, and IV
   B. I, II, and III
   C. II, III, and IV
   D. III and IV

(15:254–6)

13. The respiratory therapy practitioner is assessing a patient who has become severely distressed while receiving continuous mechanical ventilation. While the patient is being manually ventilated, the therapist performs a rapid physical examination. Auscultation at this time reveals absent breath sounds over the left apical lung field. The percussion note is dull on the right and hyperresonant on the left. Tracheal shift to the right is also noted. The most likely cause of this patient's distress is:

   A. Right-sided hemothorax
   B. Left-sided tension pneumothorax
   C. Right mainstem intubation
   D. Ventilator malfunction

(15:254–6)

14. A 72-year-old patient with steady-state chronic obstructive pulmonary disease is seen in the emergency department after being admitted in respiratory distress. His respirations are labored and he is noted to be cyanotic. Further data collected with the patient breathing room air are as follows:

pH	7.26
$Pa{CO_2}$	80 mm Hg
$Pa{O_2}$	39 mm Hg
HCO_3^-	38 mEq/L
BP	160/120
Pulse	130
Respiratory rate	35
Minute ventilation	20 L/min

Administration of 40% oxygen to this patient will most likely have which of the following results?

   I. An increase in alveolar ventilation
   II. Worsening of respiratory acidosis

III. Blunting of the hypoxic drive
IV. Worsening of cardiovascular vital signs

A. I only
B. II and IV
C. II, III, and IV
D. I and III

(9:136–40)

15. Which of the following alarms would be *least* likely to be activated in the event that the patient became disconnected from the ventilator?

A. I:E ratio
B. Apnea
C. Low pressure
D. Low tidal volume

(15:197–8)

16. A patient who has been admitted to the ICU with a diagnosis of narcotic overdose and aspiration pneumonia is on a pulse oximeter. The Sa_{O_2} reading is 90%. This correlates with a Pa_{O_2} of approximately:

A. 95–100 torr
B. 90 torr
C. 60 torr
D. 50 torr

(15:332)

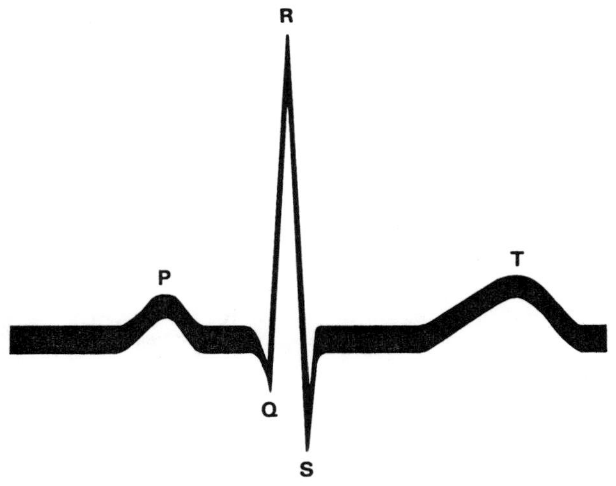

Figure 32.

17. Figure 32 illustrates a normal cardiac cycle. If there were no uniform ventricular repolarization, which of the following waves would disappear?

A. P wave
B. T wave
C. QRS complex
D. R wave

(17:220–20)

Answer Key

1. A. A satisfactory definition of respiratory insufficiency is the inability to maintain normal arterial blood gases (Pa_{CO_2} > 50 torr; Pa_{O_2} < 60 torr).
2. D. Peripheral cyanosis is caused by diminished capillary blood flow; hypoxia may not be present. Anemic patients do not become cyanotic until they are severely hypoxemic. Central cyanosis, however, is considered to be a reliable sign of hypoxemia.
3. B. Pa_{O_2} greater than 70 mm Hg on 40% oxygen and negative inspiratory force greater than 20 cm to 30 cm H_2O are both indications that weaning may begin.
4. C. VC is monitored closely in patients with neuromuscular disorders; patients who become progressively weaker, and are unable to maintain a tidal volume of 12 cc/kg, are often intubated electively.
5. A. A clinical goal of oxygen therapy is decreased myocardial work; in cor pulmonale (RV failure), this translates to less work for the RV.
6. D. A newborn in respiratory distress would not be able to cry loudly, due to dyspnea and increased work of breathing.
7. C. Pa_{CO_2} is the best indicator of ventilatory failure.
8. A. A score of 1 is given for HR < 100 beats/min; weak respiratory effort; some flexion of extremities; peripheral cyanosis; and some response to reflex irritability.
9. C. The ET tube may have entered the right mainstem (increased resonance on the right, decreased on the left). The RCP should pull back the tube slightly, and reassess.
10. D. All of these selections may cause the high-pressure alarm to sound.
11. B. A pneumothorax can be ruled out due to the flat percussion note, indicative of blood or fluid. Tracheal shift away from the affected side implicates a hemothorax on the right side.
12. C. Slippage of the ET tube into the right mainstem would cause increased aeration on the right (hyperresonant percussion), decreased aeration on the left, and decreased static compliance (same volume, increased pressure).
13. B. Hyperresonance and absent breath sounds on the left with tracheal shift to the right indicates left-sided pneumothorax.
14. C. Because 40% oxygen will be likely to minimize this patient's hypoxic drive to breathe, cardiovascular vital signs and respiratory acidosis will likely worsen.
15. A. In the event that a patient became disconnected from the ventilator, all of those alarms would sound, with the exception of I:E.
16. C. A Pa_{O_2} of 60 torr will be accompanied by Sa_{O_2} of 90%.
17. B. If there were no uniform ventricular repolarization, the T-wave would disappear.

Advanced Practitioner Pretest

According to the NBRC, 13% of the questions on the Advanced Practitioner Examination are from this content category. In addition, the Composite Examination Matrix states that questions in this category are designed to test the candidate's ability to obtain, interpret, and/or evaluate the following bedside and laboratory data on an advanced level to assess patient response to respiratory care procedures:

1. Chest x-ray
2. Mean airway pressure
3. Arterial, capillary, and mixed venous blood gas and acid-base data
4. Transcutaneous O_2/CO_2 monitoring
5. Blood chemistry data (i.e., hemoglobin, electrolytes, CBC)
6. Fluid intake and output
7. Subjective response to therapy
8. Central venous pressure, pulmonary artery pressures, pulmonary capillary wedge pressures, and/or cardiac output and cardiac index
9. Co-oximetry
10. Airway resistance
11. Exhaled CO_2 tension
12. V_D/V_T
13. $P(A\text{–}a)O_2$
14. $\dot{Q}_S/\dot{Q}_T$
15. $C(a\text{-}\bar{v})O_2$
16. Effective compliance values
17. Pulmonary and systemic vascular resistance
18. Compliance values
19. Stroke volume

The following self-study questions were developed from the NBRC Composite Examination Matrix.

1. Which of the following are known to cause the P_{50} to rise above normal?

 I. Acidosis
 II. Decreased red blood cell 2-3 DPG levels
 III. Carbon monoxide poisoning
 IV. Hypercarbia

 A. I and III
 B. I, II, and IV
 C. I, III, and IV
 D. I and IV

(19:42)

2. When a patient who has a large right-to-left intrapulmonary shunt is administered 100% oxygen for 20 min which of the following will apply?

 I. The $P(A\text{–}a)O_2$ will narrow.
 II. The PaO_2 will increase dramatically.
 III. PaO_2 will not improve.
 IV. Nitrogen washout will occur.

 A. I and IV
 B. II and IV
 C. III and IV
 D. IV only

(15:356–7; 6:87)

3. Which of the following hemodynamic measurements is believed to reflect left ventricular filling pressures (preload) most reliably?

 A. Central venous pressure
 B. Pulmonary artery systolic pressure
 C. Pulmonary wedge pressure
 D. Mean peripheral arterial pressure

(5:155–6)

4. A patient on a volume ventilator is noted to have his plateau pressure increase from 30 to 40 cm H_2O. Which of the following is (are) correct assessment(s) regarding this situation?

 I. The static effective compliance has decreased.
 II. The effective dynamic compliance has increased.
 III. There has been an increase in lung thorax distensibility.
 IV. The airway resistance has increased.

 A. I, II, and IV
 B. I and III
 C. I only
 D. I and IV

(1:175)

5. The respiratory therapy practitioner would not generally consider the PWP elevated until it exceeds:

 A. 9 cm H_2O
 B. 12 mm Hg
 C. 9 mm Hg
 D. 25 cm H_2O

(5:147)

6. Which of the following would be most helpful in assessing the adequacy of tissue oxygenation?

 A. $\dot{Q}_T$
 B. PaO_2
 C. $P\bar{v}O_2$
 D. $\dot{Q}_S/\dot{Q}_T$

(5:206–11)

7. A 37-year-old, 70-kg patient is seen in the intensive care unit following a splenectomy. The following data are gathered at this time, with the patient receiving an FIO_2 of 0.7 via a T tube setup:

PaO_2	40 mm Hg
$PaCO_2$	40 mm Hg
pH	7.33
Base excess	–3.9 mEq/L
Temperature	37° C
Tidal volume	560 cc
Respiratory rate	44/min

Based on these data, which of the following assessments are true?

 I. The patient's hypoxemia is due to a diffusion deficit.
 II. The patient's V_D/V_T is probably elevated.
 III. Refractory hypoxemia exists.
 IV. The patient is hyperventilating.

 A. II, III, and IV
 B. II and III
 C. I and II
 D. II and IV

(1:151–2; 331–2)

8. Which of the following statements regarding the arterial minus venous oxygen content difference, $C(a-\bar{v})O_2$, is (are) true?

   I. It is generally unaffected by changes in cardiac output.
   II. Accurate measurement requires placement of a pulmonary artery catheter.
   III. A value of 7.2 vol% generally indicates presence of excellent cardiovascular reserves.
   IV. The normal value for a healthy resting subject is approximately 5.0 vol%.

   A. II and IV
   B. IV only
   C. I and IV
   D. I, III, and IV

(4:247–8)

9. All four of the following patients are intubated and are receiving 100% oxygen via a volume ventilator in the control mode. In addition, each one has a PaO_2 of 50 mm Hg and an oxygen consumption ($\dot{V}O_2$) of 250 mL O_2/min. Based on this and the following information, which patient will have the largest physiologic shunt ($\dot{Q}_S/\dot{Q}_T$)?

   A. Patient A has a $C(a-\bar{v})O_2$ of 2.5 vol%.
   B. Patient B has a $C(a-\bar{v})O_2$ of 3.5 vol%.
   C. Patient C has a $C(a-\bar{v})O_2$ of 5.0 vol%.
   D. Patient D has a $C(a-\bar{v})O_2$ of 6.0 vol%.

(4:245)

10. Four patients with identical physiologic shunt fractions ($\dot{Q}_S/\dot{Q}_T$) of 20% are seen in the intensive care unit. They all have varying $C(a-\bar{v})O_2$ values as listed below. Assuming that their oxygen consumptions ($\dot{V}O_2$) are all 300 mL/min, which one of the following is likely to have the lowest PaO_2?

   A. Patient A: 2.5 vol%
   B. Patient B: 3.5 vol%
   C. Patient C: 4.5 vol%
   D. Patient D: 8.0 vol%

(4:246–8)

11. Assuming a steady-state oxygen consumption, as a patient's cardiac output falls, which of the following most likely will take place?

   I. An increase in $C(a-\bar{v})O_2$
   II. An increase in PaO_2
   III. A decrease in $P\bar{v}O_2$

   A. I and III
   B. II and III
   C. III only
   D. I and II

(5:186–92)

12. The respiratory therapy practitioner is monitoring a patient who is receiving continuous ventilatory support via a volume ventilator. At this time he notes that the pulmonary wedge pressure is 27 mm Hg. Which of the following is *least* likely to be responsible for this abnormality?

   A. Aortic stenosis
   B. Mitral valvular disease
   C. Left ventricular failure
   D. Adult respiratory distress syndrome

(5:329)

13. The respiratory therapy practitioner is monitoring a 60-kg patient who is intubated and is receiving positive pressure ventilation with an FIO_2 of 0.6 and a corrected V_T of 700 mL via a volume ventilator. Pertinent data collected with the tidal volume held constant are as follows:

	1:00 PM	2:00 PM
Peak pressure	48 cm H_2O	61 cm H_2O
Plateau pressure	26 cm H_2O	47 cm H_2O
PEEP	5 cm H_2O	10 cm H_2O
Inspiratory flow rate	40 L/min	65 L/min

True statements regarding the above include:

   I. There is a decrease in pulmonary compliance.
   II. There is an increase in airway resistance.
   III. There is a decrease in airway resistance.
   IV. There is an increase in pulmonary compliance.

   A. II and IV
   B. I, III, and IV
   C. I and III
   D. I and II

(15:39–40)

14. The respiratory therapy practitioner is monitoring a patient who is receiving continuous ventilatory support via a ventilator. Over the span of one hour, the peak pressure is noted to increase from 32 cm H_2O to 49 cm H_2O. Concurrently, the plateau pressure remains constant and unchanged. Noting that there have been no changes in tidal volume or flow rate, which of the following conditions are most likely responsible for the recorded changes?

   I. Cardiogenic pulmonary edema
   II. Bronchospasm
   III. Leak in the ventilator circuit
   IV. Upper airway obstruction
   V. Tension pneumothorax

   A. I, II, and IV
   B. II and IV
   C. II and III
   D. I, IV, and V

(15:277–9)

15. Which of the following statements regarding the central venous pressure is (are) true?

I. It is measured in the right ventricle.
II. It assesses right ventricular filling pressures.
III. It may not accurately reflect left ventricular functions.
IV. Normal value is 15–25 mm Hg.

A. II and III
B. II only
C. II, III, and IV
D. III and IV

(5: Chap 8)

16. Which of the following hemodynamic parameters may be determined through the use of a properly functioning four-channel pulmonary artery catheter?

I. Pulmonary arterial pressures
II. Cardiac output
III. $S\bar{v}O_2$
IV. Central venous pressure
V. Pulmonary wedge pressure

A. I, IV, and V
B. II, III, IV, and V
C. I, III, IV, and V
D. I, II, III, IV, and V

(5: Chap 9)

17. The respiratory therapy practitioner is monitoring a mechanically ventilated patient in the intensive care unit. The patient's PWP has just increased rapidly from 10 mm Hg to 32 mm Hg. Which of the following is the most likely cause?

A. Right ventricular failure
B. Left ventricular failure
C. Adult respiratory distress syndrome
D. Septic shock

(5:329)

18. The monitoring of end tidal carbon dioxide tensions ($P_{ET}CO_2$) is most frequently used to approximate:

A. Arterial CO_2 tensions
B. Physiologic deadspace
C. Anatomic deadspace
D. Ventilation-perfusion disorders

(19:349–52)

19. A patient with longstanding chronic obstructive pulmonary disease is being managed in the respiratory intensive care unit. Despite all efforts, he is increasingly unable to manage his upper airway secretions. Blood gases drawn just prior to the patient's being placed on a ventilator show a $Paco_2$ of 110 mm Hg and a pH of 7.16. Two hours after being placed on the ventilator, he begins to display seizure activity. The respiratory therapy practitioner would assess that the most likely cause of this phenomenon is:

A. Increased intracranial pressure
B. Rapid reduction in $Paco_2$
C. Cerebrospinal fluid acidosis
D. Central nervous system hypoxia

(19:161–3)

20. Which of the following will *not* cause increases in pulmonary vascular resistance?

A. Acidosis
B. Hypoxia
C. Pulmonary embolic disease
D. Administration of acetylcysteine

(5:292, 299)

21. All but which one of the following may be present in a patient who is suffering from severe hypovolemia?

A. Hypotension
B. Hypoxia
C. Increased tissue capillary blood flow
D. Lactic acidosis

(5:116–17, 259)

22. Which of the following disorders is (are) known to contribute to the development of hypoproteinemia?

I. Nasogastric feedings
II. Protein malnutrition
III. Parenteral alimentation
IV. Hepatic failure

A. I and III
B. II and IV
C. III and IV
D. IV only

(17:267–9, 277)

23. A 23-year-old, 70-kg patient is seen in the intensive care unit while receiving volume ventilation with an FIo_2 of 0.7 and 12 cm H_2O PEEP. Based on radiologic and clinical evidence, a diagnosis of pulmonary edema is made. Clinical data obtained at this time are as follows:

Pao_2	63 mm Hg
$P\bar{v}o_2$	33 mm Hg
PWP	28 mm Hg
CVP	15 mm Hg
Oxygen consumption	250 mL/min
$C(a\text{-}\bar{v})o_2$	2.5 vol%
Colloidal osmotic pressure	26 mm Hg
Total serum proteins	8.0 g/100 mL

Based on the above data, the respiratory therapy practitioner is able to assess that the most important contributor to this patient's pulmonary edema is:

A. Left ventricular failure
B. Increased pulmonary vascular resistance
C. Hypervolemia
D. Hypoproteinemia

(17:205)

24. The respiratory therapy practitioner is monitoring a 65-kg, 22-year-old patient in the intensive care unit. The patient is seen 24 hr following severe trauma sustained in a motorcycle accident. The following data are noted at this time with the patient receiving 60% oxygen via T-tube setup:

Pa_{O_2}	40 mm Hg
Pa_{CO_2}	50 mm Hg
P_B	760 mm Hg
$C(a\text{-}\bar{v})_{O_2}$	2.5 vol%
Oxygen consumption	250 mL/min

Which of the following assessments regarding the above information is (are) true?

I. The $P(A\text{–}a)_{O_2}$ is 200 mm Hg.
II. This patient is hyperventilating.
III. This patient's cardiovascular reserves are poor.
IV. Continuous ventilatory support is indicated at this time.

A. I, III, and IV
B. IV only
C. II and III
D. III and IV

(15:75–91)

25. A 75-year-old, 50-kg man from a nursing home is admitted in cardiorespiratory failure. He is placed on a volume ventilator, and an FI_{O_2} of 0.6 with 15 mm H_2O PEEP is required to maintain a Pa_{O_2} greater than 50 mm Hg. A radiologic diagnosis of interstitial and alveolar edema is made. The following information is subsequently gathered:

Pa_{O_2}	55 mm Hg
$S\bar{v}_{O_2}$	55%
$C(a\text{-}\bar{v})_{O_2}$	3.5 vol%
PWP	15 mm Hg
CVP	10 mm Hg
Colloidal osmotic pressure	12 mm Hg
Total serum proteins	3.0 g/dL
Oxygen consumption	250 mL/min
Cardiac output	7.1 L/min
PA systolic	38 mm Hg
PA diastolic	21 mm Hg

Based on this information, the respiratory therapy practitioner's assessment reveals which of the following as being the most important contributor to the patient's pulmonary edema?

A. Hypoproteinemia
B. Left ventricular failure
C. Right ventricular failure
D. Pulmonary hypertension

(17:205)

26. In which of the following patient groups will the central venous pressure frequently *not* reflect left ventricular function?

I. Those with increased pulmonary vascular resistance
II. All patients
III. Those with myocardial infarction

A. I and II
B. II only
C. I and III
D. III only

(5:117–8)

27. The quantity of oxygen being consumed per minute can be determined by which of the following formulas?

A. $\dfrac{Cc'_{O_2} - Ca_{O_2}}{Q_T}$
B. $(\dot{Q}_T)(Ca_{O_2})$
C. $(\dot{Q}_T)[C(a\text{-}\bar{v})_{O_2}]$
D. $(Ca_{O_2} - Cv_{O_2})(\dot{Q}_S/\dot{Q}_T)$

(4:246–7)

28. The respiratory therapy practitioner is monitoring a 53-year-old, 60-kg patient in the intensive care unit. Clinical information gathered and reported at the time is as follows:

Body weight	62 kg
V_T	490 mL
Respiratory rate	36/min
Pa_{O_2}	72 mm Hg
FI_{O_2}	0.28
Pulse	110
BP	140/100
Pa_{CO_2}	43 mm Hg

Based on the above data, select the most correct assessment.

A. The patient's hypoxemia is due to shunting.
B. The patient is hyperventilating.
C. Further oxygen administration will result in respiratory depression.
D. It is likely the patient's V_D/V_T is elevated.

(19:123)

29. While performing endotracheal suctioning on a 1500-g newborn, the respiratory therapy practitioner notes that the pulse has dropped from 175 to 90. This problem:

I. May be caused by vagal stimulation.
II. May be prevented through administration of parasympathomimetics.
III. Is uncommon in neonatal units.
IV. May be caused by hypoxia.

A. III only
B. I and III
C. II, III, and IV
D. I and IV

(14:307)

30. Which of the following parameters must be measured to calculate the intrapulmonary shunt?

I. Cao_2
II. $Paco_2$
III. $P(A\text{–}a)o_2$
IV. $C\bar{v}o_2$
V. $P\bar{v}o_2$
VI. $\dot{Q}_T$

A. I, IV, V, and VI
B. I, III, and IV
C. I, III, and V
D. I, II, III, and VI

(4:241)

31. The respiratory therapy practitioner is monitoring a serum sodium level of 142 mEq/L and a serum potassium level of 6.4 mEq/L. These values are consistent with:

I. Hypokalemia
II. Diuretic administration
III. Normal sodium levels
IV. Cushing's syndrome

A. I only
B. III only
C. III and IV
D. II, III, and IV

(17:211–2)

32. If 0.4 cc of air are required to obtain a PCWP, what can you assume?

A. The catheter tip has slipped into the RV.
B. The catheter tip is too peripheral in the pulmonary circulation.
C. Function is normal.
D. The balloon has ruptured.

(5:143–6)

Use the following hemodynamic parameters for the following three questions.

RA = 7 mm Hg	Arterial BP = 150/90 mm Hg
PA mean = 15 mm Hg	PCWP = 12 mm Hg
PA-S/D = 20/10 mm Hg	C.O. = 4 L/min

33. Which of the following represents the patient's systemic vascular resistance?

A. 1340 dyne sec/cm^{-5}
B. 1780 dyne sec/cm^{-5}
C. 2060 dyne sec/cm^{-5}
D. 2230 dyne sec/cm^{-5}

(5:157)

34. Which of the following represents the patient's pulmonary vascular resistance?

A. 30 dyne sec/cm^{-5}
B. 40 dyne sec/cm^{-5}
C. 50 dyne sec/cm^{-5}
D. 60 dyne sec/cm^{-5}

(5:158)

35. What therapy would you recommend for the above patient?

I. Vasodilators
II. Vasopressors
III. O_2
IV. Inotropic agents

A. I only
B. II, III
C. I and III
D. IV only

(5:157–8)

36. PCWP may be used to estimate the degree of pulmonary edema. A PCWP of 33 mm Hg indicates what level of pulmonary edema?

A. None
B. Mild
C. Moderate
D. Full-blown

(5:310)

37. *Optimally,* what position would the patient assume when hemodynamic data is being collected?

A. Prone
B. Supine
C. Semi-Fowler's
D. Full sitting

(5:160–1)

38. A patient is receiving mechanical ventilation and 15 cm PEEP. PCWP measures 25 mm Hg. What is the patient's true PCWP?

A. 25 mm Hg
B. 11 mm Hg

C. 18 mm Hg
D. 20 mm Hg

(5:169–70)

Answer Key

1. D. Acidosis and hypercarbia cause the oxyhemoglobin curve to shift to the right. This is accompanied by an increase in the P_{50}, with the oxygen given up more readily to the tissues.
2. C. If a true shunt exists, no matter how high the FIO_2, PaO_2 will not improve. Nitrogen washout occurs in about 7 min during breathing of 100% oxygen.
3. C. PWP is the most accurate estimation of left ventricular preload; in the normal heart, there is a good correlation between LV filling volume and LV filling pressure.
4. D. If the plateau pressure has increased by 10 cm H_2O, this indicates that airway resistance has increased. Since volume stays the same, an increased pressure represents a decrease in compliance (compliance = vol/press).
5. D. The PWP is normally 4–12 mm Hg (it is not measured in cm H_2O).
6. C. Mixed venous PO_2 is most indicative of tissue oxygenation status because if it is abnormally low, it means that oxygen demand is greater than supply; if it is too high, it means that the tissues are not able to use the oxygen that is delivered to them (cyanide poisoning).
7. B. Because the RR is 44 with a normal $PaCO_2$, there must be abnormally high deadspace ventilation. A PaO_2 of 40 mm Hg on .70 FIO_2 indicates refractory hypoxemia. To be able to make a statement that the patient is hyperventilating, the $PaCO_2$ would have to be decreased; at this point, we can only say that the patient is tachypneic.
8. A. A pulmonary artery catheter is necessary to assess arterial minus venous oxygen content difference because this is the only way to get mixed venous PO_2. Normal value is 5 vol%. If cardiac output decreases, CaO_2 will decrease, and vice versa.
9. A. As shunt (perfusion without ventilation) increases, the difference between arterial and venous oxygen content will be less, because the blood is not being oxygenated.
10. D. As the body's need for oxygen goes up (demand increases), reserves will be used from the venous system, and $C\bar{v}O_2$ will decrease. This will result in a widened $C(a\text{-}\bar{v})O_2$.
11. A. As C.O. decreases, the body will extract more oxygen from the venous reserve. This will result in a decreased $P\bar{v}O_2$, and an increased $C(a\text{-}\bar{v})O_2$.
12. C. As volume in the LV increases, pressure will increase. This increased LV diastolic pressure will be reflected in the PWP.
13. C. Compliance is decreased because both peak and plateua pressures have increased and V_T has remained constant. Airway resistance has also decreased. To calculate airway resistance, use the following formula: (PIP – Plateau pressure)/Flow. Remember to change flow to L/sec (divide ventilator flow by 60). In this example, (48 – 26)/.66 L/sec = 22/.66 = 33.3 cm H_2O/(L/sec) at 1:00. At 2:00, (61 – 47)/1.08 L/sec = 14/1.08 = 12.96.
14. B. Because the peak pressure has increased, while the plateau pressure has remained the same. This indicates that there is no problem with the lung itself; the problem must be an upper airway one (bronchospasm, obstruction). A leak would cause a decrease in pressure.
15. B. The CVP catheter sits in the RA to reflect RV filling pressure. In the event that the patient has ischemia, cor pulmonale, or valve defects, the pressure in the LV will not be the same as the pressure in the RV.
16. D. All of the parameters listed can be measured with a five-channel PA catheter. The mixed venous saturation is available only on certain brands.
17. B. A dramatic, sudden increase in PWP indicates that something is wrong with the left heart (remember that PWP is an indication of LV function).
18. A. $P_{ET}CO_2$ is often used as an estimation of $PaCO_2$, usually to observe trending.
19. B. When CO_2 is depleted quickly, the effect may be seizure activity.
20. D. Chronic hypoxia and acidemia cause vasoconstriction, which leads to increased PA pressures and PVR. Pulmonary embolus increases PVR because it represents an obstruction to blood flow.
21. C. Patients who are hypovolemic are also hypotensive and hypoxemic, and will change over to anaerobic metabolism (lactic acidosis) because the tissues are not getting enough oxygen.
22. B. Protein malnutrition and hepatic failure lead to hypoproteinemia; parenteral feedings and N/G tubes are utilized to prevent it.
23. C. Normal colloid osmotic pressure (the force that tends to move fluid out of the capillary) is 16 mm Hg. Too much fluid is leaking out of the capillary, most likely as a result of hypervolemia. Protein level is normal.
24. B. Based on both PaO_2 and $PaCO_2$, mechanical ventilation is indicated.
25. A. Plasma protein level is decreased (nl = 8 g/100 mL). Therefore, hypoproteinemia is probably the cause of this patient's pulmonary edema.
26. C. Patients who have had an M.I., those with valve defects, increased PVR, or cor pulmonale have differing pressures in their right and left ventricles due to disease. In all of these patients, CVP may not be used to estimate LV function.
27. C. $(\dot{Q}_T)$ $[C(a\text{-}\bar{v})O_2]$ is the formula for determination of oxygen consumption.
28. D. Increased RR without hyperventilation (decreased $PaCO_2$ levels) indicates deadspace ventilation.
29. D. Both vagal stimulation and hypoxia may cause bradycardia.
30. B. CaO_2, $P(A\text{–}a)O_2$, and $C\bar{v}O_2$ are needed in order to calculate intrapulmonary shunt.

31. B. Sodium is normal (135–144 mEq/L); potassium is elevated (normal = 3.5–5.5 mEq/L).
32. B. If a volume less than normal is inserted into the balloon port, and a wedge is obtained, the RCP can assume that it has floated into the periphery and should be pulled back (making sure the balloon is deflated).
33. C. $SVR = \frac{\text{Mean arterial BP} - \text{CVP}}{\text{Cardiac Output}} \times 80$

    Mean arterial pressure can be calculated as follows: $(S + 2D)/3$
34. D. $PVR = \frac{\text{Mean PA pressure} - \text{PWP}}{\text{C.O.}} \times 80$
35. A. SVR is elevated (normal 770–1500 dyne sec/cm^{-5}), which means that the LV is working against too much resistance. Vasodilators are indicated. PVR is normal (20–120 dyne sec/cm^{-5}). Cardiac output is within normal range (4–8 L/min), so positive inotropic agents are unnecessary.
36. D. A PCWP of 33 mm Hg indicates full-blown pulmonary edema.
37. B. When hemodynamic data is being collected, the patient should be supine with the transducer at heart level.
38. B. First, convert the PEEP to mm Hg (divide by 1.36), and divide by two. Next, apply the following formula: Measured PWP–PEEP value that has been converted to mm Hg and halved.

H. Modify Therapy/Make Recommendations Based on Patient's Response

Questions in this category are designed to assess the candidate's ability to make necessary modifications in therapeutic procedures based on patient response. This content category is a logical extension of the previous one, in which the practitioner was asked to assess the patient's response to therapy. Now, having made his or her assessment, the respiratory therapy practitioner must modify therapy to achieve a more optimal therapeutic response. This category represents the section on both of the NBRC examinations that contains the greatest percentage of questions.

Entry Level Pretest

According to the NBRC, 15% of the questions on the Entry Level Examination are from the modify therapy content category. In addition, the Composite Examination Matrix states that questions in this category assess the candidate's ability to properly and safely modify all respiratory therapy techniques on a basic level. The following self-study questions were developed from specific competencies listed in the NBRC Composite Examination Matrix.

1. A 69-year-old man with advanced chronic obstructive pulmonary disease is admitted to the emergency department in respiratory distress and considerable confusion. The patient's baseline $Paco_2$ is known to be in excess of 60 mm Hg. The physician wants the respiratory therapy practitioner to place the patient on low concentration oxygen and then draw a blood gas sample. Which of the following would be the *least* advisable means for the respiratory therapy practitioner to administer O_2 to this patient?

   A. One liter via nasal cannula
   B. 24% air entrainment mask
   C. Two liters via nasal cannula
   D. Three liters via nasal cannula

   (1:332–4)

2. The respiratory therapy practitioner is administering 0.5 mL metaproterenol with 2.0 mL normal saline to a 22-year-old asthmatic via hand-held nebulizer. During the treatment, the patient complains of nervousness and anxiety. At this time, the therapist observes that the patient's extremities are extremely tense and are shaking uncontrollably. The therapist should:

   A. Stop therapy and notify the physician
   B. Realize this is a cardiovascular side effect and chart it as such
   C. Stop therapy and administer only half the bronchodilator dose next time
   D. Wait until the patient calms down and then resume therapy

   (7:135–6)

3. The respiratory therapy practitioner is helping transport an apneic patient to the radiology department for a CAT scan. The patient has a tracheostomy tube in place and is being ventilated with a pressure-cycled ventilator. As the patient's transport cart is being pushed onto the elevator, the patient coughs violently, causing the tracheal tube to fall down into the elevator shaft. What action should the respiratory therapy practitioner take at this time?

   A. Run to the nearest nurses' station and call your medical director.
   B. Ventilate the patient in any way possible.
   C. Have an aide get a sterile tube.
   D. Obtain a manual resuscitation unit as rapidly as possible.

   (13:302–7)

4. During the administration of IPPB, the respiratory therapy practitioner observes his patient cough up sputum containing a moderate amount of fresh blood. The therapist should:

   A. Discontinue therapy and chart the results.
   B. Discontinue therapy and notify the physician.

C. Page the physician and inform him that hemoptysis is a contraindication to IPPB.
D. Continue therapy if the patient will agree to it.

(4:90–2)

5. While administering IPPB to a patient with advanced emphysema, the respiratory therapy practitioner observes that the patient is unable to exhale completely following assisted ventilations. The proper therapeutic modification would be to:

A. Review therapeutic instructions with patient.
B. Increase flow rate.
C. Employ expiratory retard device.
D. Decrease cycling pressure.

(2:190–5)

6 While administering IPPB the respiratory therapist notes that the patient's respiratory rate is 25 breaths/min. Which of the following is the proper therapeutic modification?

A. Make no modification.
B. Decrease the flow rate.
C. Decrease the sensitivity.
D. Instruct the patient to pause between each breath.

(4:88–9)

7. The respiratory therapist finds that due to the thickness and tenacity of tracheobronchial secretions, only scant amounts can be aspirated through a patient's orotracheal tube. Which of the following therapeutic modifications may facilitate removal of this patient's secretions?

I. Instilling 5–10 mL of distilled H_2O
II. Flexing the patient's head and neck during attempts
III. Increasing suctioning pressure to 140 mm Hg
IV. Using postural drainage techniques prior to attempts

A. I and IV
B. II and IV
C. III and IV
D. I and II

(7:218)

8. A patient is receiving 40% oxygen via heated aerosol mask following triple vein/coronary artery bypass graft. She is progressing well, and solid foods are ordered as tolerated. To prevent hypoxia the respiratory therapy practitioner would place his/her patient on ___ liters via nasal cannula while eating.

A. 2
B. 3
C. 4
D. 5

(4:129)

9. The respiratory therapy practitioner finds a patient who has a long history of chronic obstructive pulmonary disease who is apparently asleep. At this time, the therapist notes that the patient is being administered 6 L oxygen via cannula. The therapist should immediately:

A. Remove nasal oxygen.
B. Begin to ventilate.
C. Establish unresponsiveness.
D. Establish an airway.

(10:20)

10. A patient on a volume ventilator becomes acutely distressed. The high-pressure alarm is sounding with each breath, and fluctuations in the patient's arterial blood pressure are noted. Which of the following is the most appropriate therapeutic modification at this time?

A. Raise the pressure limit to 80 cm H_2O and check the ventilator for malfunctions.
B. Have a colleague manually ventilate the patient while checking the ventilator circuit for leaks.
C. Manually ventilate the patient while a colleague performs a physical examination.
D. Recommend insertion of a chest tube.

(13:16–26)

11. A respiratory therapist is administering IPPB to a patient who is 3 days post left upper lobectomy. Suddenly the patient complains of sharp chest pains. Rapid physical examination reveals that the left lung field is hyperresonant to percussion and that the trachea has shifted to the right. Which of the following therapeutic modifications must the practitioner make at this time?

A. Terminate therapy and chart the above information.
B. Terminate therapy and have a nurse notify the physician.
C. Terminate therapy and insert a chest tube.
D. Terminate therapy, call for help, and administer supplemental oxygen.

(9:287–9)

12. A patient is receiving continuous flow IMV via a volume ventilator with a 5-L reservoir bag in the system. The mandatory rate is 6 and the patient is not receiving PEEP therapy. During the patient's spontaneous respirations, the therapist notes that the system pressure manometer reads –8 cm H_2O. Based on the above information, the therapist should perform which of the following corrective actions?

A. Increase the continuous flow rate.
B. Increase the sensitivity as well as the continuous flow rate.
C. Decrease the sensitivity.
D. Use a smaller reservoir bag system.

(2:281–3)

13. The arterial blood gases of a patient who is on continuous mechanical ventilation are consistent with respiratory alkalosis. Which of the following is the *least* appropriate corrective action?

A. Switch to IMV.
B. Decrease tidal volume.
C. Sedate patient.
D. Wait for metabolic compensation to occur.

(15:240–1)

14. The respiratory therapist is administering 2.0 mL of 20% acetylcysteine and 2.0 cc distilled water via a pressure-cycled ventilator to a patient with tenacious secretions. During the therapy the patient becomes acutely dyspneic. Audible wheezes are noted throughout both lung fields. The most appropriate recommendation for the respiratory practitioner to make at this time is to:

A. Reduce the length of the treatment.
B. Discontinue this therapy.
C. Reduce acetylcysteine dosage.
D. Add a bronchodilator to the drug therapy.

(7:210–12)

15. The physician orders 0.3 cc metaproterenol diluted to a 1:4 ratio with one-half normal saline and administered every 2 hr to an asthmatic patient. During the second treatment, the pulse is noted to rise from 100 to 135. Based on this information, the respiratory therapy practitioner should:

A. Administer 0.25 cc isoproterenol next treatment.
B. Stop therapy and notify the nurse.
C. Stop therapy and notify the physician.
D. Wait until the pulse returns to baseline and resume therapy.

(7:151–7)

16. IPPB is being administered to a patient via a pressure-cycled ventilator. The therapist notices that the system pressure gauge reads –10 cm H_2O just prior to initiation of the inspiratory phase. The practitioner should make which of the following therapeutic modifications?

A. Increase the flow rate setting.
B. Check for leaks in the high-pressure line.
C. Adjust the pressure magnet and clutch assembly.
D. Increase ventilator sensitivity.

(2:195–7, 235)

17. The respiratory therapist is administering IPPB to a postoperative patient via mouthpiece. During the treatment, the patient is unable to cycle the ventilator off. The most appropriate action(s) would be:

I. Adjust the sensitivity control.
II. Check for a leak in the system.
III. Check exhalation valve function.
IV. Decrease the cycling pressure to 10 cm H_2O.

A. II and III
B. I and III
C. I and II
D. III and IV

(2:195–7, 228–35)

18. The respiratory therapy practitioner is administering oxygen via a partial rebreathing mask. Noting that the reserve bag collapses completely during inspiration, the practitioner should:

A. Replace the one-way valve between the mask and reservoir bag.
B. Tape the ambient entrainment valve shut.
C. Get a blood gas analysis stat.
D. Increase the oxygen flow rate.

(4:125)

19. The respiratory therapy practitioner is to administer oxygen therapy to a patient via simple oxygen mask. After attaching the device, he notices that the humidifier's safety valve repeatedly pops off. The practitioner should make which of the following modifications?

A. Replace the mask with a new one.
B. Tape the valve shut.
C. Leave well enough alone and get a blood gas sample.
D. Realize the oxygen tubing is obstructed and correct the problem.

(2:82; 18:149)

20. Which of the following aerosolized medications would the respiratory therapist be *least* likely to recommend for patients with croup or postextubation laryngeal edema?

A. Racemic epinephrine
B. Corticosteroids
C. Theophylline
D. Phenylephrine

(7:144, 145, 186, 259)

21. For which of the following patients could the respiratory therapy practitioner recommend the use of pressure control ventilation as a means of providing continuous ventilatory support?

A. Those with chronic obstructive pulmonary disease
B. Those with adult respiratory distress syndrome
C. Those with neuromuscular disorders who require long-term ventilatory support
D. Those with increased work of breathing

(15:173–5)

22. For patients with which of the following conditions would the respiratory therapy practitioner *not* recommend postural drainage techniques?

A. Bronchiectasis
B. Empyema
C. Lung abscess
D. Cystic fibrosis

(4:96–9)

23. The respiratory therapy practitioner is monitoring a 65-kg patient with acute neuromuscular disease. Bedside pulmonary function tests reveal the following:

Respiratory rate	44
Vital capacity	430 mL
Negative inspiratory force	12 cm H_2O

Based on the above information, which of the following is the most appropriate recommendation?

A. Administer high concentration oxygen.
B. Do a before and after bronchodilator study.
C. Administer continuous ventilatory support.
D. Administer CPAP.

(9:307–18)

24. Which of the following could the respiratory therapy practitioner recommend as a means of correcting hypocarbia in a patient who is being mechanically ventilated?

A. Decrease inspiratory flow rate.
B. Administer sodium bicarbonate.
C. Add mechanical deadspace.
D. Administer PEEP.

(15:285–6)

25. The respiratory therapy practitioner is instructed to place a patient on the level of PEEP that corresponds to the best cardiovascular function. In so doing the following data are collected on various levels of PEEP:

Level of PEEP	Sao_2	$S\bar{v}o_2$
0	70%	43%
3	72%	46%
6	76%	51%
9	82%	59%
12	84%	63%
15	86%	56%
18	87%	52%

The level of PEEP the therapist should recommend is:

A. 6 cm H_2O
B. 9 cm H_2O
C. 12 cm H_2O
D. 15 cm H_2O

(4:353)

26. Which of the following methods would the respiratory therapy practitioner be *least* likely to recommend to help stabilize the chest wall of a patient with flail chest who also requires continuous ventilatory support?

A. Pharmacologic paralysis and controlled mechanical ventilation
B. IMV with PEEP
C. PEEP
D. NEEP

(9:295–7)

27. Within minutes following extubation, a 45-year-old patient is noted to develop moderate inspiratory stridor. The patient is alert and otherwise in no distress. Which of the following recommendations would be appropriate for the respiratory therapist to make at this time?

I. Perform emergency intubation stat.
II. Administer a continuous cool aerosol.
III. Administer aerosolized decongestants and/or corticosteroids.
IV. Be prepared to reintubate.

A. I and III
B. II and IV
C. I only
D. II, III, and IV

(4:190)

28. A 39-year-old, 50-kg woman is brought to the emergency department following barbiturate overdose. She is comatose and her eyes are fully dilated. The following laboratory data are collected immediately after admission:

FIo_2	0.21
pH	7.19
Pao_2	53 mm Hg
$Paco_2$	74 mm Hg
HCO_3^-	26.2 mEq/L
Base excess	–3.0 mEq/L

Which of the following is the most appropriate recommendation regarding this patient?

A. Place on 3 L oxygen via nasal cannula and administer IPPB.
B. Intubate and place on assist/control with a V_T of 600, a backup rate of 15, and an FIo_2 of 0.30.
C. Intubate and place on a pressure-cycled ventilator with a cycling pressure of 20 cm H_2O.
D. Intubate and place on assist/control with a V_T of 1000, a backup rate of 20, and an FIo_2 of 0.3.

(15:76, 227–39)

29. An alert, 17-year-old patient is scheduled for surgery to repair tendon and ligament damage sustained in a football game. As part of a routine preoperative workup, the following data are gathered:

PaO_2	43 mm Hg
$PaCO_2$	47 mm Hg
pH	7.35
FIO_2	0.21
Respiratory rate	12
Pulse	45
BP	110/60
Temperature	37.4°C

Which of the following should the respiratory therapy practitioner recommend regarding the above data?

A. An electrocardiogram
B. Administration of 6 L oxygen via nasal cannula
C. Repeating the arterial blood gas studies
D. Intubation and continuous mechanical ventilation

(19:173–5)

30. A physician's order reads: "Administer 4 L oxygen via hood." The patient is a 2100-g newborn who was born approximately 1 month preterm. The respiratory therapy practitioner should:

A. Administer therapy as ordered.
B. Obtain a chest roentgenogram.
C. Ask the physician to specify a concentration of oxygen.
D. Refuse to administer therapy.

(14:231)

31. The respiratory therapy practitioner receives an order to administer IPPB every 2 hr to a 33-year-old patient who is recovering from upper abdominal surgery performed approximately 16 hr earlier. During the treatment, the patient consistently achieves tidal volumes in excess of 2.4 L, with a cycling pressure of 15 cm H_2O. Further investigation reveals that the patient's spontaneous vital capacity is 25 cc/kg. Based on this information, which of the following is the most appropriate recommendation?

A. Sustained maximal inspiratory therapy (incentive spirometry) every hour while awake
B. Aerosol therapy followed by postural drainage
C. All respiratory therapy should be discontinued
D. Blow bottles every other day four times a day

(4:94)

32. An order is received to administer incentive spirometry to an 84-year-old woman who is recovering from hip surgery performed 18 hr previously. However, even after thorough instructions, the therapist finds that the patient is unable to accomplish a proper sustained inspiratory maneuver. Further investigation reveals this patient's vital capacity is 12 cc/kg. Based on the above information, which of the following is the most appropriate recommendation?

A. Intubation and administration of CPAP therapy is indicated.
B. Respiratory therapy should be discontinued.
C. Postural drainage and percussion is indicated.
D. IPPB should be administered instead of incentive spirometry.

(4:94)

33. A 25-year-old patient with advanced cystic fibrosis is brought to the emergency department by her parents. She is cyanotic and distressed but is able to protect her airway. She is placed on 3 L oxygen via nasal cannula, and an intravenous line is started. Twenty minutes later arterial blood is analyzed, revealing:

PaO_2	40 mm Hg
$PaCO_2$	90 mm Hg
pH	7.12
Base excess	+8 mEq/L
HCO_3^-	30 mEq/L
Hb concentration	18.9 g/dL

Following consideration of this information, the respiratory therapy practitioner should recommend:

A. Decreasing the liter flow to 1 L/min
B. Placing patient on a 35% air entrainment mask
C. Initiation of continuous mechanical ventilation with an FIO_2 of 0.35
D. Placing the patient on 4 L oxygen via nasal cannula

(15:75–91)

34. Which of the following means of oxygen administration would the respiratory therapy practitioner recommend for a patient who has a carboxyhemoglobin concentration of 30%?

A. Nonrebeathing mask
B. Partial rebreathing mask
C. Simple oxygen mask
D. Nasal cannula

(9:212–13)

35. The physician wants the respiratory therapy practitioner to place the patient on the level of PEEP that corresponds to the best effective static compliance. With the corrected tidal volume held constant, the following data are accumulated:

Level of PEEP	Plateau Pressure
0 cm H_2O	48 cm H_2O
3 cm H_2O	50 cm H_2O
6 cm H_2O	52 cm H_2O
9 cm H_2O	51 cm H_2O
12 cm H_2O	51 cm H_2O
15 cm H_2O	52 cm H_2O
18 cm H_2O	58 cm H_2O
21 cm H_2O	66 cm H_2O

Which of the following levels of PEEP should the respiratory therapist recommend?

A. 15 cm H_2O
B. 12 cm H_2O
C. 9 cm H_2O
D. 18 cm H_2O

(15:40)

36. Which of the following would the respiratory therapy practitioner be *least likely* to recommend to help facilitate the weaning of a patient from mechanical ventilation?

A. Deflation of the tracheal tube cuff during the procedure
B. Not suctioning the patient during weaning attempts
C. Using an FIO_2 10% higher than on the ventilator
D. Positioning the patient in a sitting or semirecumbent position

(15:496–7)

37. A patient with a history of chronic obstructive pulmonary disease is brought to the emergency department after several days of increasing respiratory distress. After a baseline arterial sample is drawn, oxygen is administered via nasal cannula at a flow rate of 2 L/min. Pertinent arterial blood gas data are revealed below:

	Room Air	2 L Oxygen
PaO_2	35 mm Hg	45 mm Hg
$PaCO_2$	75 mm Hg	70 mm Hg
pH	7.24	7.31
HCO_3^-	33 mEq/L	36 mEq/L

Based on the above clinical data, the respiratory therapy practitioner should recommend which of the following changes in this patient's therapy?

A. Increase the oxygen flow to 5 L/min
B. Intubate and place on assist/control with an FIO_2 of 0.35
C. Place on a 28% air entrainment mask
D. Increase oxygen flow to 3 L/min

(9:136–40)

38. A respiratory therapy practitioner receives an order to use postural drainage techniques on a patient who underwent surgery 24 hr previously to repair a cerebral aneurysm. On reviewing the patient's chest roentgenogram the practitioner notes the presence of considerable infiltrates in the right lateral and posterior basal segments. The most appropriate course of action for the respiratory therapy practitioner to take would be to:

A. Drain the affected segments as best as possible while a nurse monitors the patient's arterial blood pressure.
B. Tell the physician that postural drainage is in fact contraindicated for this patient.
C. Refuse to perform the therapy as ordered.
D. Inform the physician of possible hazards and ask for clarification.

(4:99)

Answer Key

1. D. 3 L would deliver approximately 32% oxygen; since this represents the highest FIO_2, it would be the least advisable (higher FIO_2 levels may blunt the patient's hypoxic drive to breathe).
2. A. Treatment should be stopped, and the physician notified. The RCP may suggest lowering the dose or administering a bronchodilator with fewer β_1 effects.
3. B. The RCP's first concern is to ventilate the patient in any way possible. Never go on transport without a manual resuscitator!
4. B. Hemoptysis is *always* a reason for physician consultation; stop the treatment and call.
5. C. Expiratory retard simulates pursed-lip breathing and minimizes air trapping.
6. D. This patient is breathing too fast; RR for IPPB is ideally 6 to 8. Advise the patient to pause between breaths to avoid hyperventilation and dizziness.
7. A. To decrease the viscosity of thick secretions, instill with distilled water or try to loosen them with chest PT prior to suctioning attempts.
8. D. 5 L/min delivers approximately 40% oxygen.
9. C. Establish unresponsiveness before taking any action; the patient may really be asleep.
10. C. Because you are unsure what is causing this patient's distress, assess the patient while a colleague manually ventilates.
11. D. Always terminate treatment and get help if a patient complains of sharp chest pain. Since the RCP probably is not authorized to insert a chest tube (it is clear that the patient has a pneumothorax), oxygen should be delivered until the physician arrives.
12. A. The patient is outdrawing the system; increase the continuous flow rate.
13. B. Respiratory alkalosis (increased pH caused by a decreased $PaCO_2$) means that the patient is hyperventilating. Either the rate or tidal volume should be lowered (but make only one change at a time).
14. D. Wheezing is a complication associated with use of

acetylcysteine; add a bronchodilator to minimize this effect.

15. C. Treatment should be stopped whenever the heart rate increases more than 20% above baseline. Recommend a bronchodilator like albuterol, with less β_1 stimulation.
16. D. The patient is exerting too much effort to get a breath (the pressure should not go below −2 cm H_2O). Increase the sensitivity.
17. A. If a pressure-cycled machine will not cycle off, either there is a leak in the system or the exhalation valve is malfunctioning.
18. D. The reservoir bag should never collapse; it should always remain at least one-third full on maximal inhalation.
19. D. The humidifier's 2 psi pop-off is sounding because there is an obstruction; the tubing is probably kinked. If the tubing is unkinked, and the pop-off continues to sound, replace the humidifier.
20. C. All of the drugs listed have decongestant or anti-inflammatory effects (helpful in treating airway inflammation that occurs with post-extubation laryngeal edema), with the exception of theophylline.
21. D. PCV allows demand flow to occur as the patient inspires, so it may be beneficial for patients with a high work of breathing.
22. B. An empyema is pus in the pleural space, so postural drainage will have no effect on it. The other diseases are characterized by a large amount of sputum production, and represent indications for chest PT.
23. C. Vital capacity and NIF (very low) and high RR indicate that the patient probably cannot sustain his own breathing for very much longer; intubate and mechanically ventilate.
24. C. The addition of mechanical deadspace (usually done in 50 cc increments) will cause the patient to retain CO_2.
25. C. 12 cm H_2O PEEP is accompanied by the smallest difference between arterial and venous oxygen saturation, indicating that the patient is not depleting venous oxygen reserves.
26. D. Negative end expiratory pressure may cause airway collapse and is not indicated.
27. D. Because the patient is in no distress, intubation at this time would be too aggressive. Try the other suggestions first, but always be prepared to intubate.
28. B. ABGs indicate that the patient should be intubated and mechanically ventilated. Tidal volume should be 500–750 cc (10–15 mL/kg); assist control is indicated until the patient "wakes up." This patient will require low levels of oxygen; her hypoxemia is secondary to ventilatory respiratory failure.
29. C. Nothing in this patient's history supports the ABG results. Get another sample; this one is probably venous.
30. C. The concentration of oxygen must be specified; the capability of the hood is 21–100%.
31. A. IS is indicated; the patient has an adequate VC (> 15 cc/kg), and is not a candidate for IPPB.
32. D. Because this patient cannot perform IS, and her VC is low, IPPB is indicated.
33. C. This patient's ABGs indicate that she is in respiratory failure. She needs to be intubated and mechanically ventilated.
34. A. 100% oxygen is indicated; hyperbaric oxygen therapy would bring the carboxyhemoglobin level down even more quickly.
35. B. 15 cm H_2O offers the lowest plateau minus PEEP number. This number, divided into the tidal volume, represents static compliance.
36. A. The cuff should *not* be deflated during weaning attempts; deflation results in inadequate delivery of tidal volume (from IMV, SIMV, or PSV), and may cause secretions pooled above the cuff to enter the patient's lung.
37. D. Oxygenation and ventilation are improving on 2 L, but moderate hypoxemia still exists. Try increasing the flow to 3 L.
38. D. Postural drainage is relatively contraindicated in patients with high intracranial pressure; let the physician know this, and make another suggestion (like the PEP mask, vest therapy, etc.).

Advanced Practitioner Pretest

According to the NBRC, 30% of the questions on the Advanced Practitioner Examination are from the modify therapy content category. In addition, the Composite Examination Matrix states that questions in this category assess the candidate's ability to properly and safely modify all respiratory therapy techniques on an advanced level. The following self-study questions were developed from specific competencies listed in the NBRC Composite Examination Matrix.

1. The respiratory therapist notes that even with proper hyperinflation and hyperoxygenation, a 1650-g newborn repeatedly experiences bradycardia shortly after initiation of tracheal suctioning through a 3.5-mm endotracheal tube. Which of the following therapeutic modifications would be *least* helpful in preventing this side effect?

   A. Use of pulmonary drainage techniques
   B. Lavage with physiologic saline to thin secretions
   C. Administration of sympathomimetics prior to therapy
   D. Use of smaller size suction catheter

   (14:286–9)

2. Which of the following pediatric patients should the respiratory therapy practitioner monitor with great caution because of the danger of oxygen-induced hypoventilation?

   I. Those with infant respiratory distress syndrome
   II. Those with bronchiolitis

III. Those with cystic fibrosis
IV. Those with patent ductus arteriosus
V. Those with bronchial asthma

A. III only
B. II and III
C. III and IV
D. I, II, and V

(9:167–71)

3. The high-pressure alarm of a volume-cycled ventilator is sounding with each breath and the patient is acutely distressed. The respiratory therapist begins manually hyperinflating while a colleague performs a rapid chest physical examination. The practitioner notes that each manual breath takes a great deal of effort and is accompanied by a musical inspiratory note. Severely diminished aeration is noted bilaterally, and tracheal shift is not noted. Which of the following corrective actions should the respiratory therapist perform at this time?

A. Recommend insertion of a chest tube.
B. Retract the airway slightly.
C. Change the airway.
D. Deflate the tracheal tube cuff.

(15:197–8)

4. The respiratory therapy practitioner is asked to place a 90-year-old patient on a volume-cycled ventilator with an FIo_2 of 0.4 following orthopaedic surgery. The following arterial blood gas study was reported on the above FIo_2 with the alert patient in the assist/control mode:

Pao_2	59 mm Hg
$Paco_2$	40 mm Hg
pH	7.43
Base excess	–0.4 mEq/L

Which of the following therapeutic modifications should the respiratory therapy practitioner make at this time?

A. Increase the FIo_2 to 0.6.
B. Place the patient on 5 cm H_2O PEEP.
C. Increase the minute ventilation.
D. No setting changes are indicated.

(19:221)

5. The respiratory therapy practitioner is caring for a patient with myasthenia gravis who is receiving continuous ventilatory support via a volume-cycled ventilator. Because of excessive parasympathetic activity, the volume of secretions above the tracheal tube cuff is usually considerable. Which of the following is the *least* acceptable method of managing these secretions?

A. Instruct the patient to suction his pharynx on a p.r.n. basis.
B. Suction below the cuff, above the cuff, then deflate the cuff and manually sigh the patient to help expel any remaining secretions.
C. Recommend the administration of parasympatholytics.
D. Deflate the endotracheal tube cuff prior to suctioning the trachea.

(13:215–16)

6. A 20-year-old, apneic, 100-kg patient with considerable neurologic trauma sustained in a suicide attempt is brought to the emergency department and immediately placed on a volume ventilator in the control mode (RR-24). The following data were collected half an hour later with an FIo_2 of 0.45:

Pao_2	52 mm Hg
$Paco_2$	30 mm Hg
pH	7.50
HCO_3^-	20 mEq/L
Base excess	–1.4 mEq/L
V_T	900 mL
Respiratory rate	24
Peak flow rate	60 L/min

Which of the following modifications should the respiratory therapy practitioner make at this time?

A. Decrease the tidal volume and increase the RR.
B. Decrease the respiratory rate and add PEEP.
C. Increase the the FIo_2.
D. Add 200 cc mechanical deadspace and increase the FIo_2.

(13:633–40)

7. The physician asks the respiratory therapy practitioner to begin weaning a 50-kg patient who has a vital capacity of 440 mL and a negative inspiratory force of 14 cm H_2O. The patient is currently on a volume ventilator in the assist/control mode. His blood gases on an FIo_2 of 0.4 are as follows:

Pao_2	78 mm Hg
$Paco_2$	34 mm Hg
pH	7.49
HCO_3^-	27.3 mEq/L

The most appropriate modification would be to:

A. Switch the patient to SIMV with a mandatory rate of 5
B. Place the patient on a T tube setup with an FIo_2 of 0.4
C. Switch the patient to SIMV with a mandatory rate of 12
D. Place the patient on a T tube setup with an FIo_2 of 0.5

(13:652–5)

8. The physician writes an order asking the respiratory therapist to make whatever ventilator changes are necessary to keep a 1200-g newborn's arterial blood gases within normal limits. The most recent results show a $Pa{O_2}$ of 42 mm Hg and a $Pa{CO_2}$ of 40 mm Hg on an $FI{O_2}$ of 0.7. Which of the following therapeutic modifications is most appropriate at this time?

A. Increase the PEEP.
B. Increase the $FI{O_2}$.
C. Increase the ventilator rate.
D. Get another blood gas sample.

(14:303–26)

9. Following traumatic nasotracheal intubation, the respiratory therapist notes that a patient is bleeding profusely from upper airway soft tissues. The proper action for the respiratory therapy practitioner to take at this time is to:

A. Page the physician and recommend orotracheal intubation
B. Apply 1:100 epinephrine topically to achieve hemostasis
C. Deflate the cuff periodically and carefully suction blood and secretions
D. Notify the physician, keep the cuff inflated, and suction the pharynx as needed

(3:489–96)

10. The respiratory therapy practitioner is administering continuous ventilatory support to an apneic 70-kg patient. The following information is charted with the patient receiving a tidal volume of 600 cc, an $FI{O_2}$ of 0.5, and a respiratory rate of 14:

$Pa{O_2}$	156 mm Hg
$Pa{CO_2}$	52 mm Hg
pH	7.33
HCO_3^-	26 mEq/L

Which of the following therapeutic modifications should the practitioner make at this time?

A. Decrease the $FI{O_2}$ and increase the tidal volume.
B. Increase the respiratory rate.
C. Increase the tidal volume to 800 cc.
D. Add mechanical deadspace and lower the $FI{O_2}$.

(13:650–2)

11. During tracheal suctioning of a 30-year-old patient, the onset of bigeminal and multifocal premature ventricular contractions is noted on the cardiac monitor. The patient's color becomes ashen and he complains of dizziness. At this time, the respiratory therapy practitioner should take which of the following actions?

A. Lower the suctioning pressure and resume therapy.
B. Page the physician stat.
C. Stop therapy, and ensure ventilation and oxygenation.
D. Let the patient rest and then continue suctioning.

(4:181–2)

12. A spontaneously breathing 55-year-old patient with noncardiogenic pulmonary edema is intubated and placed on a volume ventilator with an $FI{O_2}$ of 0.6 and 5 cm H_2O PEEP. Twenty minutes later the following blood gas and acid-base data are charted:

$Pa{O_2}$	40 mm Hg
$Pa{CO_2}$	36 mm Hg
pH	7.40
HCO_3^-	24.0 mEq/L
Base excess	−1.1 mEq/L

Based on the above information, which of the following ventilator modifications needs to be made at this time?

A. Leave settings unchanged.
B. Increase $FI{O_2}$ to 0.7.
C. Decrease ventilator sensitivity.
D. Increase PEEP to 10 cm H_2O.

(3:826–7)

13. Which of the following modifications could the respiratory therapy practitioner use as a method to reduce condensation of water in the ventilatory circuit of a newborn who is on a Baby Bird ventilator?

A. Using a disposable circuit
B. Decreasing the proximal airway temperature to 32° C
C. Using a heated wire circuit
D. Using a thick-walled, narrow-bore tubing

(14:351, 3)

14. One hour after being placed on a volume ventilator, an apprehensive 68-year-old patient with chronic obstructive pulmonary disease is experiencing ventricular arrhythmias and generalized seizures. Arterial blood gas analysis at this time in the assist/control mode with an $FI{O_2}$ of 0.4 reveals a $Pa{O_2}$ of 62 mm Hg, a $Pa{CO_2}$ of 42 mm Hg, a pH of 7.65, and an HCO_3^- of 34 mEq/L. Which of the following is the correct modification of this patient's respiratory therapy?

A. Add 400 cc mechanical deadspace and pharmacologically paralyze.
B. Adjust ventilator to allow $Pa{CO_2}$ to return to baseline values.
C. Increase the backup rate and administer acetazolamide (Diamox®) to control metabolic alkalosis.

D. Place patient on 5 cm H_2O PEEP and pharmacologically paralyze.

(19:207–8)

15. The respiratory therapist is performing nasotracheal suctioning on a patient in the intensive care unit. Looking at the cardiac monitor, the therapist notes the onset of ventricular tachycardia. Which of the following is the most acceptable sequence of actions?

A. Stop therapy and notify the physician at once.
B. Leave the catheter in place and administer 6–10 L oxygen through it.
C. Call for help, establish an airway, and ensure ventilation with supplemental oxygen.
D. Place patient on nasal oxygen and wait for arrhythmia to subside.

(10:46, 260)

16. After 9 days on continuous ventilatory support in the assist/control mode, a 53-year-old patient regains consciousness. Because of an improving clinical picture, the respiratory therapy practitioner is asked to gather the following data for weaning purposes:

Weight	75 kg
$Pa{O_2}$	96 mm Hg
$Pa{CO_2}$	29 mm Hg
$FI{O_2}$	0.4
pH	7.48
Vital capacity	13 cc/kg
Negative inspiratory force	21 cc/kg
Resting spontaneous minute volume	16 L/min

Based on the above data, which of the following would be the most appropriate recommendation?

A. Place on PSV with an $FI{O_2}$ of 0.7.
B. Add 200 cc deadspace and get an arterial sample.
C. Place on SIMV with an $FI{O_2}$ of 0.4.
D. Place on T tube with an $FI{O_2}$ of 0.6.

(13:652–5)

17. The respiratory therapy practitioner is administering IPPB to a patient in the cardiac care unit when he notes the rhythm on a cardiac monitor shown in Figure 33.

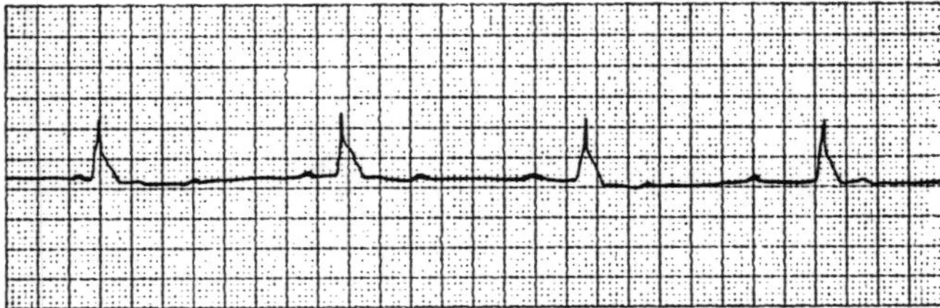

Figure 33.

Which of the following therapeutic modalities should the therapist recommend at this time?

A. Lidocaine
B. Morphine
C. Pacemaker
D. Sodium bicarbonate

(10:133)

18. The respiratory therapist is asked to help correct a neonatal condition in which the $Pa{O_2}$ is 45 mm Hg while breathing 35% oxygen via Isolette. At the same time, a pH of 7.42 and a $Pa{CO_2}$ of 40 mm Hg are noted. Which of the following is to be recommended?

A. Administer 60% oxygen via Isolette.
B. Administer 50% oxygen via hood.
C. Intubate and place on 4 cm H_2O CPAP with an $FI{O_2}$ of 0.5.
D. Administer 100% oxygen via hood

(14:231, 234)

19. A comatose 37-year-old patient is admitted to the emergency department following a suicide attempt involving ingestion of an unknown quantity of secobarbital. The following data are obtained at this time with the patient breathing room air:

$Pa{O_2}$	35 mm Hg
$Pa{CO_2}$	78 mm Hg
pH	7.11
Base excess	−6.8 mEq/L

Based on the above data, which of the following would the respiratory therapy practitioner *not* recommend as part of this patient's management?

A. Continuous ventilatory support
B. Naloxone
C. Supplemental oxygen
D. Emergency airway

(7:390–1)

20. Cardiopulmonary resuscitation is in progress for a 60-year-old patient in the cardiac care unit, and she is being ventilated via manual resuscitator. The monitor shows a fine ventricular fibrillation. Two initial attempts at defibrillation with 200J are unsuccessful in treating this arrhythmia. Which of the following should the advanced respiratory therapy practitioner *not* recommend at this time?

A. Emergency intubation
B. Ventilation with 100% oxygen
C. $NaHCO_3$ administration
D. Additional attempts at defibrillation with 360J

(10:146)

21. A 63-year-old asthmatic who has developed adult respiratory distress syndrome and gram-negative hypotensive shock is placed on volume ventilation with an FIO_2 of 0.6 and 8 cm H_2O PEEP. Subsequently the decision is made to paralyze the patient pharmacologically and control her ventilation. Which one of the following drugs should the therapist recommend to accomplish this goal?

A. Succinylcholine
B. Pancuronium bromide
C. Morphine
D. Sodium pentothol

(15:321)

22. An 18-year-old, 40-kg woman is seen in the intensive care unit 2 days after being found comatose by friends at home. She is on a volume ventilator in the assist/control mode with an FIO_2 of 0.4. Because she has regained consciousness and is fighting the ventilator, the physician asks the respiratory therapist to collect appropriate weaning data. The following information is charted at this time:

PaO_2	88 mm Hg
$PaCO_2$	24 mm Hg
Vital capacity	1760 mL
Negative inspiratory force	58 cm H_2O
pH	7.56

The respiratory therapist would most likely be correct in recommending which of the following?

A. Placing the patient on a T tube system with an FIO_2 of 0.5
B. Sedating the patient to prevent her from fighting the ventilator
C. Placing the patient on IMV with an FIO_2 of 0.4
D. Adding 200 cc mechanical deadspace and obtaining a blood gas analysis

(13:252–5)

23. The respiratory therapy practitioner is monitoring a hemodynamically stable 1200-g (32-week gestation) newborn who is being ventilated by a time-cycled controller in the continuous flow IMV mode. Umbilical arterial blood gases on an FIO_2 of 0.9, a mandatory rate of 20, 3 cm H_2O PEEP, and an I:E ratio of 1:3 are as follows:

PaO_2	40 mm Hg
$PaCO_2$	65 mm Hg
pH	7.20
Base excess	–5.1 mEq/L
HCO_3^-	15.6 mEq/L

Based on the above information, which of the following should the respiratory therapy practitioner recommend?

A. Increase the PEEP and use an I:E ratio of 1:4.
B. Increase the PEEP and the FIO_2.
C. Increase the PEEP and the IMV rate.
D. Increase the FIO_2 and use inverse I:E ratios.

(14:304–6)

24. Which of the following size (I.D.) endotracheal tubes should the respiratory therapy practitioner recommend for an average-size patient who is 8 years old?

A. 4.0 mm
B. 6.0 mm
C. 7.5 mm
D. 8.0 mm
E. 9.0 mm

(14:287)

25. A 30-year-old patient received a vagotomy and partial pyloroplasty 8 days previously. Three days postoperatively, he became septic and was taken back to the operating room to repair a perforated ileum. Since that time he has been on a volume ventilator with high levels of PEEP and FIO_2s of 0.7 or greater. Because of the danger of oxygen toxicity, the pulmonary physician makes the decision to raise the patient's PEEP to 28 cm H_2O and at the same time lower his FIO_2 to 0.5. Concurrent and pertinent information is noted below:

	20 cm H_2O PEEP	28 cm H_2O PEEP
PaO_2	46 mm Hg	46 mm Hg
$S\bar{v}O_2$	57%	47%
$C(a\bar{v})O_2$	3.5 vol%	5.8 vol%
$\dot{Q}_s/\dot{Q}_T$	34%	28%
FIO_2	0.7	0.5
PWP (on ventilator)	6 mm Hg	9 mm Hg
Oxygen consumption	250 mL/min	250 mL/min

Further orders are to leave the FIO_2 at the 0.5 level despite any cardiovascular depression noted at 28 cm H_2O PEEP. At this time, which of the following should the advanced respiratory therapy practitioner recommend to treat this patient's hypoxia?

A. Lower the PEEP to 15 cm H_2O.
B. Raise the PEEP to 30 cm H_2O.
C. Induce hypothermia to lower metabolic demands.
D. Expand intravascular volume.

(5:259)

26. A 12-year-old boy sustains trauma including a long-bone fracture and is admitted to the emergency department in shock. After appropriate fluid resuscitation, he is hemodynamically stable. The chest roentgenogram on admission is unremarkable. Twelve hours later the following data are obtained while the patient is receiving an FIO_2 of 0.6 via T tube setup:

PaO_2	40 mm Hg
$PaCO_2$	27 mm Hg
pH	7.42
HCO_3^-	12 mEq/L
Base excess	−7.4 mEq/L

Based on the above information, which of the following is the most appropriate recommendation?

A. Obtain a stat chest roentgenogram.
B. Place on 5 cm CPAP with an FIO_2 of 0.5.
C. Place on controlled mechanical ventilation with an FIO_2 of 1.0.
D. Place on assist/control with 8 cm H_2O PEEP.

(13:650–5)

27. A 1650-g (33-week gestation) newborn is seen in the nursery 5 hours after an uneventful delivery. The following is noted with the patient breathing room air:

Respiratory rate	75
Pulse	195
Blood pressure	65/35
Expiratory grunt	Audible with stethoscope
Sternal retractions	Some noted
Color	Peripheral cyanosis

Which of the following should the respiratory therapy practitioner recommend at this time?

A. Intubate and place on 2 cm H_2O CPAP.
B. Place patient on 4 cm H_2O nasal CPAP.
C. Place on 60% oxygen via hood.
D. Place on 40% oxygen via Isolette.

(14:227–335)

28. The intern is unable to pass an oral endotracheal tube despite repeated attempts. In desperation, he asks someone to give him the antidote for the succinylcholine he has administered to facilitate tracheal intubation. The respiratory therapist should promptly hand him:

A. Neostigmine
B. Pancuronium bromide (Pavulon)
C. Edrophonium chloride (Tensilon®)
D. A bag-valve-mask unit

(15:321)

29. A 20-year-old, 60-kg patient is seen in the emergency department during a severe asthma attack. The following information is noted at that time with the patient receiving 3 L oxygen via nasal cannula:

PaO_2	60 mm Hg
$PaCO_2$	40 mm Hg
pH	7.34
HCO_3^-	20 mEq/L
Vital capacity	20 cc/kg

Regarding the above information, which is the correct recommendation?

A. The patient should be given intramuscular and aerosolized sympathomimetics and admitted to a medical ward immediately.
B. The patient should be intubated and transferred to the intensive care unit.
C. Isoetharine should be administered via IPPB and the patient sent home.
D. Appropriate bronchodilator and oxygen therapy should be administered and the patient transferred to the intensive care unit.

(9:155–7)

30. A 43-year-old patient is admitted to the progressive care unit with a diagnosis of acute bronchial asthma. On admission, he is ordered "IPPB every 2 to 3 hours while awake and p.r.n. at night with 0.3 cc metaproterenol." Because of the complaint that this therapy is not providing significant benefit, his physician asks the respiratory therapy practitioner to recommend methods to evaluate therapeutic effectiveness. Which of the following will provide the physician with the information he needs when the patient is monitored both before and after therapy?

I. FEV_1%/FVC
II. Pulse
III. Forced vital capacity
IV. Blood pressure
V. Chest physical findings

A. I, IV, and V
B. I, II, and IV
C. I, III, and V
D. I only

(13:586–94)

31. Which of the following delivered energy settings should the respiratory therapy practitioner recommend for initial attempts at defibrillation when performed on adult patients?

A. 200 J
B. 300 J
C. 400 J
D. 1–4 J/kg

(10:146)

32. The respiratory therapy practitioner is monitoring a hemodynamically stable 1100-g newborn who is being ventilated with a conventional time-cycled controller in the continuous flow IMV mode. Umbilical arterial blood gases on an FIO_2 of 0.7 and 4 cm H_2O PEEP, a mandatory rate of 15, and an I:E of 1:3.5 are as follows:

PaO_2	41 mm Hg
$PaCO_2$	38 mm Hg
pH	7.32
Base excess	–4.8
HCO_3^-	15.9 mEq/L

Based on the above information, which of the following is the most appropriate recommendation?

A. Increase the PEEP to 6 cm H_2O.
B. Increase the FIO_2 to 1.0 and decrease mandatory rate.
C. Decrease the PEEP and increase the mandatory rate.
D. Place on high-frequency jet ventilation.

(14:324–44)

33. Following a gunshot wound to the head, a 16-year-old patient develops adult respiratory distress syndrome and requires continuous ventilatory support, PEEP, and high concentrations of oxygen. Six days later the patient is still comatose. A resolving radiologic picture and improving effective static compliance are indications for the following blood gas study drawn with an FIO_2 of 0.4 and 10 cm H_2O PEEP:

PaO_2	148 mm Hg
$PaCO_2$	35 mm Hg
pH	7.46
HCO_3^-	24.8 mEq/L
Ventilator mode	Assist/control

Which of the following should the respiratory therapist recommend at this time?

A. Place on SIMV.
B. Decrease the backup rate.
C. Decrease the PEEP to 6 cm H_2O.
D. Decrease the FIO_2 to 0.3.

(13:267–70)

34. The respiratory therapy practitioner is performing tracheal suctioning on a patient in the intensive care unit when he notes the rhythm shown in Figure 34 on the cardiac monitor:

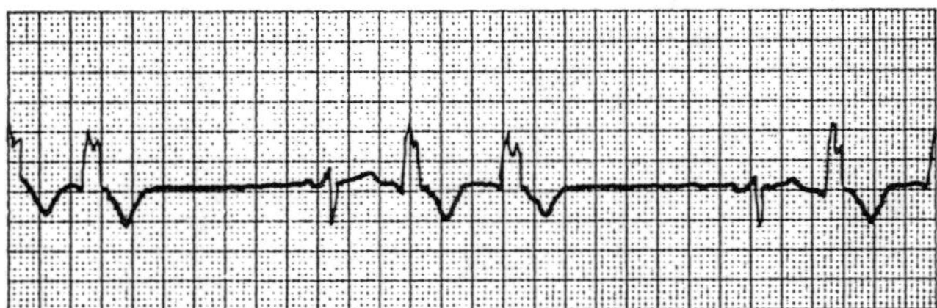

Figure 34.

Which of the following therapeutic modalities should the practitioner recommend at this time?

A. Epinephrine
B. Defibrillation with 360 J
C. Lidocaine
D. Intubation and mechanical ventilation

(10:185)

35. A severely distressed patient is removed from a volume-cycled ventilator and manually ventilated while a physical examination is performed. Dullness to percussion is noted over the right lung field and hyperresonance is present on the left. Additionally, the trachea and the apical pulse are noted to be shifted to the right. Based on the above information, the RCP should:

A. Insert a chest tube
B. Advance the endotracheal tube slightly
C. Recommend insertion of a chest tube
D. Recommend reinsertion of the endotracheal tube

(13:30, 661–2)

36. Which of the following should the respiratory therapist recommend on the basis of noting that a patient has a $PaCO_2$ of 40 mm Hg and a $P_{ET}CO_2$ of 30 mm Hg?

A. Continuous ventilatory support
B. Incentive spirometry
C. No therapy is indicated
D. Oxygen therapy

(13:601–3)

37. A patient is seen in the cardiac care unit while receiving continuous mechanical ventilation. Pertinent clinical data are presented below:

PaO_2	84 mm Hg
$PaCO_2$	40 mm Hg
pH	7.54
Base excess	+8.6 mEq/L
Na^+	145 mEq/L
Cl^-	74 mEq/L
K^+	2.9 mEq/L
Total CO_2	34 mEq/L

Which of the following should the respiratory therapist recommend to treat the above acid-base abnormality?

A. Add mechanical deadspace.
B. Administer NH_4Cl.
C. Administer acetazolamide.
D. Administer KCl.

(17:211–12)

38. For which of the following newborns would the respiratory therapy practitioner be *most* likely to recommend the use of nasal CPAP prongs?

A. Those with a cleft palate
B. Those with bilateral choanal artresia
C. Those who weigh less than 1200 grams
D. Those who weigh more than 1200 grams

(14:279–82)

39. A 14-year-old is brought to the emergency department following an automobile accident. The paramedics say that the patient's legs were on fire when they arrived. He is comatose, cyanotic, and noted to have very weak respiratory efforts. Carotid pulses are palpable, and a blood pressure of 60/20 is obtained. Gross observation reveals extensive thoracic and abdominal trauma from which there is considerable bleeding. Based on the above information, which of the following must be performed first in order to save the patient's life?

A. Control hemorrhage immediately.
B. Administer 50 mEq $NaHCO_3$ stat.
C. Establish an airway.
D. Check pupil response to light.

(10: Chap 1)

40. A 32-year-old man is brought to the emergency department in a coma. The following blood gas results are noted at this time with the patient breathing room air:

Pao_2	104 mm Hg
$Paco_2$	18 mm Hg
pH	7.09
Base excess	–18 mEq/L
HCO_3^-	4 mEq/L

Based on the above data, which of the following is (are) appropriate therapeutic recommendations?

I. Intubate and place on 10 cm H_2O CPAP.
II. Monitor vital signs.
III. Place on 8 L O_2 via simple oxygen mask.
IV. Intubate and place on 5 cm H_2O PEEP.
V. Place an oropharyngeal airway.

A. I and II
B. II and IV
C. III only
D. II and V

(1:461–3)

41. Which of the following methods is (are) recommended to improve cardiac performance?

I. Administering negative inotropic agents
II. Optimizing venous return
III. Increasing left ventricular afterload

A. I and III
B. II only
C. II and III
D. III only

(5:257–8)

42. A 72-year-old patient with a long history of chronic obstructive pulmonary disease is brought to the emergency department following several days of increasing respiratory distress. Arterial blood gas analysis is performed on room air and 2 L nasal oxygen. These data appear below:

	Room Air	2 L Oxygen
Pao_2	35 mm Hg	45 mm Hg
$Paco_2$	75 mm Hg	78 mm Hg
pH	7.21	7.30
HCO_3^-	31 mEq/L	38 mEq/L
Base excess	+6 mEq/L	+13 mEq/L

Based on the above data, which is the most appropriate therapeutic recommendation?

A. Place on a 28% air entrainment mask.
B. Intubate and support ventilation with an FIo_2 of 0.3.
C. No change in therapy is indicated.
D. Increase oxygen liter flow to 3 L/min.

(9:136–8)

43. Which of the following could the respiratory therapy practitioner safely recommend for emergency treatment of acute congestive heart failure?

I. 100% oxygen administration
II. Norepinephrine administration
III. Administration of diuretics
IV. KCl administration

A. I and III
B. II and III
C. I and IV
D. I, III, and IV

(5:324–5)

44. The respiratory therapy practitioner is monitoring a patient who has the following serum laboratory values:

Sodium	125 mEq/L
Chloride	85 mEq/L
Potassium	5.0 mEq/L
Total osmolality	255 mOsmol/L

Which of the following should the respiratory therapy practitioner recommend at this time?

A. KCl
B. NaCl
C. 15 g albumin
D. Diuretic

(17:210–13)

45. The respiratory therapy practitioner is monitoring a patient who has the following serum laboratory values:

Sodium	140 mEq/L
Chloride	105 mEq/L
Potassium	5.0 mEq/L
Blood sugar	400 mg%

Based on the above information, which of the following is the most appropriate recommendation?

A. Mannitol administration
B. KCl
C. 10% dextrose with 0.9% NaCl
D. Insulin administration

(17:210–13)

46. The respiratory therapy practitioner would recommend the use of a fenestrated tracheostomy tube for which of the following reasons?

I. To prevent aspiration of oropharyngeal secretions
II. To assist in tracheostomy tube weaning
III. To provide for better upper airway humidification
IV. To force the patient to ventilate via upper airway

A. II and IV
B. I and IV
C. I and II
D. III and IV

(1:477–8)

47. Tracheostomy buttons may be recommended for all but which one of the following purposes?

A. To wean patients with tracheostomies
B. To maintain stoma patency
C. To provide continuous ventilatory support
D. To ensure a patent suction port

(1:478–80)

48. A COPD patient is receiving 80% helium/20% oxygen therapy via nonrebreather. If the desired flow rate is 12 L/min, what is the actual flow rate that should be set on a standard oxygen flowmeter?

A. 7 L
B. 10 L
C. 12 L
D. 18 L

(1:294–5)

49. An ICU patient diagnosed with ARDS is on a mechanical ventilator in the pressure control mode. Which of the following is the *least* appropriate setting for pressure control ventilation?

A. High respiratory rates
B. Low control pressure
C. Inverse I:E ratio
D. High levels of PEEP

(1:523–4)

50. A patient diagnosed with obstructive sleep apnea has been prescribed CPAP at a level of 12 cm H_2O. After 4 weeks of this therapy, the patient still complains of daytime somnolence and morning headaches. Reevaluation in the sleep lab reveals dysrhythmias, desaturation, and apneic periods every 10–15 min. What therapy should the RCP recommend?

A. Increased level of CPAP
B. Chest cuirass
C. BiPAP®
D. Intubation and mechanical ventilation

(14:437)

51. An HIV-positive patient has been receiving outpatient pentamidine treatments for the past 2 days. During each treatment, the patient develops a persistent cough with expiratory wheeze. What should the RCP suggest at this time?

A. Administer a bronchodilator with the pentamidine treatment.
B. Administer a bronchodilator before the pentamidine treatment.
C. Administer half the dose of pentamidine.
D. Monitor the patient for 3 more days to see if the side effects continue.

(7:290–3)

52. A mechanically ventilated infant with severe RSV has been ordered to receive ribavirin therapy via the small particle aerosol generator (SPAG). Which of the following problems is least likely to occur?

A. Expiratory valve occlusion
B. Occlusion of the endotracheal tube
C. Occlusion of the patient interface
D. Occlusion of expiratory sensors

(7:301–3)

53. Which category of bronchodilator may contribute to dehydration in the COPD patient?

A. Sympathomimetics
B. Parasympatholytics
C. Xanthines
D. Corticosteroids

(7:437)

54. The RCP would be *least* likely to recommend surfactant therapy for which of the following conditions?

A. COPD
B. Pneumonia

C. ARDS
D. IRDS

(7:237)

55. Which of the following recommendations is most effective for the patient who wishes to stop smoking?

A. Hypnosis
B. Nicotine patch with behavior modification
C. Aversive conditioning
D. Acupuncture

(12:134–6)

Answer Key

1. C. Administration of a bronchodilator prior to suctioning would not be expected to minimize bradycardia.
2. A. Cystic fibrosis is the only obstructive disease process listed. Only CF patients may be expected to breathe on a hypoxic drive.
3. D. The tube cuff may have herniated over the end of the tube, blocking airflow and causing the high-pressure alarm to sound. The patient is distressed because he is not receiving adequate tidal volume.
4. D. No changes are necessary; Pa_{O_2} is normal for a 90-year-old (Pa_{O_2} decreases about 1 mm Hg/year from age 60 to 90).
5. D. Never deflate the cuff prior to suctioning; secretions pooled here will drain into the lung.
6. B. The Pa_{CO_2} is too low; drop the rate (it's on the high side at 24). This patient is moderately hypoxemic; add PEEP so you don't run the risk of oxygen toxicity.
7. C. Switch the patient to SIMV to begin weaning. Because his NIF is not great, support him initially at a RR of 12.
8. A. Because the patient's Pa_{O_2} is so low on an FI_{O_2} of .70 (refractory), try increasing the PEEP.
9. D. Notify the physician to assess the bleeding, keep the cuff inflated so that the blood is not aspirated, and suction the pharynx as needed.
10. A. Decrease the FI_{O_2} and increase the tidal volume; 600 cc is inadequate for a 70-kg patient.
11. C. Stop suctioning, administer oxygen, and ventilate if necessary.
12. D. This patient is still severely hypoxemic; increase the PEEP level.
13. C. Use of a heated wire circuit minimizes condensation in the ventilator tubing, and also requires it to be changed less often.
14. B. This patient's CO_2 levels have been reduced too quickly, and too much; allow the Pa_{CO_2} to return to baseline values.
15. C. In the event that v-tach occurs, the RCP should call for help, establish an airway, and ensure ventilation with supplemental oxygen.
16. C. Place this patient on SIMV to begin weaning; he is not hypoxemic, so high concentration of O_2 is not indicated.
17. C. This rhythm is third degree heart block; put in a pacemaker.
18. B. Increase the FI_{O_2}, and try an oxyhood to assure more consistent oxygen delivery. Each time patient care is performed on a baby in an isolette, the FI_{O_2} potentially drops.
19. B. Naloxone is indicated to reverse the effects of narcotics, not babiturates.
20. C. No indication for bicarb administration exists.
21. B. Pancuronium bromide is longer-acting than succinylcholine; the other choices are not paralyzing agents.
22. A. Ventilatory parameters are good; this patient can likely support her own ventilation. Try a T-piece before extubating.
23. C. Increase the PEEP to get the Pa_{O_2} up; increase the rate to lower Pa_{CO_2}.
24. B. An average size 8-year-old should have a size 6.0 mm ET tube.
25. D. By giving the patient fluids, his cardiac output may increase. This will hopefully prevent him from using his venous oxygen reserves, and improve oxygenation to the tissues.
26. D. This patient is hyperventilating and is suffering from severe hypoxemia. Add PEEP, and assist his ventilation.
27. D. The baby is probably hypoxic; administer 40% via Isolette and reassess.
28. D. There is no antidote for succinylcholine; give him/her a bag/mask! It will wear off in 2–10 min.
29. D. Give the patient bronchodilator and oxygen therapy; transfer him to the intensive care unit.
30. C. In order to assess ventilatory improvement, measure FEV_1/FVC%, FVC, and perform chest physical assessment for percussion note, wheezing, etc.
31. A. The respiratory therapy practitioner should recommend 200 joules for initial attempts at defibrillation for adult patients.
32. A. Increase the PEEP to treat the hypoxemia.
33. C. Begin weaning the patient from PEEP because the Pa_{O_2} is high.
34. C. Lidocaine is the standard treatment for significant ventricular ectopy.
35. C. Recommend chest tube insertion to treat the pneumothorax.
36. C. Don't recommend anything; these are normal values.
37. D. Potassium and chloride levels are both low (3.5–5.5 mEq/L; 95–105 mEq/L, respectively). Administer KCl.
38. C. Nasal CPAP is indicated in the newborn (newborns are obligate nose breathers) who weighs > 1200 grams.
39. C. The order of importance is airway, breathing, circulation.
40. D. An oropharyngeal will establish an airway; the comatose patient tolerates this type of airway. Be alert for possible deterioration of vital signs.

41. B. Optimization of venous return will improve cardiac performance by preventing hypovolemia.
42. D. Increase the liter flow to 3 in an effort to increase the Pa_{O_2}.
43. A. CHF may be treated with 100% oxygen (to decrease myocardial work) and diuretics (to increase the efficiency of the ventricles).
44. D. Patient suffers from sodium, potassium and chloride depletion. BUN is low (normal = 9–25 mg/L); don't give diuretics.
45. D. All levels are normal except the markedly elevated blood sugar. This patient needs insulin.
46. A. fenestrated trach tubes will make it easier to wean the patient, and will force the patient to use his/her upper airway to breathe.
47. C. Continuous mechanical ventilation cannot be provided through a tracheostomy button!
48. A. Divide by the He/O_2 correction factor: 12/1.8 = 7 L.
49. D. Reduced PEEP levels (<10 cm H_2O) and inflation pressures are used with PCV, while still increasing mean airway pressures.
50. C. BiPAP is often used successfully in patients with obstructive sleep apnea who cannot tolerate high levels of CPAP.
51. B. To minimize the side effect of wheezing, administer a bronchodilator before the pentamidine treatment.
52. C. Occlusion of the patient interface has not been reported; it's large enough that occlusion is highly unlikely.
53. C. Xanthines have a diuretic effect and are similar to caffeine in structure, benefits, and side effects.
54. A. Surfactant therapy is not indicated for COPD.
55. B. The nicotine patch with behavior modification is associated with the greatest success rate of the choices listed.

I. Perform Cardiopulmonary Resuscitation (Entry Level Only)

According to the NBRC, this content category is assessed only on the Entry Level Examination. Questions in this category are designed to assess the candidate's ability to initiate, conduct, or modify basic cardiopulmonary and respiratory therapy techniques in an emergency setting.

According to the NBRC, 3.6% of the questions on the Entry Level Examination are from the initiate cardiopulmonary resuscitation content category. In addition, the Composite Examination Matrix states that questions in this category assess the candidate's ability to perform the following related tasks:

1. Recognize the need for emergency resuscitation.
2. Call for help.
3. Establish a patent airway.
4. Use mouth-to-mouth, bag-mask, and/or mouth-to-valve mask ventilation.
5. Perform external cardiac compressions.
6. Check pulse.
7. Provide supplemental oxygen.
8. Observe chest excursion.
9. Recommend obtaining an arterial blood gas sample.

The following self-study questions were developed from the NBRC Composite Examination Matrix.

1. The respiratory therapy practitioner is treating a patient who is in a Stryker frame because of trauma involving the cervical spine. During therapy the patient becomes apneic. Which of the following methods should the therapist employ to establish a patent airway?

   A. Place head in "sniffing" position.
   B. Flex head slightly.
   C. Use a modified jaw thrust maneuver.
   D. Hyperextend head and neck.

   (10: Chap 10)

2. According to the American Heart Association, the condition of pulselessness in an infant victim can best be assessed by palpating which of the following pulses?

   A. Apical
   B. Carotid
   C. Pedal
   D. Femoral

   (13:297)

3. All but which one of the following are part of the procedure for relieving upper airway obstruction in the unconscious infant?

   A. Back blows
   B. Heimlich maneuver
   C. Chest thrusts
   D. Attempts to ventilate

   (13:299)

4. Which of the following statements regarding rescue breathing in the infant respiratory arrest victim is (are) true?

   I. The rate should be 25/min.
   II. Hyperextension of the head and neck is recommended.
   III. Gastric distention is a known hazard.

   A. I and III
   B. II only
   C. I, II, and III
   D. III only

   (13:299)

5. The respiratory therapy practitioner finds a patient with advanced chronic obstructive pulmonary disease who has apparently fallen asleep while receiving IPPB. The patient does not respond to being shaken. After calling for help, the therapist should immediately:

A. Check the patient's FIO_2
B. Open the airway
C. Give two slow breaths
D. Give four slow breaths

(13:299)

6. During the performance of cardiopulmonary resuscitation, which of the following is believed to be a contraindication to external cardiac compressions?

A. Fracture of three or more ribs
B. Development of tension pneumothorax
C. Presence of a carotid pulse
D. Fracture of the sternum

(10: Chap 1)

7. Which of the following statements regarding external cardiac compression in the adult victim is (are) true?

I. The single rescuer rate is 80–100/min.
II. The midportion of the sternum should be depressed.
III. The recommended compression depth is 1½ to 2 inches.

A. II and III
B. I, II, and III
C. I only
D. I and III

(13:299)

8. According to the American Heart Association, the proper rate for external cardiac compressions in the newborn is:

A. 60/min
B. 80/min
C. 100/min
D. 120/min

(13:299)

9. Which of the following is most consistent with a diagnosis of partial airway obstruction with poor gas exchange?

A. Marked sternal and intercostal retractions without air movement
B. Weak cough, inspiratory stridor, and cyanosis
C. Inability of rescuer to ventilate after opening the airway
D. Inspiratory stridor, effective cough, and a complaint of "sore throat"

(10: Chap 1)

10. Abdominal thrusts are generally *not* recommended as part of the procedure to relieve complete airway obstruction in which of the following patients?

I. Infants
II. Children
III. Conscious victims
IV. Pregnant victims
V. Obese victims

A. I and III
B. II and III
C. I, IV, and V
D. II, III, IV, and V

(13:299)

11. According to the American Heart Association, which of the following is the most effective technique for administering external cardiac compressions to a newborn?

A. Two fingers placed on the lower third of the sternum
B. One finger placed midsternum
C. Two thumbs placed midsternum with the hands encircling the chest
D. Two fingers placed midsternum

(13:299)

12. According to the American Heart Association, during cardiopulmonary resuscitation, properly performed cardiac compressions will result in a carotid artery blood flow that is approximately what percentage of normal?

A. 10–20
B. 15–25
C. 25–30
D. 40–50

(13:296)

13. The respiratory therapy practitioner has just delivered two slow breaths to an unconscious and apneic adult patient. Now, while carefully palpating the area between the thyroid cartilage and the sternocleidomastoid muscle, he feels a weak but distinct carotid pulse. The practitioner should:

A. Spend another 5 sec palpating the pulse
B. Begin rescue breathing at a rate of 16/min
C. Begin external cardiac compressions
D. Begin rescue breathing at a rate of 12/min

(13:299)

14. The respiratory therapy practitioner is assisting in the delivery of a 2000-gram (34-week gestation) newborn. At approximately 1 min postpartum the following vital signs are noted:

Heart rate	90 beats/min
Respirations	Absent
Muscle tone	Flaccid
Reflex irritability	Absent
Color	Central cyanosis

Based on the above information, what is the proper therapeutic recommendation?

A. Suction the pharynx: dry patient and place under radiant heat warmer.
B. Place patient on nasal CPAP of 10 cm H_2O.
C. Suction upper airway and ventilate with 100% oxygen via bag-valve-mask unit.
D. Hyperoxygenate, intubate, and ventilate with 100% oxygen.

(14:37, 55–9)

15. Which of the following represents the concentration of oxygen in expired gas during performance of mouth-to-mouth resuscitation?

A. 7–9%
B. 10–12%
C. 14–17%
D. 16–19%

(13:294)

Answer Key

1. C. Use a modified jaw thrust maneuver to establish a patent airway in a patient with cervical spine injury.
2. D. Palpate the brachial or femoral artery of an infant; their short, fat neck makes carotid artery palpation difficult.
3. B. The Heimlich maneuver is not part of the procedure for relieving upper airway obstruction in the unconscious infant.
4. C. RR should be 20/min. Gastric distension is a known hazard of rescue breathing.
5. C. Give 2 slow breaths to the unconscious adult who is not breathing.
6. C. Only the presence of a carotid pulse is a contraindication to chest compressions; all other complications are treatable.
7. A. Depress the lower half of the sternum; other statements are correct.
8. C. The proper rate for external cardiac compressions in the newborn is at least 100/min.
9. B. Weak cough, inspiratory stridor, and cyanosis characterizes partial airway obstruction.
10. C. Abdominal thrusts are generally *not* recommended as part of the procedure to relieve complete airway obstruction in infants or obese or pregnant victims; use chest thrusts instead.
11. A. Two or three fingers placed on the lower third of the sternum is the method of choice for performing cardiac compressions on an infant.
12. C. Properly performed cardiac compressions will result in a carotid artery blood flow that is approximately 25–30% of normal.
13. D. Begin rescue breathing at a rate of 10–12/min.
14. D. APGAR = 1; intubate, ventilate, and hyperoxygenate.
15. D. There is 16–19% oxygen in expired gas.

J. Perform Emergency Procedures (Advanced Level Only)

According to the NBRC, this content category is assessed only on the Advanced Level Examination. Questions in this category are designed to assess the candidate's ability to initiate, conduct, or modify basic cardiopulmonary and respiratory therapy techniques in an emergency setting.

According to the NBRC, 7% of the questions on the Advanced Level Examination are from this content category. In addition, the Composite Examination Matrix states that questions in this category assess the candidate's ability to perform the following related tasks:

1. Initiate ECG monitoring.
2. Observe pupillary size and reactivity.
3. Recommend administration of bicarbonate.
4. Recommend defibrillation.
5. Perform endotracheal intubation.
6. Recommend capnography to confirm adequacy of CPR.
7. Participate in land/air patient transport.
8. Recommend instillation of medication through the endotracheal tube.

The following self-study questions were developed from the NBRC Composite Examination Matrix.

1. All but which of the following are necessary in order to perform oral endotracheal intubation?

A. Laryngoscope
B. Magill forceps
C. Flexible stylet
D. Oxygen source

(13:309–10)

2. The RCP has initiated capnography in order to determine adequacy of cardiac compressions. Optimal performance would be characterized by which of the following?

A. $P_{ET}CO_2 > 15$ torr
B. $P_{ET}CO_2 < 15$ torr
C. Extended phase I
D. B and C

(13:603)

3. ECG monitoring would be *least* important in which of the following circumstances?

   A. Cardiac arrest
   B. Post cardiac arrest
   C. Pulmonary function testing
   D. Stress testing

   (13:317–8)

4. Which of the following condition(s) calls for defibrillation?

   A. Ventricular tachycardia with pulse
   B. Pulseless ventricular tachycardia
   C. Ventricular fibrillation
   D. B and C

   (13:319–20)

5. Which of the following drugs can be instilled through the endotracheal tube?

   I. Atropine
   II. Epinephrine
   III. Lidocaine
   IV. Phenylephrine

   A. I, II, III, and IV
   B. II, III, and IV
   C. I, II, and III
   D. I, III, and IV

   (13:325)

6. Which of the following are guidelines for endotracheal tube medication infusion?

   I. Drug dose is the same as IV dose.
   II. Drug should be diluted in 10 cc of normal saline.
   III. Instillation should be immediately followed by delivery of several large breaths.
   IV. Chest compressions should continue uninterrupted throughout the process.

   A. I, II, III, and IV
   B. II, III, and IV
   C. I, II, and IV
   D. II and III

   (13:325)

7. All but which of the following are true about the administration of sodium bicarbonate?

   A. It is a first-line drug during CPR.
   B. It inhibits the release of oxygen.
   C. It does not improve survival rates when given during CPR.
   D. The initial dose given is 1 mEq/kg.

   (13:332–3)

8. Which of the following statements about pupillary size is correct?

   A. Dilated pupils indicate satisfactory cerebral perfusion.
   B. Constricted pupils indicate satisfactory cerebral perfusion.
   C. Pupils become nonreactive 30 min after cardiac arrest.
   D. Pupil size does not correlate with cerebral perfusion.

   (13:334)

9. Which of the following would a RCP be *least* likely to take on transport?

   A. Oxygen cylinders
   B. Self-inflating resuscitation bag
   C. Assorted syringes
   D. Assorted endotracheal tubes

   (14:385–9)

Answer Key

1. B. Magill forceps are not necessary for oral endotracheal intubation; they are often used for nasotracheal intubation to guide the tube through the oropharynx.
2. A. $P_{ET}CO_2$ > 15 torr increases the likelihood of successful resuscitation.
3. C. ECG monitoring is not necessary during PFT.
4. D. Pulseless ventricular tachycardia and ventricular fibrillation are indications for defibrillation.
5. C. Atropine, lidocaine, and epinephrine can be instilled through an ET tube.
6. D. Dose is 2–2.5 times IV dose; dilute in 10 cc saline; stop compressions and give several large tidal volumes to enhance distribution in the lung.
7. A. Sodium bicarb is *not* a first-line drug during cardiac resuscitation; other statements about bicarb are true.
8. B. Constricted pupils indicate satisfactory cerebral perfusion.
9. C. An RCP would probably not take assorted syringes on transport; the other items listed are important components needed by the therapist on transport.

K. Maintain Records and Communication

Questions in this category assess the candidate's ability to maintain proper patient records and communicate effectively relevant information to other members of the health care team. For instance, if the respiratory therapy practitioner were to use terms such as *windpipe* or *stomach* in his or her charting instead of the proper terms, *trachea* and *abdomen,* it would only serve to arouse suspicion as to the competence of that practitioner among other members of the health team.

Entry and Advanced Level Pretest

According to the NBRC, 1–2% of the questions on the Entry Level Examination are from the maintain records and communication content category. In addition, the Composite Examination Matrix states that questions in this category assess the candidate's ability to perform the following related tasks:

1. Note and interpret all subjective and objective responses to care procedures (including vital signs, auscultatory findings, cough and sputum production, and adverse reactions).
2. Specify therapy administered, including date, time, frequency of therapy, medication administered, and pertinent ventilatory data.
3. Communicate pertinent information regarding the patient's clinical status to appropriate members of the health care team.
4. Communicate pertinent information relevant to coordinating patient care (scheduling, avoiding conflicts, and proper sequencing of therapies).
5. Verify computations.

In addition to the competencies listed above, the Advanced Level Examination candidate is expected to perform the following:

6. Delineate discharge planning information.
7. Give information about smoking cessation.

The following self-study questions were developed from the NBRC Composite Examination Matrix.

1. Which of the following abbreviations would be *least* likely to be considered acceptable for use in a patient's chart?

   A. q.o.d.
   B. Bronk.
   C. 1/4 N.S.
   D. gtts

   (1:106–9)

2. A respiratory therapy practitioner has just completed tracheobronchial suctioning of a patient who has multiple lung abscesses. Regarding this procedure, which of the following clinical diagnostic data should be charted as being valid?

   I. Sputum quantity
   II. Sputum color
   III. Sputum viscosity
   IV. Sputum odor

   A. I only
   B. II only
   C. I and III
   D. I, II, III, and IV

   (1:106–9)

3. A 24-year-old woman is admitted to the emergency department following an automobile accident in which she suffered multiple abrasions and contusions. She is subsequently transferred to the progressive care unit where 3 L nasal oxygen is ordered along with monitoring of vital signs every 30 min. As the respiratory therapy practitioner places this patient on supplemental oxygen, he observes that the patient sleeps when not disturbed but responds brisky and appropriately in response to mild stimuli. Which of the following terms would be the most appropriate for use in charting this patient's level of consciousness?

   A. Drowsy or somnolent
   B. Disoriented to time and place
   C. Deeply comatose
   D. Deeply stuporous

   (1:211–17)

4. While auscultating the posterior basal segments of a patient who was admitted in congestive heart failure, the respiratory therapy practitioner notes that the patient's expiratory breath sounds are equal in length and intensity to the patient's inspiratory breath sounds. Which of the following terms should the therapist record in the patient's chart to describe these sounds?

   A. Vesicular breath sounds
   B. Amphoric breath sounds
   C. Decreased breath sounds
   D. Bronchovesicular breath sounds

   (1:222–7)

5. Shortly after endotracheal extubation, a 48-year-old postgastrectomy patient is heard making medium-pitched crowing sounds synchronous with labored inspiratory efforts. Which of the following terms should the respiratory care practitioner record in the patient's chart to describe this sound?

   A. Stertorous breathing
   B. Barking cough
   C. Tussive breathing
   D. Stridorous breathing

   (1:224–5)

6. Following a cardiac arrest requiring approximately 30 min of basic and advanced cardiopulmonary resuscitation, a patient is transported to the cardiac care unit and placed on a volume-cycled ventilator. In assessing this patient the respiratory therapy practitioner notes that the patient does not respond at all to painful stimuli. Which of the following should the practitioner record in the chart to describe this patient's sensorium?

   A. Somnolence
   B. Deep coma
   C. Stupor
   D. Light coma

   (1:211–17)

7. Following placement on a volume-cycled ventilator, an 82-year-old patient is noted to have significant

depressions in her systolic blood pressure that are synchronous with delivered mechanical breaths. Which of the following terms should the respiratory therapy practitioner use to record the above finding in the patient's chart?

A. Pulsus alternans
B. Pulsus paradoxus
C. Pulsus obliternans
D. Arterial hypotension

(5:68)

8. It has been recommended that the respiratory therapy practitioner record all pertinent data regarding any administered therapeutic procedure in the patient's chart. Most respiratory therapy department protocols require the charting of which of the following data with every volume IPPB treatment?

I. Ventilator sensitivity
II. Occurrence of all adverse effects
III. Pulse rate
IV. Auscultatory findings
V. Delivered volume
VI. Source gas or delivered FIO_2

A. I, II, III, V, and VI
B. II, III, and IV
C. II, III, IV, and V
D. II, III, IV, V, and VI

(13:223–9)

Answer Key

1. B. Bronk. is not an acceptable abbreviation to chart.
2. D. All of the sputum characteristics listed are appropriate to include in charting.
3. A. This patient is not disoriented, only sleepy.
4. D. The breath sounds described here are bronchovesicular.
5. D. Inspiratory difficulty accompanied by crowing noises describes stridor.
6. B. No response to painful stimuli is characteristic of deep coma.
7. B. Pulsus paradoxus describes a decrease in pulse volume during inspiration, and an increase during expiration.
8. C. Everything except ventilator sensitivity should be charted.

Advanced Level Only

1. Which of the following is *least* likely to be addressed in the process of discharge planning?

A. Financial resources of the patient
B. Air travel for the COPD patient
C. Home health care agencies
D. Vocational services

(12:291–6)

2. Financial assistance appropriate for COPD patients about to be discharged from the hospital may include all but which of the following?

A. Food stamps
B. Social security
C. Medicare
D. Veteran's benefits

(12:294–5)

3. Behavior modification techniques that should be discussed within the realm of smoking cessation include which of the following?

I. Self-management
II. Aversive conditioning
III. Support groups
IV. Hypnosis

A. I, II, III, and IV
B. I, II, and IV
C. II, III, and IV
D. I, II, and III

(12:134–6)

Answer Key

1. B. Air travel for the COPD patient would be an unlikely discharge planning item.
2. A. Food stamps do not provide financial assistance, as do the other selections.
3. D. Aversive conditioning, self-management, and support groups are all types of behavior modification that have been used in nicotine intervention.

L. Assist Physician with Special Procedures and Conduct Pulmonary Rehabilitation and Home Care (Advanced Level Only)

According to the NBRC, the assist physician with special procedures/conduct pulmonary rehab and home care content category is assessed only on the Advanced Practitioner Examination. Questions in this category are designed to assess the candidate's ability to assist the physician with special procedures in a clinical laboratory procedure room or operating room setting, and to initiate and carry out pulmonary rehabilitation and/or home care within a prescription.

Advanced Practitioner Pretest

According to the NBRC, 5% of the questions on the Advanced Practitioner Examination are from this category. In addition, the Composite Examination Matrix states that questions in this category assess the candidate's ability to assist the physician in performing the following special procedures:

1. Bronchoscopy
2. Transtracheal aspiration

3. Thoracocentesis
4. Tracheostomy
5. Stress testing
6. Transtracheal oxygen catheter placement
7. Sleep studies
8. Cardioversion
9. Intubation

Questions in this category further assess the candidate's ability to initiate and conduct pulmonary rehabilitation and home care as follows:

1. Establish therapeutic goals.
2. Implement and monitor graded exercise.
3. Monitor and maintain home respiratory care equipment.
4. Assure safety and infection control.
5. Modify respiratory care procedures for home use.
6. Evaluate patient's progress.
7. Explain and instruct therapeutic goals to patient and family.
8. Maintain apnea monitors.

The following self-study questions were developed from the NBRC Composite Examination Matrix.

1. Which of the following is believed to be the most acceptable method of preventing hypoxemia during transnasal fiberoptic bronchoscopy?

   A. Administration of nasal oxygen
   B. Administration of intermittent positive pressure ventilation
   C. Administration of mask oxygen
   D. Inotropic stimulation

   (1:691–95)

2. All of the following are intraoperative and postoperative complications of tracheotomy. Which is most commonly seen?

   A. Hemorrhagic shock
   B. Tension pneumothorax
   C. Onset of life-threatening arrhythmias
   D. Subcutaneous emphysema

   (4:171–4)

3. Which of the following complications is *not* associated with the use of tracheostomy tubes?

   A. Pulmonary infection
   B. Dysphagia
   C. Laryngeal edema
   D. Glottic edema

   (4:171–4)

4. Which of the following statements is (are) true regarding the technique of elective tracheotomy?

   I. A vertical incision is invariably used.
   II. The trachea is usually incised between the second and third tracheal rings.
   III. Hemostasis may be aided by infiltrating the operative site with a dilute epinephrine solution.

   A. I only
   B. II and III
   C. I, II, and III
   D. III only

   (16:497)

5. Which of the following is the most frequent hazard associated with needle biopsy of the lung?

   A. Severe hemorrhage
   B. Pneumothorax
   C. Death
   D. Air embolism

   (16:437–8)

6. Tracheal intubation with the fiberoptic laryngoscope is frequently recommended in which of the following circumstances?

   A. Prior to induction of general anesthesia
   B. Emergency airway placement in the patient with suspected cervical spine fracture
   C. Management of the severely asphyxiated newborn
   D. Management of the patient with croup

   (16:831–2)

7. Bronchoscopy may be used to do all of the following *except:*

   A. Determine the source of hemoptysis
   B. Tracheobronchial toilet
   C. Determine the cause of atelectasis
   D. Transthoracic biopsy

   (1:691–5)

8. Which of the following should the respiratory therapist *not* recommend as part of the home care plan for a patient with chronic bronchitis who also has cor pulmonale?

   A. Chest physical therapy
   B. Oxygen therapy
   C. Adequate hydration
   D. Mask CPAP therapy

   (9:136–8)

9. The respiratory therapy practitioner is asked to help set up a home care plan for a patient who is to be discharged with a permanent tracheostomy. Because the patient sustained a midcervical spinal column transection, some diaphragmatic function remains. This is evidenced by a vital capacity of 8 cc/kg. Based on the above information, which of

the following would be the *least* appropriate therapeutic recommendation?

A. Teaching the patient to suction himself
B. Teaching the patient's family pulmonary drainage techniques
C. Instructing the patient in breathing retraining techniques
D. Instructing the patient in incentive spirometry

(9:316–17)

10. The RCP has been asked to prepare to defibrillate a patient in ventricular fibrillation. Which of the following is *not* indicated?

A. Use "unsynchronized" mode.
B. Remove nitroglycerine patch from patient's chest.
C. Set defibrillator to deliver 400 J.
D. Assure that the area is clear before discharging the paddles.

(10:144–7)

11. Prior to implementation of a progressive exercise program, all patients:

I. Should be instructed on diaphragmatic and PLB
II. Should perform general muscle reconditioning/ROM exercises
III. Should be given oxygen at a minimum flow of 2 L/min
IV. With asthma should use their bronchodilator 15–30 min prior to beginning exercise

A. I, II, and IV
B. I, II, and III
C. II, III, and IV
D. I, II, III, and IV

(20:26–7, 499–501)

12. Exercise testing should be stopped under which of the following circumstances?

I. Patient's systolic blood pressure increases more than 20 mm Hg from baseline.
II. Patient has chest pain.
III. Patient complains of dizziness.
IV. Patient's perceived level of exertion becomes "severe."

A. I, II, III, and IV
B. I, II, and III
C. II, III, and IV
D. I, II, and IV

(20:493–6)

13. Why is exercise testing done?

A. To identify physiologic reasons for exercise-related symptoms
B. To identify psychologic reasons for exercise-related symptoms
C. To determine how the patient is limited by his disease
D. A and C

(20:42)

14. Patient is 60 years old with COPD. What is an acceptable training dyspnea (effort) rating?

A. Very easy to easy
B. Somewhat hard to hard
C. Very hard to very very hard
D. Until exhaustion

(20:484–6)

15. You are responsible for educating a 4-year-old patient about his nasal cannula. In order to be effective, you should do all but which of the following?

A. Keep your session short.
B. Tell a story.
C. Hold the child responsible for the material.
D. Review the normal range of acceptable flow rates.

(20:72–84)

16. Guidelines related to the four components of the exercise prescription include all but which of the following?

A. Daily strength training
B. Aerobic activity 3–5 times/week
C. Maintaining target heart rate for 20–30 minutes each day that the patient exercises
D. Letting the patient choose his/her mode of exercise

(20:500–1)

17. The incision for a transtracheal oxygen catheter is made:

A. Horizontally through the trachea
B. With a needle puncture through the trachea
C. At the sternal notch
D. Through the vocal cords

(16:1166)

18. Measurements taken during a sleep study include:

I. EEG
II. ECG
III. Electrodes to detect chest/abdominal movement
IV. Hemoglobin

A. I, II, III, and IV
B. I, II, and IV
C. II and III
D. I, II, and III

(9:56–7)

19. The clinically ideal ventilator patient pre-discharge meets which of the following criteria?

    I. 2–4 weeks of stable ABGs
    II. 2–4 weeks of stable ventilatory parameters
    III. No acute problems
    IV. No chronic problems

    A. I, II, III, and IV
    B. I, II, and III
    C. II and III
    D. I and IV

    (13:355–6)

20. RT equipment should be cleaned at home with

    A. Baking soda and H_2O
    B. 70% ethyl alcohol and H_2O
    C. Undiluted vinegar
    D. Vinegar/water solution (1:3)

    (13:350–1)

21. Initial evaluation of the home care patient's house should include all but which of the following?

    A. Enough electrical outlets
    B. Minimal dust
    C. Adequate space for cleaning and storage of equipment
    D. Carpeting

    (13:350–1)

22. Home care patients should be instructed to recognize which of the following signs of infection in their home, so that they can seek medical attention?

    I. Increased WBC
    II. Change in color of sputum
    III. Increased temperature
    IV. Redness/swelling

    A. I, II, III, and IV
    B. II, III, and IV
    C. I, II, and IV
    D. II and III

    (13:356–7)

23. When a patient goes home on a ventilator, which of the following should be taken care of by the RCP?

    I. Notify the port authority.
    II. Notify the electric company.
    III. Notify the local EMS.
    IV. Notify the gas company.

    A. I, II, III, and IV
    B. II and IV
    C. II and III
    D. I, II, and IV

    (20:379–82)

24. Which of the following characteristics of respiratory home care equipment is *least* important?

    A. Apparatus should have loud alarms.
    B. Equipment should be easy to operate.
    C. It should be easy to manipulate settings.
    D. Electrical devices should have an internal battery.

    (20: Chap 20)

25. Types of mechanical ventilators used in the home include which of the following?

    I. Oxygen conserving devices
    II. Noninvasive ventilation (BiPAP)
    III. Positive pressure ventilation
    IV. Negative pressure ventilation

    A. I, II, III, and IV
    B. II, III, and IV
    C. I, II, and III
    D. II and III

    (20: Chap 20)

26. Which of the following techniques is best for obtaining an anaerobic sputum sample from a nonintubated patient?

    A. Transtracheal aspirate
    B. Nasotracheal suction
    C. Sputum induction with hypotonic saline
    D. Thoracentesis

    (9:28)

27. Which of the following types of patients would be *least* likely to require an apnea monitor?

    A. Siblings of infants who have died of SIDS
    B. Infants who have had documented periods of apnea
    C. Infants with cystic fibrosis
    D. Infants with tracheostomies

    (14:428–9)

Answer Key

1. C. Mask oxygen is the most acceptable method of providing oxygen during transnasal bronchoscopy.
2. D. Subcutaneous emphysema, which resolves spontaneously, is the most common complication of tracheotomy.
3. D. Glottic edema is not associated with tracheostomy tube use.
4. B. The trachea is usually incised between the second and third tracheal rings. Hemostasis may be aided by infiltrating the tracheostomy site with a dilute epinephrine solution.
5. B. Pneumothorax is the most common complication of thoracentesis.
6. B. Emergency airway placement in the patient with suspected cervical spine fracture is best accomplished using a fiberoptic laryngoscope.

7. D. A transthoracic biopsy cannot be performed via a bronchoscope.
8. D. All of the therapies with the exception of mask CPAP should be included in the home care plan of a patient with chronic bronchitis and cor pulmonale.
9. D. Incentive spirometry is the least appropriate therapy for the trach patient at this time.
10. C. Initially, the defibrillator should be set to deliver 200 joules.
11. A. Not all patients who are beginning a pulmonary rehab exercise program require supplemental oxygen.
12. C. Any one who exercises should experience an increase in systolic blood pressure. All other choices are indications for discontinuing the exercise test.
13. D. Psychologic reasons for exercise-related symptoms cannot be determined through exercise testing.
14. B. Patients should exercise in the somewhat hard to hard range, as measured by effort or perceived exertion.
15. D. When preparing patient education for the pediatric patient, keep your session short, tell a story, and hold the child responsible for the material.
16. A. Daily strength training is not recommended; patients should wait at least 24 hr between strength training sessions. Other statements are correct.
17. B. The incision for a transtracheal oxygen catheter is made by a needle puncture through the trachea.
18. D. Hemoglobin is generally not assessed during a routine sleep study. All other items are monitored.
19. B. Patients who will be receiving ventilator care in the home should have no acute problems (infection, atelectasis, etc.), and should be fairly stable both hemodynamically and ventilatorily.
20. D. RT equipment should be cleaned at home with vinegar and water (1:3) solution.
21. D. The patient's house should be clean, have enough space, and have enough electrical outlets for necessary equipment.
22. B. The patient can observe all of the signs/symptoms listed, with the exception of WBC.
23. C. The electric company and the local EMS should both be notified when a patient goes home with a ventilator.
24. C. To avoid problems, patients should not be able to easily or accidentally change their settings.
25. B. Ventilators available for home use include BiPAP, positive pressure, and negative pressure ventilators.
26. A. Transtracheal aspiration is best for obtaining an anaerobic sputum sample from a nonintubated patient.
27. C. Infants with cystic fibrosis would be least likely, of the disorders listed, to be monitored with an apnea monitor.

II

EXAMINATION POSTTEST AND MASTERY

UNIT I

Entry Level Examination Posttest

The following full-length Entry Level Examination posttest was constructed according to specifications outlined in the current NBRC Composite Examination Matrix. The examination categories and the number of questions the NBRC has allotted to each are listed in the table below. In addition, *the answer key at the end of this test is referenced to the examination matrix so the candidate may further identify his or her weak areas.* For a more thorough discussion of the NBRC Composite Examination Matrix, please refer to the Introduction of this book and to the Examination Category Review and Pretest.

TABLE 1. ENTRY LEVEL EXAMINATION CONTENT MATRIX

	Examination Category	Number of Questions	Percentage of Questions
I.	***Clinical Data***	60	30
A.	Review patient records	9	4.5
B.	Collect and evaluate clinical information	21	10.5
C.	Recommend and obtain diagnostic procedures	6	3
D.	Perform and evaluate laboratory procedures	12	6
E.	Assess therapeutic plan	12	6
II.	***Equipment***	50	25
A.	Select, assemble, check, and correct malfunctions of equipment	42	21
B.	Ensure cleanliness, calibration, and quality control	8	4
III.	***Therapeutic Procedures***	90	45
A.	Educate patients	3	1.5
B.	Control infection	4	2
C.	Maintain airway	8	4
D.	Mobilize and remove secretions	9	4.5
E.	Ensure ventilation	11	5.5
F.	Ensure oxygenation	11	5.5
G.	Assess patient response to therapy	11	5.5
H.	Modify therapy	10	5
I.	Recommend modifications in therapy	8	4
J.	Initiate cardiopulmonary resuscitation	11	5.5
K.	Maintain records and communication	3	1.5

Examination for Entry Level Respiratory Therapy Practitioners

Time: 3 hours

Directions: Each of the questions or incomplete statements below is followed by four suggested answers. Select the one that is best in each case and then mark accordingly.

1. The drop in Pa_{O_2} that may accompany administration of isoproterenol has been attributed to:

   I. A β_1 side effect
   II. Increased ventilation to underperfused lung units
   III. Increased perfusion to underventilated lung units
   IV. Pulmonary vasodilatation

   A. I and III
   B. II and III
   C. II and IV
   D. III and IV

2. A 39-year-old man presents to the emergency department with fever, respiratory distress, and a cough that is productive of copious quantities of thick, green-tinged sputum. The patient states that he raises several dozen teaspoons of these secretions daily and that he has had recurrent bouts with bronchopneumonia since childhood. Physical examination reveals mild clubbing of digits and a remarkable variety of rhonchi over both lung fields. Based on the above information, which of the following disorders is most likely responsible for this patient's distress?

   A. Bronchogenic carcinoma
   B. Anaerobic lung abscess
   C. Chronic bronchitis
   D. Bronchiectasis

3. Which of the following clinical disorders are commonly known to involve or lead to pulmonary edema?

   I. Left ventricular failure
   II. Hypovolemia
   III. Right ventricular failure
   IV. Adult respiratory distress syndrome

   A. I and IV
   B. I, II, III, and IV
   C. II and IV
   D. III and IV

4. For every 10 mm Hg acute increase in Pa_{CO_2}, the pH of the blood will drop approximately:

   A. 0.5
   B. 0.05
   C. 0.10
   D. 0.15

5. An all-purpose jet type nebulizer is being used on a patient in the intensive care unit. Although it is set to deliver 40% oxygen, a properly calibrated analyzer placed at the patient's proximal airway repeatedly reads 46%. Which of the following is (are) the most probable cause(s) for this occurrence?

   I. Humidity is affecting analyzer accuracy.
   II. There is a leak in the system.
   III. Backpressure is affecting air entrainment valve function.

   A. II only
   B. I, II, and III
   C. III only
   D. I only

6. Which of the following *cannot* be determined through the analysis of pulmonary function data obtained by simple spirometry?

   A. FEF_{50}
   B. $\frac{FEV_1}{FVC}\%$
   C. $FEF_{200-1200}$
   D. Expiratory reserve volume

7. A ventilator that is classified as being pressure cycled is generally so termed because:

   A. The inspiratory phase is initiated after preset conditions of pressure have been achieved.
   B. The expiratory phase is initiated after preset conditions of flow have been achieved.
   C. The expiratory phase is initiated after preset conditions of pressure have been achieved.
   D. The inspiratory phase is initiated after preset conditions of flow have been achieved.

8. Which of the following is *least* likely to lead to retrolental fibroplasia in the preterm infant?

   A. Perfusion of the retina with Pa_{O_2}s greater than 100 mm Hg
   B. Administration of 40% or less oxygen
   C. Intermittent bagging with 100% oxygen
   D. Administration of 100% oxygen directly to the eye itself

9. Mild gastric inflation is observed in a cardiac arrest victim who is being ventilated via a manual resuscitator and mask unit. Without interrupting cardiopulmonary resuscitation, the most appropriate action for the respiratory therapy practitioner to take at this time would be to:

   A. Apply pressure to the abdomen during the performance of external cardiac compressions

B. Reposition the airway
C. Roll the victim to his side and apply pressure to the upper abdomen
D. Use two hands to compress the bag-valve unit

10. A 68-year-old man is brought to the emergency department in severe distress. An oral history of severe chronic obstructive pulmonary disease is consistent with barrel chest, pursed lipped breathing, and the cyanosis that accompany his presentation. Room air blood gases are as follows:

Pa_{O_2}	45 mm Hg
Pa_{CO_2}	75 mm Hg
pH	7.32
HCO_3^-	34 mEq/L
BP	170/120
Pulse	110
Respiratory rate	30

Administration of 24% oxygen to this patient will most likely have which of the following effects?

I. Marked increase in minute ventilation
II. Worsening of cardiovascular vital signs
III. Improvement in cardiovascular vital signs
IV. Appreciable relief of hypoxia

A. I and IV
B. III and IV
C. I and II
D. I and III

11. In which of the following patients might percussion and vibration techniques be contraindicated?

I. Those with osteoporosis
II. Those with fractured ribs
III. Those with resectable lung tumors

A. II only
B. I only
C. I and III
D. I, II, and III

12. Ventilator weaning attempts are in progress for a 68-year-old patient who is recovering from pneumonia caused by *Klebsiella pneumoniae.* The patient has a history of pulmonary emphysema and has required continuous ventilatory support for the past 5 days. He has been receiving supplemental oxygen via T tube setup for the past hour. Arterial blood gas data gathered during this process appear below:

	After 5 Minutes on T tube	After 30 Minutes on T tube	After 60 Minutes on T tube
FI_{O_2}	0.5	0.5	0.5
Pa_{O_2}	62 mm Hg	56 mm Hg	55 mm Hg
Pa_{CO_2}	65 mm Hg	69 mm Hg	74 mm Hg
pH	7.40	7.33	7.20

Based on the above information, what is the correct recommendation?

A. Extubate at once.
B. Support ventilation at this time.
C. Increase the FI_{O_2}.
D. Obtain an arterial sample.

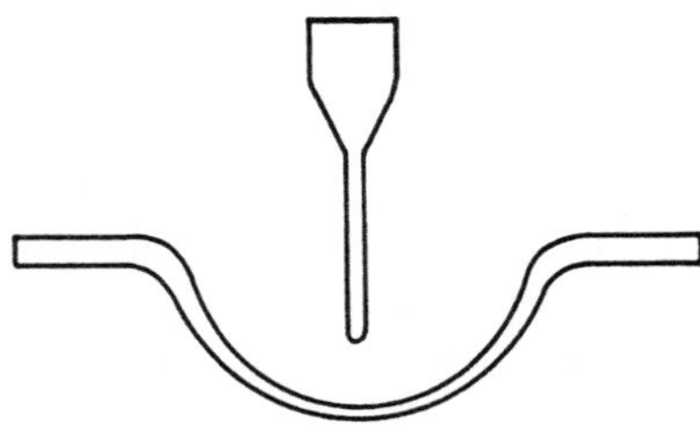

Figure 35.

13. Figure 35 shows:

A. A normal unit
B. A shunt unit
C. A deadspace unit
D. A silent unit

14. True statements regarding humidifiers in general include:

I. They produce particulate water only.
II. They produce water vapor only.
III. They are incapable of transmitting bacteria.
IV. They are incapable of delivering gases at conditions of BTPS.

A. II and IV
B. II and III
C. I and II
D. II only

15. A respiratory care practitioner is administering IPPB to a patient who has suffered a recent myocardial infarction. Which of the following signs and symptoms would be most likely to lead the respiratory therapy practitioner to assess that cardiovascular embarrassment is taking place?

I. Dyspnea
II. Appearance of sonorous rhonchi
III. Distended neck veins
IV. Rapid, thready pulse

A. I, II, and IV
B. I, II, and III
C. I, III, and IV
D. I only

16. The respiratory therapy practitioner is assigned to a neurotrauma patient in the intensive care unit. Gross observation of this patient reveals the fact that he pauses for several seconds at the end of every inspiration. Which of the following terms should the practitioner record in the patient's chart to describe this ventilatory pattern?

A. Biot's breathing
B. Hypopnea
C. Apneustic breathing
D. Cluster breathing

17. How long must equipment contaminated by *Mycobacterium tuberculosis* be immersed in a commercial glutaraldehyde solution to ensure that all these organisms have been killed?

A. 12 hr
B. 1 hr
C. 10–20 min
D. 3–10 hr

18. True statements regarding tracheal tube cuff herniation include:

I. Cuff overinflation may lead to its occurrence.
II. It is associated with high-pressure cuff usage.
III. It may lead to upper airway obstruction.
IV. Presence of tracheal shift is diagnostic.

A. I and II
B. I and III
C. II and IV
D. III and IV

19. A 32-year-old woman is brought to the emergency department in a diabetic coma. The following arterial blood gas data were obtained on admission:

FIO_2	0.21
PaO_2	105 mm Hg
$PaCO_2$	19 mm Hg
pH	7.07
HCO_3^-	4 mEq/L
Base excess	–17 mEq/L

The most correct interpretation of the above results is:

A. Partially compensated metabolic alkalosis
B. Partially compensated metabolic acidosis
C. Partially compensated respiratory acidosis
D. Fully compensated respiratory acidosis

20. Which of the following is *not* part of the normal or resident flora of the upper respiratory tract?

A. *Candida albicans*
B. *Hemophilus* species
C. *Klebsiella* species
D. Streptococci

21. Instructions in which of the following techniques would be *least* likely to enhance the deposition of aerosolized medication within the respiratory tract?

A. End inspiratory breath holding
B. Mouth breathing
C. Slow, deep inspirations
D. Use of accessory muscles during exhalation

22. In reading the admission note of a patient with severe pulmonary emphysema, the respiratory therapy practitioner would expect the patient's historical data to reveal a chief complaint of:

A. Platypnea
B. Dyspnea
C. Cough with copious sputum production
D. Somnolence

23. From which of the following devices may *true* mixed venous blood be obtained under most clinical circumstances?

A. Central venous catheter
B. Pulmonary venous catheter
C. Subclavian catheter
D. Pulmonary artery catheter

24. The administration of high concentrations of oxygen (greater than 60%) to patients with adult respiratory distress syndrome would most likely result in which of the following occurrences?

I. Narrowing of the patient's $P(A–a)O_2$
II. Oxygen-induced hypoventilation
III. Little improvement in arterial hypoxemia
IV. Congestive heart failure

A. I and II
B. II and IV
C. III only
D. III and IV

25. Which of the following would be the preferred method of maintaining airway patency for a semiconscious patient who is not in respiratory distress?

A. Oral endotracheal intubation
B. Nasopharyngeal airway
C. Oropharyngeal airway
D. Tracheostomy

26. Excessive delay in the running of a sample of arterial blood may result in which of the following sampling errors?

I. High pH
II. Low PO_2
III. Low PCO_2
IV. High PO_2
V. High PCO_2

A. II and V
B. III and IV
C. I, III, and IV
D. I, II, and IV

27. After delivering two slow breaths to an unconscious and apneic 5-year-old child, the respiratory therapy practitioner is able to palpate a weak carotid pulse. Which is the proper action to take at this time?

A. Begin rescue breathing at a rate of 16/min.
B. Begin rescue breathing at a rate of 20/min.
C. Begin external cardiac compressions.
D. Begin rescue breathing at a rate of 12/min.

28. Which of the following airways should the respiratory therapy practitioner select for an unconscious patient who is breathing spontaneously and adequately?

A. Nasopharyngeal airway
B. Endotracheal tube
C. Tracheostomy tube
D. Oropharyngeal airway

29. Following upper abdominal surgery, the respiratory therapy practitioner finds a 44-year-old male patient completely unwilling to perform deep breathing and coughing exercises. Which of the following are the most appropriate actions under these circumstances?

I. Synchronize therapy with analgesic administration if possible.
II. Restrain the patient's arms and administer IPPB via mask.
III. Attempt to further instruct the patient.
IV. Support the incision during therapy.

A. I, III, and IV
B. II and IV
C. I and IV
D. I, II, and IV

30. The physician wants the respiratory therapy practitioner to place the patient on the level of PEEP that corresponds to the best effective static compliance. With the corrected tidal volume held constant, the following data are accumulated:

Level of PEEP	Plateau Pressure
0 cm H_2O	48 cm H_2O
3 cm H_2O	50 cm H_2O
6 cm H_2O	52 cm H_2O
9 cm H_2O	51 cm H_2O
12 cm H_2O	51 cm H_2O
15 cm H_2O	52 cm H_2O
18 cm H_2O	58 cm H_2O
21 cm H_2O	62 cm H_2O

Which of the following levels of PEEP should the respiratory therapist recommend?

A. 9 cm H_2O
B. 12 cm H_2O
C. 15 cm H_2O
D. 18 cm H_2O

31. While auscultating the chest of a patient with chronic obstructive pulmonary disease, the respiratory therapy practitioner notes the presence of high-pitched musical, squeaking, and bubbling sounds confined primarily to the expiratory phase. Which of the following terms could the practitioner record in the patient's chart to describe these sounds?

A. Rales
B. Wheezes
C. Pleural friction rub
D. Sonorous rhonchi

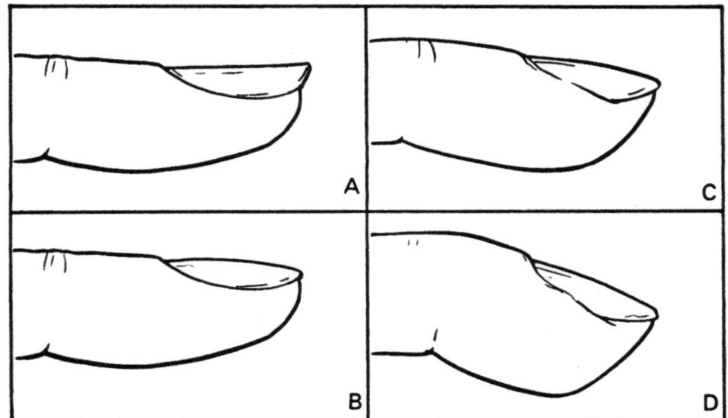

Figure 36.

32. Figure 36 shows normal nails in *A* and *B* and clubbed nails in *C* and *D*. All of the following are true about the physical sign of clubbing *except:*

A. It can often be seen in patients with chronic obstructive pulmonary disease.
B. It may be caused by chronic hypoxia.
C. It involves soft tissue swelling at the terminal phalanx.
D. It is rarely noted in patients with cystic fibrosis.

33. When an entrainment mask is administering 24% oxygen to a patient, it is entraining how many liters of room air for each liter of driving (source) gas?

A. 3
B. 10
C. 20
D. 25

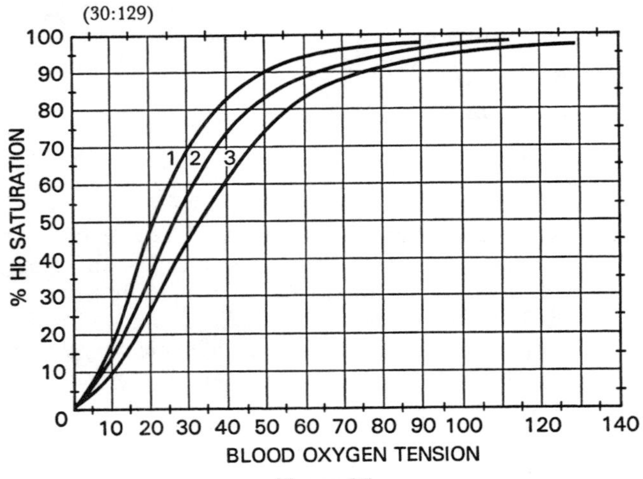

Figure 37.

34. For Figure 37, which of the following statements is *not* true?

 A. The P_{50} is highest in curve number 3.
 B. Curve number 1 displays the highest oxygen affinity.
 C. Curve number 2 represents the normal position of the oxyhemoglobin dissociation curve.
 D. Alkalosis would most likely result in curve number 3.

35. The respiratory therapy practitioner has discovered an unconscious and apneic patient. After calling for help and delivering four quick breaths, the therapist now is attempting to establish pulselessness. According to the American Heart Association, how much time should he or she devote to this effort?

 A. 0–5 seconds
 B. 5–10 seconds
 C. 10–15 seconds
 D. 15–20 seconds

36. On a pressure-cycled ventilator an increase in lung thorax compliance will most likely result in:

 A. A decrease in delivered volume
 B. An increase in peak airway pressure
 C. Altered machine sensitivity
 D. An increase in delivered volume

37. A respiratory therapy practitioner is administering continuous ventilatory support to a patient in the coronary care unit using a pressure-cycled ventilator. Suddenly he notices that the inspiratory phase has become extremely short. Which of the following might be responsible for the above occurrence?

 I. The patient's tidal volume may have increased.
 II. The problem may be caused by a leak in the circuit.
 III. The patient may need to be suctioned.
 IV. The endotracheal tube may have slipped into the right mainstem bronchus.
 V. A tension pneumothorax may be present.

 A. I, IV, and V
 B. II, III, and V
 C. II, III, IV, and V
 D. II, IV, and V

38. Which of the following breath sounds are *always* considered abnormal when heard while auscultating the chest?

 I. Vesicular
 II. Amphoric or cavernous
 III. Bronchial
 IV. Bronchovesicular

 A. II and IV
 B. I and III
 C. III and IV
 D. II only

39. True statements regarding external cardiac compressions when applied to children include:

 I. The sternum should be depressed 1–1½ inches.
 II. A rate of 100/min should be employed.
 III. The upper portion of the sternum should be depressed.
 IV. The heel of one hand may be used.

 A. I and III
 B. II and IV
 C. III and IV
 D. I, II, and IV

40. Which of the following statements regarding the radial artery is (are) true?

 I. It is usually accessible among inpatient and outpatient populations.
 II. It generally possesses adequate collateral blood flow.
 III. It is not proximal to nervous or periosteal tissue.
 IV. It is not considered a superficial artery.

 A. I and II
 B. II and IV
 C. I, II, and IV
 D. I and III

41. The respiratory therapy practitioner is reviewing the chart of an extremely obese patient who has been diagnosed as having the classic Pickwickian syndrome. Which of the following findings would the therapist be *least* likely to note in this patient's chart?

 A. Somnolence
 B. Anemia

C. Hypercapnia
D. Cor pulmonale

42. The narrowest portion of the newborn's upper airway is at the level of the:

A. Trachea
B. Thyroid cartilage
C. Oropharynx
D. Cricoid cartilage

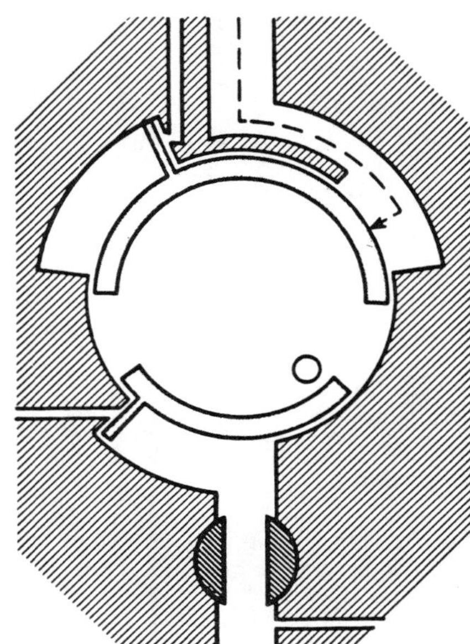

Figure 38.

43. Figure 38 shows the Bennett valve in which position?

I. Open
II. Closed
III. With the sensitivity control on
IV. With peak flow at the minimum setting

A. I and III
B. II only
C. I, III, and IV
D. I and II

44. A 35-year-old woman is brought to the emergency department in distress. Historical data include a high fever, shaking, chills, and severe pleuritic chest pain. The patient has a harsh cough that is productive of moderate quantities of rusty-colored sputum. Arterial blood gas analysis reveals hypoxemia and hypocarbia. Based on the above information, which of the following is the most probable cause of this patient's distress?

A. Gram-negative bacterial pneumonia
B. Bacterial endocarditis
C. Bronchiectasis
D. Pneumococcal pneumonia

45. The breath sounds heard over most of the lung fields in a normal subject are termed:

A. Vesicular
B. Bronchovesicular
C. Tracheal
D. Tubular

46. When administering oxygen to a premature newborn, umbilical arterial oxygen tensions of ___ are usually considered safest.

A. 20–40 mm Hg
B. 30–70 mm Hg
C. 40–80 mm Hg
D. 80–100 mm Hg

47. The administration of excessive doses of oxygen to premature newborns is believed to result in the development of which of the following disorders?

I. Retrolental fibroplasia
II. Alveolar hypoventilation
III. Massive pulmonary hemorrhage
IV. Bronchopulmonary dysplasia
V. Wilson-Mikitty syndrome

A. I and III
B. I and IV
C. II, IV, and V
D. I, III, and V

48. Which of the following physical signs are most typically noted in patients with cor pulmonale?

I. Rales
II. Neck vein distention
III. Mediastinal shift
IV. Peripheral edema

A. I and III
B. III and IV
C. I and IV
D. II and IV

49. The deleterious side effects of PEEP on the cardiovascular system are *least* likely to be pronounced in which of the following patients?

A. Those with normal pulmonary compliance
B. Those with decreased pulmonary compliance
C. Those with pulmonary emphysema
D. Those who are hypovolemic

50. A 38-year-old patient is seen in the intensive care unit after being admitted with a severe right-sided infiltrate that occurred as a result of aspiration of gastric contents. Because of severe hypoxemia, this patient is placed on 7 cm H_2O PEEP with an FIO_2 of 1.0. Hypoxemia persists, however, despite PEEP therapy and cardiovascular support. The respiratory therapy practitioner would recommend which of the following positions as being most likely to improve this patient's oxygenation status?

A. Supine
B. High Fowler's
C. Lying on left side
D. Lying on right side

51. Which of the following must be known to calculate the minute alveolar ventilation?

I. Respiratory rate
II. Anatomic deadspace
III. Tidal volume
IV. $PaCO_2$
V. V_D/V_T

A. I, III, and IV
B. I, III, IV, and V
C. I, II, and III
D. I, III, and V

52. The lung is the most common site of postoperative complications. Which of the following types of surgical procedures is associated with the highest incidence of postoperative pulmonary complications?

A. Neurologic
B. Lower abdominal
C. Orthopaedic
D. Upper abdominal

53. Use of which of the following agents or methods is *not* capable of achieving complete sterilization?

I. Alcohols
II. Alkaline glutaraldehyde
III. Pasteurization
IV. Acid glutaraldehyde

A. I and III
B. III only
C. III and IV
D. II and IV

54. Figure 39 shows the patient lying on his right side in Trendelenburg. In this position, which segment will drain?

A. Lower lobe, lateral basal segment on the left
B. Upper lobe, apical posterior segment on the right
C. Lower lobe, posterior basal segment on the right
D. Lower lobe, posterior basal segment on the left

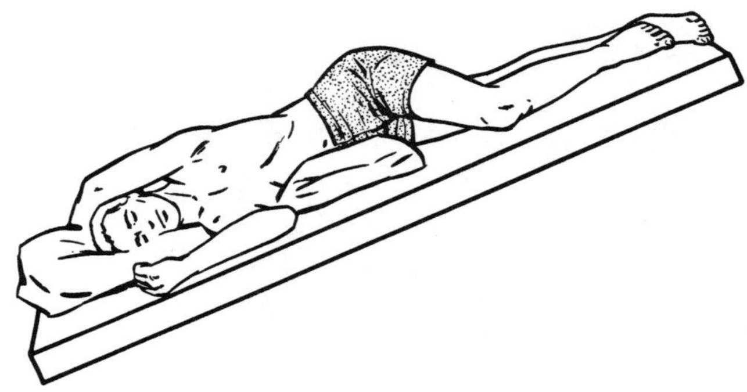

Figure 39.

55. According to the American Heart Association, which of the following are indications for the initiation of basic cardiac life support during the first few minutes of life?

I. Apgar score of 4–6
II. Prolonged periods of apnea
III. Presence of meconium staining
IV. Absent cardiac rate

A. II and IV
B. III and IV
C. I and III
D. II and III

56. Which of the following best describes consolidated lung tissue?

I. Porous, well-aerated structure
II. Relatively poor transmitter of sound
III. Relatively firm, semisolid structure
IV. Relatively good transmitter of sound

A. II only
B. I and IV
C. I and II
D. III and IV

57. True statements regarding postextubation edema include:

I. Development of respiratory distress shortly after extubation is an unfavorable sign.
II. Even mildly distressed individuals should be reintubated.
III. Aerosolization of decongestants and corticosteroids may be helpful.
IV. Unfavorable response to pharmacologic agents is an indication for immediate tracheotomy.

A. I and II
B. II and III
C. I and III
D. II, III, and IV

58. For sterilization to occur, which of the following actions must an agent or method possess?

I. Bacteriocidal
II. Sporicidal

III. Viricidal
IV. Tuberculocidal
V. Fungicidal

A. I, II, III, and IV
B. I, III, IV, and V
C. II, III, IV, and V
D. I, II, III, IV, and V

59. Which of the following statements regarding the ratio of compressions to ventilations during basic cardiopulmonary resuscitation (CPR) is (are) true?

I. During two-rescuer infant CPR it is 5:1.
II. During one-rescuer adult CPR it is 15:2.
III. During two-rescuer CPR to children it is 5:2.

A. I only
B. I and II
C. II and III
D. III only

60. During auscultation of the chest, the respiratory therapy practitioner frequently asks the patient to cough. Which of the following chest sounds will most frequently disappear following this maneuver?

A. Rales
B. Rhonchi
C. Pleural friction rub
D. Egophony

61. Patients with refractory hypoxemia accompanied by which of the following presentations are frequently *not* considered good candidates for PEEP therapy?

I. Diffuse bibasal pulmonary infiltrates
II. Unilateral pulmonary infiltrates
III. Decreased functional residual capacities
IV. Severely diminished cardiovascular reserves

A. I and IV
B. II and III
C. I and II
D. II and IV

62. The respiratory therapy practitioner is teaching a patient the techniques of taking an IPPB treatment. Proper instructions include:

I. Exhale through pursed lips only.
II. Initiate inspiration and let the lungs fill and empty passively.
III. Pause for a few seconds between each breath.
IV. Force as much air in and out of the lungs as possible with each breath.

A. II and IV
B. I and III
C. III and IV
D. II and III

63. In reviewing a patient's chart, the respiratory therapy practitioner notes that the patient's most recent acid-base study revealed a base deficit of 6.8 mEq/L. This value is most consistent with the presence of:

A. Alveolar hyperventilation
B. Metabolic acidosis
C. Mixed respiratory and metabolic acidosis
D. Severe respiratory acidosis

64. A 48-year-old man in moderate respiratory distress is brought to the emergency department by his wife. His chief complaint is of progressive numbing and weakness of his extremities that has progressed over the past several days to the point where dyspnea and fatigue are noted on even mild exertion. This was preceded by a severe upper respiratory infection. Based on the above information, the most likely cause of distress is:

A. Guillain-Barré syndrome
B. Idiopathic thrombocytopenic purpura
C. Myasthenia gravis
D. Chronic obstructive pulmonary emphysema

65. Before a pleural effusion may be diagnosed on the basis of physical signs of decreased breath sounds and abnormal percussion note, how much fluid must be present?

A. 0–50 mL
B. 300–500 mL
C. 400–800 mL
D. 50–150 mL

66. In reviewing the chart of a 20-year-old patient with allergic bronchial asthma, the respiratory therapy practitioner would expect to see evidence of which of the following?

I. Mucopurulent or mucoid sputum
II. Polycythemia
III. Wheezing on auscultation
IV. Considerable improvement following bronchodilator administration

A. I, III, and IV
B. II and III
C. III only
D. I and III

67. A patient is being given oxygen via a properly fitting 24% air entrainment mask. Which of the following ventilatory patterns will result in the lowest FIO_2?

A. Minute ventilation, 12 L; frequency, 18/min
B. Minute ventilation, 14 L; frequency, 6/min
C. Minute ventilation, 12 L; frequency, 24/min
D. The FIO_2 will not vary with the ventilatory pattern.

68. If during the performance of external cardiac compressions the rescuer's hands inadvertently depress the area over the xiphoid process, which of the following may occur?

A. Lung contusion
B. Laceration of the liver
C. Myocardial contusion
D. Damage to the rescuer's hands

69. In which of the following types of hypoxia is oxygen administration *least* likely to be of benefit?

A. Hypoxemic
B. Anemic
C. Circulatory
D. Histotoxic

70. Which of the following conditions is *most* likely to be associated with the presence of barrel chest?

A. Pectus excavatum
B. Emphysema
C. Old age
D. Middle age

71. During the performance of basic cardiopulmonary resuscitation, which of the following is believed to *best* indicate the fact that external cardiac compressions are producing adequate cerebral blood flow?

A. Improvement in patient's color
B. Constriction of the pupils in response to light
C. A palpable carotid pulse
D. Presence of rib fractures

72. Which of the following statements are true regarding the performance of external cardiac compressions to the infant who has suffered a cardiac arrest?

I. The sternum should be depressed ½ to 1 inch.
II. The rate should be at least 100/min.
III. The middle of the sternum should be depressed.
IV. The heel of one hand should be used.

A. II and III
B. I and II
C. I and IV
D. III and IV

73. After performance of a tracheotomy and the insertion of a cuffed tracheal tube, a reasonable estimate of a 50-kg patient's anatomic deadspace would be:

A. 25 cc
B. 55 cc
C. 75 cc
D. 100 cc

74. Which of the following are true statements regarding the color-coding of medical gas cylinders?

I. The system was designed by the Compressed Gas Association.
II. It should be followed *exclusively* in identifying the contents of the cylinder.
III. If color code and cylinder label information are in conflict, the cylinder should not be used.

A. I and II
B. II only
C. I and III
D. I only

75. True statements regarding the $P(A\text{–}a)O_2$ when measured with the patient breathing 100% oxygen include:

I. Values greater than 400 mm Hg indicate the presence of oxygenation failure.
II. Values greater than 400 mm Hg indicate that hypoxemia is probably due to shunting.
III. Values greater than 100 mm Hg are a contraindication for oxygen therapy.
IV. The normal value for a healthy 20-year-old person is 100 mm Hg.

A. I and II
B. III and IV
C. II and IV
D. III only

76. The respiratory therapist receives an order to administer sustained maximal inspiratory therapy (incentive spirometry) to a 34-year-old, 100-kg patient who is recovering from a laminectomy performed 4 days previously. The following data are collected by the therapist at the patient's bedside:

BP	120/80
Pulse	88
Respiratory rate	18
Vital capacity	50 cc/kg
Breath sounds	Normal
V_T	750 mL

The therapist should recommend that:

A. Therapy be performed as ordered
B. Therapy be discontinued
C. The patient be discharged from the hospital
D. IPPB be administered instead

77. Which of the following statements about cromolyn sodium is (are) true?

I. It is not effective against allergic asthma.
II. It is a synthetic corticosteroid.
III. It inhibits the release of slow-reacting substance of anaphylaxis from the mast cell.
IV. It is a potent bronchodilator.

A. II and III
B. III and IV
C. III only
D. II, III, and IV

78. A 1340-g male infant is delivered following a 30-week gestation. At approximately 1 min of life the following vital signs are noted:

Heart rate	110
Respirations	Absent
Muscle tone	Flaccid
Reflex irritability	No response
Color	Systemic cyanosis

Based on the above information, which of the following actions should the respiratory therapy practitioner recommend at this time?

A. Administer intracardiac epinephrine
B. Start an intravenous line stat
C. Intubate and ventilate with 100% oxygen
D. Continue to monitor closely

79. Which of the following will likely cause the FIO_2 delivered by an air entrainment device to decrease significantly?

I. If the humidity of the driving gas is decreased
II. If the jet is made smaller
III. If the jet is made larger
IV. If the entrainment ports are made smaller
V. If the entrainment ports are made larger

A. I and III
B. II and V
C. II and IV
D. III and IV

80. In reading his patient's chart prior to IPPB therapy, the therapist notes that the patient had 5+ ankle edema when admitted to the hospital. Which of the following disorders would most likely be responsible for this physical sign?

A. Bronchial asthma
B. Adult respiratory distress syndrome
C. Cor pulmonale
D. Drug overdose

81. Which of the following abnormalities can usually be treated by increasing alveolar ventilation?

I. Hypercarbia
II. Metabolic acidosis
III. Hypoxia
IV. Alveolar hypoventilation
V. Respiratory acidosis

A. I, II, and V
B. I, IV, and V
C. II, III, and V
D. II and III

82. Which of the following will enhance the tendency of medical aerosols to "rain out" before entering the patient's smaller airways?

I. Ninety-degree bends in the delivery tubing
II. Use of isotonic solutions
III. Administration with the patient "nose breathing"
IV. Rapid, shallow patient ventilatory pattern
V. Administration of aerosol particles greater than 10µ in diameter

A. I and V
B. II, III, IV, and V
C. I, III, IV, and V
D. I, II, and V

83. For which of the following pulmonary disorders would a hyperresonant percussion note be a common physical finding?

I. Pleural effusion
II. Pneumothorax
III. Emphysema
IV. Hemothorax

A. II and III
B. I, II, and IV
C. II only
D. III only

84. Which of the following is the normal value for $FEV_1\%$?

A. Greater than 40% FVC
B. Greater than 60% FVC
C. Greater than 75% FVC
D. Greater than 90% FVC

85. When using a Wright respirometer, the respiratory therapy practitioner should be aware that flow rates below which of the following levels can produce inaccurate readings?

A. 3 L/min
B. 30 L/min
C. 10 L/min
D. 15 L/min

86. An elderly man is brought to the emergency department after being found unconscious. He is febrile and appears extremely malnourished. He is immediately placed on 8 L oxygen via simple oxygen mask, and a sample of arterial blood is drawn and analyzed. These data appear below:

PaO_2	70 mm Hg
$PaCO_2$	27 mm Hg
pH	7.36
HCO_3^-	12 mEq/L
Base excess	–9 mEq/L

Which of the following is the most correct interpretation of the above results?

A. Fully compensated metabolic acidosis
B. Fully compensated respiratory acidosis
C. Acute respiratory alkalosis
D. Acute metabolic acidosis

87. Which of the following bronchodilators is believed to have the shortest duration of action?

A. Isoproterenol
B. Isoetharine
C. Terbutaline
D. Metaproterenol

88. For which of the following patients could the respiratory therapy practitioner recommend the use of cromolyn sodium?

A. An allergic asthmatic during an acute episode
B. A nonallergic asthmatic during an asthmatic episode
C. An asthmatic who is in remission
D. A nonallergic asthmatic who is not receiving bronchodilator therapy

89. Which of the following clinical signs would be most likely to accompany massive unilateral pulmonary atelectasis?

I. Dull percussion note over the affected area
II. Tracheal shift to the unaffected side
III. Vesicular breath sounds over the affected area
IV. Egophony over the affected area

A. III only
B. II and IV
C. I and IV
D. III and IV

90. Which of the following disorders is *least* likely to be associated with the production of copious amounts of purulent sputum?

A. Pulmonary emphysema
B. Aspiration pneumonia
C. Anaerobic lung abscess
D. Bronchiectasis

91. A P_{50} of ___ would indicate the normal positioning of the oxyhemoglobin dissociation curve.

A. 26.5 mm Hg
B. 25 mm Hg
C. 40 mm Hg
D. 97 mm Hg

92. Which of the following formulas would be most useful in helping the respiratory therapy practitioner establish the initial tidal volume for a patient who is to receive continuous ventilatory support?

A. 15–20 cc/kg
B. 7–10 cc/kg
C. 10–15 cc/lb
D. 10–12 cc/kg

93. Which of the following common household agents would the respiratory therapy practitioner recommend to decontaminate respiratory therapy equipment prescribed for home use?

A. Common household bleach
B. Sodium bicarbonate
C. Acetic acid (vinegar)
D. Baking soda

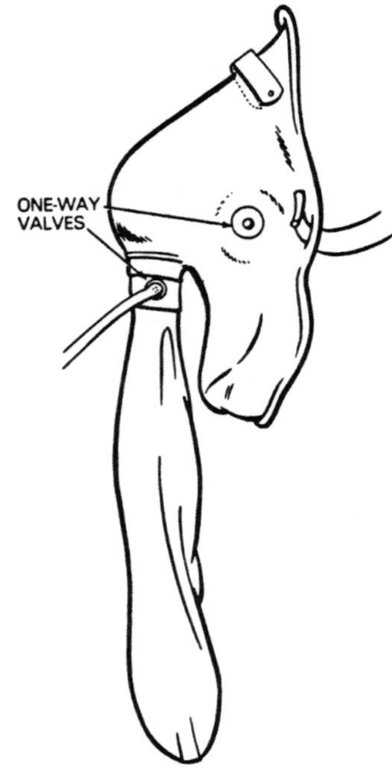

Figure 40.

94. Figure 40 shows:

A. Simple oxygen mask
B. Partial rebreathing mask
C. Nonrebreathing mask
D. Rebreathing mask

95. A satisfactory definition of *respiratory failure* is:

A. Inability to maintain normal venous blood gases
B. Inability to sustain internal respiration
C. Inability to sustain external respiration
D. Inability to maintain normal oxygen saturation

96. Recognized complications that may result from the use of a resuscitator bag, mask, and oral airway combinations include which of the following?

I. Inadequate tidal volumes
II. Hyperventilation
III. Gastric distention

A. II and III
B. I and III
C. I and II
D. II only

97. Which of the following aerosolized bronchodilators is known to have the least amount of β_1 activity?

A. Isoetharine
B. Racemic epinephrine
C. Metaproterenol
D. Albuterol

98. Which of the following are believed to be advantages of anesthesia bag type manual resuscitation devices?

I. Delivery of any desired concentration of oxygen is possible.
II. They are truly self-inflating.
III. Their design allows for "feel" of patient lung mechanics.
IV. They need not be used by highly trained personnel.

A. I and II
B. II and III
C. I and III
D. III and IV

99. Which of the following procedures would be most useful in establishing the existence of a tracheo-esophageal fistula in a patient who is receiving continuous ventilatory support?

A. Arterial blood gas analysis
B. Barium bronchogram
C. Methylene blue (dionosil dye) test
D. Chest physical examination

100. Sympathomimetic bronchodilators are frequently ineffective when administered to:

I. Patients who are severely acidotic
II. Patients with intrinsic asthma
III. Patients with extrinsic asthma

A. I only
B. I, II, and III
C. I and II
D. II and III

101. Whenever significant adverse effects occur involving any respiratory therapeutic modality, the respiratory therapy practitioner must immediately terminate the procedure and notify the ordering physician. Which of the following is the *least* appropriate means of communicating this information?

A. Ask the charge nurse to relay the information.
B. Ask the shift supervisor to page the physician.
C. Page the physician yourself.
D. Chart the information and wait for the physician to read it.

102. All of the following are reportedly reasons why disposable oxygen delivery equipment is desirable. From the standpoint of the respiratory therapy practitioner, which is most significant?

A. They decrease the cost of sterilization procedures.
B. They are more cost-effective overall.
C. Their use allows the therapist to spend more time at the patient's bedside.
D. They decrease the incidence of cross-contamination.

103. An average arterial oxygen tension (Pa_{O_2}) for a healthy 60-year-old would be:

A. 50 mm Hg
B. 60 mm Hg
C. 70 mm Hg
D. 80 mm Hg

104. Which of the following is *not* a recognized hazard of oxygen administration?

A. Hyperventilation
B. Absorption atelectasis
C. Pulmonary edema
D. Retrolental fibroplasia

105. Retrolental fibroplasia:

I. Will result when the newborn's Pa_{O_2} is greater than 50 mm Hg
II. Is related to the PI_{O_2}, not the Pa_{O_2}
III. Is almost invariably seen in the premature newborn

A. I and III
B. III only
C. II only
D. I, II, and III

106. Clubbing of the digits is a physical sign that is known to accompany all of the following disorders *except:*

A. Bronchogenic carcinoma
B. Cystic fibrosis
C. Infant respiratory distress syndrome
D. Chronic bronchitis

107. For which of the following disorders is cyanosis *least* likely to be a clinical sign?

A. Neonatal asphyxia
B. Methemoglobinemia
C. Carbon monoxide poisoning
D. Tetralogy of Fallot

108. Which of the following factors reportedly contribute(s) to the incidence of cuff-related side effects of continuous mechanical ventilation?

I. Arterial hypertension
II. Tracheal infection
III. Use of low-pressure cuffs
IV. Tube movement in the trachea
V. Prolonged artificial ventilation

A. II, IV, and V
B. V only
C. I, II, and IV
D. IV and V

109. Factors that have been held responsible for the extremely high mortality rate among patients developing gram-negative nosocomial pulmonary infections include:

I. Frequent occurrence among immunosuppressed hosts
II. Concurrent administration of continuous ventilatory support
III. Use of broad-spectrum antibiotics
IV. Concurrent development of adult respiratory distress syndrome

A. I and III
B. I, III, and IV
C. I, II, III, and IV
D. II, III, and IV

110. The respiratory therapy practitioner is asked to help set up a home care program for a quadriplegic patient with a vital capacity of 7 cc/kg. The practitioner notes that the patient is unable to cough effectively. Instruction in which one of the following techniques would be most likely to help improve this patient's cough effort?

A. Diaphragmatic breathing
B. Glossopharyngeal ("frog") breathing
C. Pursed lip breathing
D. Chest vibration

111. Which of the following would be the emergency airway modality of choice for an unconscious patient on whom attempts at intubation have failed?

A. Tracheotomy
B. Oropharyngeal airway
C. Cricothyroidotomy
D. Modified jaw thrust

112. The term *pectus excavatum* is most synonymous with which of the following terms?

A. Pigeon chest
B. Barrel chest
C. Funnel chest
D. Bell chest

113. The respiratory therapy practitioner is monitoring a 30-year-old patient who is intubated and receiving an FI_{O_2} of 0.7 via a T tube setup, and acid-base data obtained at that time are as follows:

Pa_{O_2}	34 mm Hg
Pa_{CO_2}	48 mm Hg
HCO_3^-	19 mEq/L
Base excess	−3.8 mEq/L
Respiratory rate	48/min

Which of the following modifications in therapy should the practitioner recommend at this time?

A. Raise the FI_{O_2} to 1.0
B. Place on 5 cm H_2O CPAP with an FI_{O_2} of 0.9
C. Place on assist/control with an FI_{O_2} of 0.8
D. Place on 5 cm H_2O PEEP with an FI_{O_2} of 0.8

114. Which of the following conditions is *least* likely to be associated with the presence of barrel chest?

A. Infancy
B. Emphysema
C. Old age
D. Middle age

115. Which of the following is the *least* likely cause of respiratory alkalosis?

A. Metabolic alkalosis
B. Acute hypoxemia
C. Third-trimester pregnancy
D. Intracranial hypertension

116. The respiratory therapy practitioner can most readily check the accuracy of an oxygen blender device by:

A. Checking the air and oxygen lines to lines on the blender on a regular basis
B. Checking the flow rate from the blender
C. Measuring the patient's arterial oxygen tension every hour
D. Employing an oxygen analyzer

117. Which of the following most correctly describes the term *iatrogenic infection?*

A. One that results from the use of immunosuppressive agents
B. One that occurs postoperatively
C. One that results from the activities of medical or surgical personnel
D. One that occurs in the hospital

118. Which of the following statements are true regarding wheezing heard while auscultating the chest?

I. It is considered to be a type of rale.
II. It may be described as a musical, whistling, or squeaking sound.

III. It is a frequent finding in patients with congestive heart failure.
IV. It always denotes the presence of asthma.

A. I, II, III, and IV
B. I, II, and IV
C. I and IV
D. II and III

119. Common effects of mild to moderate hypoxia include all but which of the following pathophysiologic actions?

A. Increased cardiac output
B. Pulmonary vasoconstriction
C. Increased arterial blood pressure
D. Decreased cardiac output

120. The respiratory therapy practitioner's therapeutic goal is to mobilize secretions in a 68-year-old postoperative patient. Which of the following modalities would the therapist consider as a last resort?

A. Aerosol therapy
B. Instruction in cough technique
C. Nasotracheal suctioning
D. Aerosolized mucokinetic agents

121. Which of the following are recommended methods of keeping ventilator tubing system compliance as low as possible?

I. Using thick-walled tubing
II. Keeping humidifiers filled
III. Keeping gases at BTPS
IV. Using minimal tubing length

A. I, III, and IV
B. I, II, and IV
C. I and IV
D. II, III, and IV

122. The respiratory therapy practitioner would be most likely to employ a nonrebreathing type mask on patients with which one of the following disorders?

A. Bronchiectasis
B. Cystic fibrosis
C. Anemia
D. Carbon monoxide poisoning

123. If the gas flow through an unheated bubble humidifier is increased from 2 L/min to 6 L/min, which of the following will occur?

I. The percent body humidity of gases delivered will decrease.
II. The temperature within the device will increase.
III. The absolute humidity of the gases will increase.
IV. The temperature within the unit will decrease.

A. I and IV
B. I and II
C. III and IV
D. II and IV

124. Which of the following are advantages associated with the use of high-flow oxygen delivery systems?

I. Changes in ventilatory pattern are less likely to affect the delivered FIO_2.
II. The temperature and absolute humidity of the inspired gases may be more easily controlled.
III. The incidence of nosocomial infection is known to be lower with their use.
IV. Alveolar ventilation tends to increase with their use.

A. I and II
B. III and IV
C. I, II, and III
D. I, II, and IV

125. Which of the following pulmonary disorders is *not* associated with shifts of the mediastinal contents to the unaffected side?

A. Massive atelectasis
B. Pleural effusion
C. Tension pneumothorax
D. Hemothorax

126. In reading a patient's chart, the respiratory therapy practitioner notes the attending physician's statement that the patient's primary pathology involves the loss of pulmonary parenchymal elastic recoil. This observation is most consistent with:

A. Chronic bronchitis
B. Emphysema
C. Bronchiectasis
D. Bronchial asthma

127. All of the following methods have been recommended to help prevent a patient from fighting a ventilator. Which method reportedly provides fewest hindrances to the weaning process?

A. Use of mechanical hyperventilation
B. Use of analgesics
C. Use of SIMV
D. Use of paralyzing agents

128. A 17-year-old girl is brought to the emergency department by her father after she suffered an asthma attack that did not respond to metered-dose isoetharine at home. The patient's respiratory rate is 25/min and her pulse is 100. Arterial blood sampled at this time with an FIO_2 of 0.21 would most likely reveal:

A. Partially compensated respiratory acidosis with moderate hypoxemia
B. Respiratory alkalosis with moderate hypoxemia
C. Fully compensated metabolic acidosis with mild hypoxemia
D. Respiratory alkalosis with very severe hypoxemia

Directions: Each group of questions below concerns a certain situation. In each case, first study the description of the situation, then choose the one best answer to each question following it and mark the answer accordingly.

Questions 129–131

A 70-year-old patient with longstanding COPD and cor pulmonale is admitted to the respiratory intensive care unit. Historical data reveals progressive deterioration despite an aggressive home respiratory care program.

129. Twelve hours post admission, the physician decides to intubate and begin continuous ventilatory support. Which of the following formulas should the RCP use to help determine the patient's tidal volume?

 A. 5 cc/kg
 B. 12 cc/kg
 C. 15 cc/lb
 D. 18 cc/kg

130. Which of the following is *least* likely to contribute to difficulties in weaning the patient with chronic obstructive pulmonary disease from continuous ventilatory support?

 A. Ventilatory muscle discoordination
 B. Psychologic dependence
 C. Sleep deprivation
 D. Use of IMV

131. Because a prolonged course of continuous ventilatory support is anticipated, this patient is intubated with an endotracheal tube using a low pressure, high residual volume type cuff. Also anticipated are the following complications of prolonged tracheal intubation. Which is *least* preventable?

 A. Tracheal necrosis
 B. Bacterial contamination of the airways
 C. Tracheal dilatation
 D. Tracheal stenosis

Questions 132–134

A 31-year-old patient is admitted to the respiratory intensive care unit for intensive respiratory therapy. Fourteen months ago he sustained neurologic and spinal cord damage while in the line of duty as a police officer. Weaned after 4 weeks of continuous ventilatory support, his pulmonary rehabilitation was slow. Vigorous respiratory and physical therapy were required to increase his pulmonary reserves. Five months ago he was sent home with a tracheostomy button in place. However, despite the suction port, loss of upper airway reflexes has resulted in a chronic aspiration problem. Two weeks prior to admission, he developed a low-grade fever and began coughing productively. Symptoms have gradually increased in severity. At the time of admission a diagnosis of pulmonary abscess was made.

132. True statements about a tracheal button airway include:

 I. It may facilitate suctioning.
 II. It is a type of fenestrated tracheostomy tube.
 III. It may be used to maintain a patent tracheal stoma.
 IV. It can be used to administer continuous ventilatory support.
 V. When "plugged," it may allow the patient to talk.

 A. I, II, and IV
 B. II, IV, and V
 C. III, IV, and V
 D. I, III, and V

133. The hallmark of anaerobic lung abscess is:

 A. Massive air trapping
 B. Pink frothy sputum
 C. "Currant jelly" sputum
 D. Copious amounts of foul-smelling sputum

134. Which of the following is (are) known to complicate the clinical picture of the patient with lung abscess?

 I. Empyema
 II. Pneumothorax
 III. Centrilobular emphysema

 A. I and III
 B. I and II
 C. I, II, and III
 D. III only

Questions 135–137

A 52-year-old woman is brought to the emergency department in respiratory distress. She is 4 feet, 6 inches tall and weighs approximately 40 kg. She has had kyphoscoliosis since late adolescence but has only become symptomatic in the past decade or so. This is her third admission in as many years. Each one has been precipitated by a respiratory infection. At present, she is in the intensive care unit where she is receiving supportive care.

135. Pulmonary laboratory tests on a patient with kyphoscoliosis generally reveal:

 I. Restrictive defect
 II. Decreased vital capacity
 III. Increased RV/TLC%
 IV. Decreased FRC

 A. I, III, and IV
 B. II only
 C. I, II, and IV
 D. I only

136. True statements regarding kyphoscoliosis include:

 I. It is defined as lateral and posterior curvature of the spine.

II. Its incidence is higher in females.
III. Primary pulmonary pathosis involves thickening of the alveolar-capillary membrane.
IV. Definitive treatment consists of performing a laminectomy.

A. III and IV
B. I, II, and IV
C. I and II
D. I and III

137. Mechanical ventilation in the patient with marked kyphoscoliosis:

A. Is contraindicated
B. May worsen V/Q relationships
C. Should always be used in conjunction with PEEP
D. May result in volume-related side effects

Questions 138–140

A 51-year-old woman is admitted to the intensive care unit after falling at home. Admission roentgenograms show a compound fracture of the pelvis. Physical examination reveals an extremely obese woman with a complaint of shortness of breath and easy fatigability. She is only 62 inches tall and weighs 228 kg. Gross observation also reveals large and pendulous breasts. Neck veins are distended, her respiratory rate is 32, her pulse is 110, and her blood pressure is 170/130. Arterial blood is analyzed, revealing the following data:

FIO_2	0.21
PaO_2	53 mm Hg
$PaCO_2$	59 mm Hg
pH	7.37
Base excess	+8.3 mEq/L
HCO_3^-	32.9 mEq/L
Hb concentration	21.6 g/dL

Based on this information and the patient's relevant history, a diagnosis of Pickwickian syndrome is made.

138. Which of the following is the correct interpretation of this patient's arterial blood gas data?

A. Fully compensated respiratory acidosis
B. Partially compensated metabolic alkalosis
C. Fully compensated metabolic alkalosis
D. Fully compensated metabolic acidosis

139. The patient's hemoglobin concentration most likely represents:

A. Erythrocytopenia
B. Primary polycythemia
C. Idiopathic thrombocytopenic purpura
D. Secondary polycythemia

140. One hour postoperatively, the patient is in the recovery room on a Bennett MA-I ventilator. Arterial blood gas and other data obtained on an FIO_2 of 0.6 with the patient in the control mode are as follows:

PaO_2	43 mm Hg
$PaCO_2$	26 mm Hg
pH	7.42
Base excess	−6.3 mEq/L
V_T	1200 cc

Based on the foregoing information, which of the following would be the most appropriate modification in the ventilator settings?

A. Increase the FIO_2 to 0.8, decrease the tidal volume, and place on 20 cm H_2O PEEP.
B. Increase the tidal volume and add 5 cm H_2O PEEP.
C. Place on 5 cm H_2O PEEP, increase the FIO_2 to 0.8, and decrease the tidal volume.
D. Place on 15 cm H_2O PEEP and place on IMV.

Answer Key and NBRC Examination Matrix Categories

1. D, IIIA
2. D, IB
3. A, IIIC
4. B, IIIB
5. C, IIB
6. A, IC
7. C, IIB
8. D, IIID
9. B, IIIG
10. B, IIIE
11. D, IIIB
12. B, IIIF
13. D, IIID
14. D, IIB
15. C, IIIE
16. C, IIIA
17. C, IIA
18. B, IIIB
19. B, IC
20. C, IIIA
21. D, IIIA
22. B, IA
23. D, IIID
24. C, ID
25. A, 3B
26. A, IC
27. D, IIIG
28. A, IIIB
29. A, IIIF
30. C, IIIF
31. B, IIIA
32. D, IB

33. D, IIB
34. D, IC
35. B, IIIG
36. D, IIB
37. D, IIIE
38. D, IB
39. D, IIIG
40. A, IC
41. B, IA
42. D, IIIB
43. B, IIB
44. D, ID
45. A, IB
46. C, IIID
47. B, ID
48. D, IB
49. B, ID
50. C, IIIF
51. D, IIIC
52. D, IIIC
53. A, IIA
54. A, IIIB
55. A, IIIG
56. D, IB
57. C, IIIB
58. D, IIA
59. B, IIIG
60. B, IB
61. D, ID
62. D, IIIA
63. B, IA
64. A, ID
65. B, IB
66. A, IA
67. D, IIID
68. B, IIIG
69. D, IIID
70. D, IB
71. C, IIIG
72. B, IIIG
73. B, IIIB
74. C, IIB
75. A, IIIE
76. B, IIIF
77. C, IIIB
78. C, IIIG
79. B, IIB
80. C, IA
81. B, IIIC
82. C, IIIB
83. A, IB
84. C, IA
85. A, IIB
86. A, IC
87. A, IIIB
88. C, IIIF
89. C, IB
90. A, IB
91. A, IIID
92. D, IIIC
93. C, IIA
94. C, IIB
95. C, IIIE
96. B, IIIB
97. D, IIB
98. C, IIB
99. C, IC
100. A, IIIB
101. D, IIIA
102. D, IIB
103. D, IIIE
104. A, IIID
105. B, IIID
106. C, IB
107. C, IB
108. A, IIIB
109. C, IIIA
110. B, IIIA
111. C, IIIB
112. C, IB
113. D, IIIF
114. D, IB
115. A, IC
116. D, IIB
117. C, IIIA
118. D, IB
119. D, IIID
120. C, IIIB
121. B, IIB
122. D, IIB
123. A, IIB
124. A, IIB
125. A, IB
126. B, IA
127. C, IIIC
128. B, IC
129. D, IIIC
130. D, IIIC
131. B, IC
132. D, IIB
133. D, ID
134. B, ID
135. C, IC
136. C, ID
137. B, IIIC
138. A, ID
139. D, IC
140. C, IIIF

UNIT II

Advanced Practitioner Examination Posttest

The following full-length Advanced Practitioner Examination posttest was constructed according to specifications outlined in the current NBRC Composite Examination Matrix. The examination categories and the number of questions allotted to each by the NBRC are listed in the table below. In addition, *the answer key at the end of this test is referenced to the examination matrix so the candidate may further identify his or her weak areas.* For a more thorough discussion of the NBRC Composite Examination Matrix, please refer to the Introduction of this book and to the Examination Category Review and Pretest.

TABLE 2. ADVANCED PRACTITIONER EXAMINATION CONTENT MATRIX

	Examination Category	Number of Questions	Percentage of Questions
I.	***Clinical Data***	25	25
A.	Review patient records	10	10
B.	Collect and evaluate clinical information	5	5
C.	Perform and evaluate laboratory procedures	10	10
II.	***Equipment***	10	10
A.	Select, assemble, check, and correct malfunctions of equipment	6	6
B.	Ensure cleanliness of equipment	1	1
C.	Perform quality control and calibration procedures	3	3
III.	***Therapeutic Procedures***	65	65
A.	Maintain airway	3	3
B.	Ensure ventilation	7	7
C.	Ensure oxygenation	3	3
D.	Assess patient response to therapy	20	20
E.	Modify therapy	7	7
F.	Recommend modifications in therapy	22	22
G.	Assist physician with special procedures	3	3

Examination for Advanced Level Respiratory Therapy Practitioners

Time: 2 hours

Directions: Each of the questions or incomplete statements below is followed by four suggested answers. Select the one that is best in each case and then mark accordingly.

1. A 79-year-old patient is seen in the intensive care unit while receiving continuous ventilatory support with an FIO_2 of 0.6 and 10 cm H_2O PEEP. The following data are noted at this time:

PaO_2	58 mm Hg
$PaCO_2$	42 mm Hg
pH	7.35
HCO_3^-	23 mEq/L
Colloidal osmotic pressure	14 mm Hg
Total serum proteins	3.0 g/dL
Na^+	140 mEq/L
Cl^-	103 mEq/L
K^+	5.0 mEq/L

The physician decides fluid administration is indicated. Which of the following should the therapist recommend?

A. 5% dextrose in H_2O
B. Lactated Ringer's solution
C. NaCl
D. KCl

2. After breathing 100% oxygen for 15 min, which of the following patients would be *least* likely to have had all the nitrogen washed out of his lungs?

A. An asthmatic patient in remission
B. A patient in congestive heart failure
C. A patient with normal lungs
D. A patient with advanced stage emphysema

3. Following thoracocentesis, approximately 500 mL of a thick, milky-white fluid is drained from the pleural space. This fluid most likely represents a:

A. Pleural transudate
B. Chylothorax
C. Hemothorax
D. Empyema

4. Pulmonary function studies on a 60-year-old patient reveal an FEF_{25-75} of 0.3 L/min. Which of the following statements best describes this patient's pulmonary status?

A. Mild restrictive lung disease exists.
B. Mixed obstructive and restrictive lung disease exists.
C. Mild obstructive disease exists.
D. Severe obstructive disease exists.

5. Following orthopaedic surgery, a 65-kg, 82-year-old woman develops respiratory failure. She is placed on a volume ventilator, immediately after which depression in the arterial blood pressure is noted to occur. The following findings are charted at this time with the patient in the assist mode:

Respiratory rate	32/min
Tidal volume	900 mL
Peak flow rate	55 L/min
Peak pressure	48 cm H_2O

The *least* appropriate therapeutic modification for the therapist to make at this time would be to:

A. Recommend appropriate sedation
B. Recommend fluid administration
C. Decrease the tidal volume
D. Decrease the flow rate

6. All but which of the following describe high-frequency oscillatory ventilation (HFOV)?

A. Tidal volumes less than deadspace are delivered.
B. Respiratory rates as high as 3000 can be delivered.
C. Tracheal tissue damage is a commonly seen side effect.
D. Expiration is active.

7. The respiratory therapy practitioner is monitoring a 1250-g (30-week gestation) newborn in the neonatal intensive care unit who is receiving 70% oxygen via hood. The following information is charted at this time:

PaO_2	40 mm Hg
$PaCO_2$	36 mm Hg
pH	7.30
Respiratory rate	85
Appearance	Peripheral cyanosis noted
Heart rate	210/min

Which of the following would be the most correct recommendation for the therapist to make regarding the above information?

A. Initiate continuous ventilatory support with 4 cm H_2O PEEP and an FIO_2 of 0.5.
B. Place on 15 cm H_2O CPAP with an FIO_2 of 1.0.
C. Place on 4 cm H_2O CPAP with an FIO_2 of 0.8.
D. Place on 100% oxygen via hood.

8. A 54-year-old woman with a history of bronchiectasis dating back to her adolescence is brought to the hospital by paramedics. The patient is cyanotic and her respirations are labored, but she does not complain of dyspnea. Admission blood gases on 2 L oxygen via cannula are as follows:

PaO_2	45 mm Hg
$PaCO_2$	72 mm Hg
pH	7.36
HCO_3^-	38.7 mEq/L

Based on these data, the most appropriate modification in this patient's therapy would be to:

A. Intubate the patient and place on SIMV with an FIO_2 of 0.4.
B. Decrease liter flow to 1 L/min.
C. Intubate the patient and administer 40% oxygen via heated aerosol.
D. Increase liter flow to 3 L/min.

9. Which of the following devices use(s) transducers as part of normal function and operation?

I. Fleish pneumotachometer
II. Certain volume ventilators
III. Pulmonary artery catheter
IV. Heat transfer pneumotachometer

A. I and III
B. III only
C. I, II, III, and IV
D. II, III, and IV

10. An 80-kg, 30-year-old patient with flail chest and bilateral lung contusion is pharmacologically paralyzed and placed on a Bourns Bear II ventilator in the control mode with a tidal volume of 700 mL. Arterial blood gases drawn on an FIO_2 of 0.6 yield the following data:

PaO_2	40 mm Hg
$PaCO_2$	23 mm Hg
pH	7.52
HCO_3^-	16 mEq/L
Base excess	–4 mEq/L

Which of the following therapeutic modifications should the respiratory therapy practitioner make at this time?

A. Place the patient on IMV mode and increase the FIO_2 to 0.8.
B. Decrease the tidal volume, add 250 cc mechanical deadspace and 5 cm H_2O PEEP.
C. Add 400 cc mechanical deadspace and increase the FIO_2 to 1.0.
D. Decrease the respiratory rate and add 5 cm H_2O PEEP

11. Which of the following statements are true of high-frequency jet ventilation (HFJV)?

I. Respiratory rates up to 150 breaths per minute are utilized.
II. The expiratory phase is passive.
III. It requires the use of a special catheter or endotracheal tube.
IV. Most ventilators can deliver HFJV.

A. I, III, and IV
B. I, II, and III
C. II and IV
D. II and III

12. Which of the following causes of hypoxemia is (are) believed to always be accompanied by an abnormal $P(A–a)O_2$ when the patient is breathing room air?

I. Shunting
II. Low V/Q
III. Hypoventilation
IV. Diffusion defect

A. I and IV
B. II, III, and IV
C. I, II, and IV
D. IV only

13. Which of the following is *not* a recognized hazard of the use of negative pressure tank type ventilators (iron lung)?

A. Venous pooling
B. Patient inaccessibility
C. Lack of patient assisting capability
D. Necrosis of tracheal mucosa

14. Eight days post hepatic resection, the following blood gas and acid-base data are obtained on an alert patient who is on a Servo 900 C ventilator in the assist/control mode with 10 cm H_2O PEEP:

PaO_2	183 mm Hg
$PaCO_2$	26 mm Hg
pH	7.59
HCO_3^-	24 mEq/L
Base excess	+4.0 mEq/L
FIO_2	0.7

Which of the following would be the most acceptable modification of this patient's mechanical ventilatory therapy?

A. Decrease the PEEP and place on SIMV.
B. Decrease the FIO_2 and add 300 cc mechanical deadspace.
C. Decrease the PEEP and decrease the minute volume.
D. Decrease the FIO_2 and place on SIMV.

15. Pulmonary function tests performed on a patient with pulmonary fibrosis would most likely reveal all of the following *except:*

A. Decreased D_LCO
B. Normal $\frac{FEV_1}{FVC}$ %
C. Normal ERV
D. Decreased TLC

16. Which of the following types of hypoxia is most frequently associated with elevations in mixed venous oxygen tensions?

A. Hypoxemic
B. Anemic
C. Circulatory
D. Histotoxic

17. Which of the following statements are true of Bi-PAP?

I. Both IPAP and EPAP are used.
II. It is classified as a form of noninvasive ventilation.
III. It is well tolerated in patients with neuromuscular respiratory insufficiency.
IV. It is well tolerated in children.

A. I, II, III, and IV
B. I, II, and IV
C. II, III, and IV
D. II and III

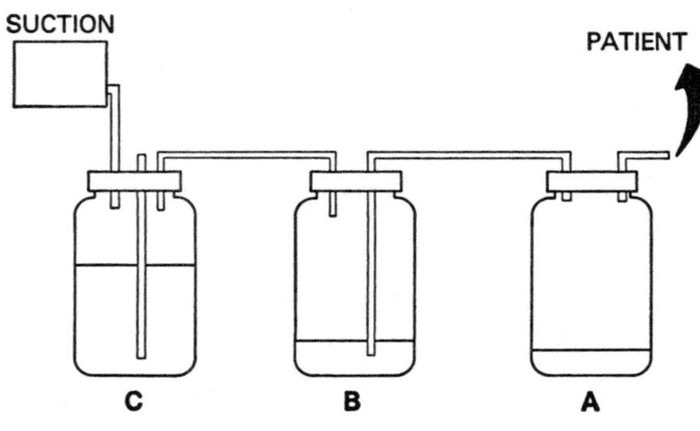

Figure 41.

18. Which of the following statements regarding three-chamber chest suction systems such as that in Figure 41 is (are) true?

I. Constant bubbling in the suction control bottle indicates evacuation of air from the pleural space.
II. The tube should be placed 15–20 cm below the surface in the water-seal chamber.
III. The tube in the suction control bottle should be placed approximately 2 cm below the surface of the water.
IV. Bottle B is the water-seal chamber.

A. IV only
B. II and IV
C. III and IV
D. I and III

19. The respiratory therapy practitioner is monitoring a critically ill patient who has just received 12 units of stored ACD blood. Results of blood gas analysis are reported and show that the patient's P_{50} has dropped from 27 mm Hg to 20 mm Hg. Which of the following statements regarding this situation is (are) true?

I. The patient's oxyhemoglobin dissociation curve has shifted to the left.
II. The amount of oxygen available to the tissues has increased.
III. 2-3 DPG deficient blood may be responsible.

A. I only
B. I and III
C. II only
D. I and II

20. Which of the following chest radiologic findings may be considered evidence of the presence of congestive heart failure?

I. Cardiothoracic ratio less than 50%
II. Presence of increased radiolucency
III. Presence of Kerley-B lines
IV. Evidence of mediastinal shift

A. II and III
B. III only
C. I and IV
D. I and II

21. Positive pressure ventilators used in the home should possess all but which of the following characteristics?

A. Portability
B. Easy to operate
C. Internal battery
D. All of the above

E. I and IV
(36:91)

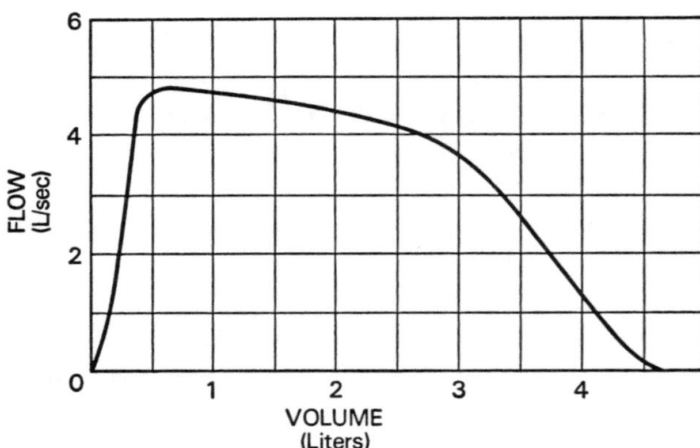

Figure 42.

22. The flow-volume loop in Figure 42 was obtained from a 48-year-old, 62-kg patient. The best interpretation of this loop would be:

A. Mild restrictive lung disease
B. Severe chronic obstructive lung disease
C. Combined obstructive-restrictive pulmonary disease
D. Large airway obstruction

23. The respiratory therapy practitioner is monitoring a patient who is receiving continuous ventilatory support. Pertinent data are listed below:

	Time	
	9:00 AM	10:00 AM
PEEP	8 cm H_2O	12 cm H_2O
Peak pressure	38 cm H_2O	55 cm H_2O
Plateau pressure	31 cm H_2O	48 cm H_2O
Tidal volume	930 mL	980 mL
Inspiratory flow rate	0.67 L/sec	40 L/min

Which of the following assessments is (are) true regarding the above information?

I. There is an increase in pulmonary elastance.
II. There is an increase in effective static compliance.
III. The airway resistance is unchanged.
IV. The patient probably needs to be suctioned.

A. I and III
B. II and III
C. I and IV
D. II and IV

24. Eight days after being placed on continuous mechanical ventilation, a patient who inhaled toxic gas in an industrial accident displays the following clinical data:

FIO_2	0.4
PEEP	15 cm H_2O
PaO_2	130 mm Hg
$PaCO_2$	34 mm Hg
Ventilator mode	Assist/control

What ventilator change(s) should the respiratory therapist recommend at this time?

A. Decrease the PEEP to 10 cm H_2O.
B. Decrease the PEEP to 5 cm H_2O and reduce the FIO_2 to 0.3.
C. Decrease the FIO_2 to 0.35 and place on IMV.
D. Add 100 cc mechanical deadspace and lower the FIO_2 to 0.3.

25. Following thoracotomy and chest tube placement, approximately 800 cc of a thick, yellowish liquid is drained. This fluid most likely represents:

A. Pleurisy
B. A pleural transudate
C. An empyema
D. Chylothorax

26. An 1850-g newborn is seen in the nursery 4 hr post partum. The infant is evaluated by the respiratory therapy practitioner at this time and the following information is charted:

Pulse	185
Respiratory rate	78/min
Muscle tone	Good
Expiratory grunting	Audible with stethoscope
FIO_2	0.35

Based on the above information, which of the following is the most correct recommendation for the respiratory therapy practitioner to make at this time?

A. Increase FIO_2 to 0.5.
B. Perform arterial blood gas analysis stat.
C. Place on 5 cm H_2O nasal CPAP.
D. Intubate and place on 5 cm H_2O CPAP.

27. A ventilator designed for out-of-hospital transport should possess all but which of the following characteristics?

A. Ability to operate over extremes of temperature
B. Uses minimal gas flow above the patient's minute ventilation
C. Must be able to provide IMV
D. Consume minimal power

28. In reviewing a patient's chart prior to performing pulmonary drainage techniques, the respiratory therapy practitioner notes that the patient's intracranial pressure is 10 mm Hg. This finding is most consistent with:

A. Intracranial hypertension
B. Normal intracranial pressure
C. Cerebral anoxia
D. Cerebral infarction

29. A patient is seen in the intensive care unit following the development of severe oxygenation failure. He is currently on a Servo 900 C ventilator with an FIO_2 of 0.8 and 18 cm H_2O PEEP. A radiologic diagnosis of pulmonary edema is made. Pertinent data are as follows:

PaO_2	53 mm Hg
$S\bar{v}O_2$	45%
PWP	39 mm Hg
Oxygen consumption	250 mL/min
Serum albumin	5.0 g/dL
$C(a-\bar{v})O_2$	7.7 vol%
Total serum proteins	8.0 g/dL
Colloidal osmotic pressure	25 mm Hg

Based on the above information, the respiratory therapy practitioner can assess that the most probable cause of this patient's pulmonary edema is:

A. Left ventricular failure
B. Hypervolemia
C. Hypoproteinemia
D. Right ventricular failure

30. The respiratory care practitioner is asked to help set up a home care program for a 74-year-old woman with advanced chronic obstructive pulmonary disease. Which of the following daily activities could the therapist recommend to help this patient rebuild her cardiopulmonary reserves?

I. Gardening
II. Sewing
III. Walking
IV. Racquetball
V. Driving an automobile
VI. Household chores

A. I and II
B. I, II, III, V, and VI
C. I, III, and VI
D. II, III, IV, V, and VI

31. The most common usage of double lumen endotracheal tubes is:

A. In the neonatal ICU
B. By paramedics in the field
C. In the emergency room
D. In the operating room

32. A 45-year-old patient is seen in the intensive care unit by a respiratory care practitioner. The patient's pulmonary wedge pressure is 30 mm Hg. To determine whether left ventricular dysfunction or hypervolemia is responsible for this abnormality, which of the following should be measured?

A. Q_T (cardiac output)
B. Pulmonary vascular resistance
C. Pao_2
D. Effective static compliance

33. In reviewing a patient's chart prior to administering IPPB, the respiratory therapy practitioner notes that the patient's "normal" electrocardiogram is one of atrial fibrillation. While taking this patient's pulse, the therapist will most likely note its:

A. Regularity
B. Rapidity
C. Strength
D. Irregularity

34. Which of the following would the respiratory therapy practitioner recommend as criteria for initiation of continuous ventilatory support in the newborn?

I. Hypoxemia on 60% oxygen and 2 cm H_2O CPAP
II. Hypoxemia on 60% oxygen via hood
III. Hypoxemia on 100% oxygen and 12 cm H_2O CPAP
IV. $Paco_2$ of 70 mm Hg on 30% oxygen

A. II and III
B. I and II
C. I and IV
D. III and IV

35. Which of the following statements about the procedure of neonatal intubation is (are) true?

I. A curved laryngoscope blade is invariably preferred.
II. When a straight laryngoscope blade is used, the tip may be placed in the vallecula.
III. Hyperextension of the head and neck should be avoided.
IV. The No. 2 laryngoscope blade is preferred for preterm newborns.

A. II only
B. II and III
C. II, III, and IV
D. I and IV

36. True statements regarding pulmonary hypertension include:

I. It is defined as an abnormally high pulmonary wedge pressure.
II. It is generally believed to exist whenever the pressures in the pulmonary circuit (systolic/diastolic) rise above 35/15 (mm Hg).
III. It is usually caused by right ventricular failure.
IV. It may be caused by increases in pulmonary vascular resistance.

A. I and IV
B. II and IV
C. II, III, and IV
D. I and III

37. In reading a patient's chart prior to therapy, the respiratory care practitioner notes that the patient's white blood cell count is 2000/µL. This value is most consistent with:

A. Leukocytosis
B. Normal value
C. Leukocytopenia
D. Nosocomial infection

38. Venous return is believed to be impaired shortly after initiation of continuous ventilatory support on a 20-year-old man. The patient was admitted following hemorrhage sustained in a motorcycle accident. Which of the following should the respiratory therapist recommend to help lessen the severity of this side effect?

I. Chronotropic stimulation
II. Administration of propranolol
III. Intravascular volume expansion
IV. Administration of morphine

A. III only
B. II only
C. I and IV
D. II, III, and IV

39. Which of the following is *not* associated with the formation of subcutaneous emphysema?

A. Peripheral venipuncture
B. Positive pressure ventilation
C. Tracheotomy
D. Traumatic intubation

40. An unconscious patient is noted to become agitated, diaphoretic, and dusky while receiving continuous ventilatory support. Pertinent findings include the appearance of bibasal rales, an increase in the ventilator plateau pressure from 35 cm H_2O to 48 cm H_2O, and an increase in the PWP from 10 mm Hg to 38 mm Hg. Based on the above information, the most likely cause of this patient's distress is:

A. Acute pulmonary embolus
B. Cardiogenic pulmonary edema
C. Upper airway secretions
D. Intestinal rupture

41. Results of a single breath diffusion study reveal a D_LCO of 5 mL/min/mm Hg. This value is most consistent with:

A. Normal study
B. Increased diffusion capacity
C. Decreased diffusion capacity
D. Small airways disease

42. The physician asks the respiratory therapy practitioner to help evaluate the following pulmonary function data obtained on a 53-year-old patient with pneumonia who is in need of bronchial hygiene therapy:

	Before Bronchodilator	After Bronchodilator
FVC	2.43 L	2.48 L
$FEF_{200-1200}$	64% of normal	62% of normal
FEV_1	53%	55%
FEF_{25-75}	40%	43%

Based on the above information, which of the following should the therapist recommend?

A. IPPB four times a day with 0.5 cc metaproterenol
B. Aerosol therapy followed by postural drainage and percussion four times a day
C. 0.5 cc isoetharine four times a day via hand-held nebulizer
D. Breathing retraining every day

43. Pharmacologic paralysis and sedation would most likely be recommended when continuous ventilatory support is required in the management of:

A. Guillain-Barré syndrome
B. Advanced stage emphysema
C. Narcotic overdose
D. Status asthmaticus

44. A patient is seen in the intensive care unit. He is on a volume ventilator and is receiving an FIO_2 of 0.6 along with 12 cm H_2O PEEP. A diagnosis of pulmonary edema is made following review of clinical and radiologic data. Additional pertinent information is listed below:

PaO_2	44 mm Hg
$P\bar{v}O_2$	28 mm Hg
PWP	29 mm Hg
Oxygen consumption	250 mL/min
$C(a-\bar{v})O_2$	2.7 vol%
Colloidal osmotic pressure	25 mm Hg
Total proteins	8.0 g/dL

Based on the above information, the respiratory therapy practitioner should assess that the most probable cause of this patient's pulmonary edema is:

A. Adult respiratory distress syndrome
B. Right ventricular failure
C. Left ventricular failure
D. Hypervolemia

45. Which one of the following is *most* likely to be abnormal in a 45-year-old man who is free of cardiopulmonary symptoms but has smoked one pack of cigarettes daily for 20 years?

A. FEF_{25-75}
B. $FEF_{200-1200}$
C. FEV_1
D. Airway resistance (R_{AW})

46. A patient in respiratory failure has been orally intubated in the emergency room. Exhaled CO_2 measures 0.5%. What should the RCP recommend?

A. Extubate the patient and reintubate.
B. Secure the tube as it is.
C. Obtain a chest x-ray to assure proper placement.
D. Perform an emergency tracheotomy.

47. Which of the following are true statements regarding laryngoscope devices?

I. The No. 0 and No. 1 blades are designed for neonatal use.
II. They are designed to be inserted in the right side of the mouth.
III. The tip of the adult straight laryngoscope blade is designed to be placed under the epiglottis.
IV. Laryngoscopes with both adult and pediatric size handles are available.

A. I, III, and IV
B. II, III, and IV
C. I and II
D. I, II, III, and IV

48. An 18-year-old woman is seen in the emergency department. She is deeply comatose and there are needle tracks on her arms. Results of arterial blood gas analysis on room air are as follows:

$Pa{O_2}$	45 mm Hg
$Pa{CO_2}$	80 mm Hg
pH	7.10
Base excess	–6.3 mEq/L
HCO_3^-	22 mEq/L

Which of the following assessments is (are) true regarding this patient's status?

I. Low V/Q is responsible for the hypoxemia.
II. The $P(A\text{-}a)O_2$ is within normal limits.
III. The hypoxemia is due to hypoventilation.
IV. Oxygen therapy would not be of benefit.

A. I, III, and IV
B. III only
C. II and III
D. II, III, and IV

49. The respiratory therapy practitioner is monitoring a hemodynamically stable 70-kg patient who is receiving controlled mechanical ventilation with a rate of 14 and a tidal volume of 700 mL. If the patient's tidal volume were increased to 1200 mL with other settings unchanged, which of the following would be most likely to occur?

I. An increase in alveolar ventilation
II. A decrease in physiologic deadspace
III. A decrease in $Pa{CO_2}$

A. I and III
B. III only
C. II only
D. II and III

50. When a straight laryngoscope blade is being used to intubate the trachea of an adult patient, which of the following should *not* be done?

A. The patient's head and neck should be placed in the sniffing position.
B. The patient's teeth should not be used as a fulcrum.
C. The tip of the blade should be placed under the epiglottis.
D. The blade should be inserted into the left side of the patient's mouth.

51. Transcutaneous oxygen monitoring devices use which of the following principles?

I. Polarographic principle
II. Paramagnetism of oxygen
III. Use of heat to "arterialize" capillary blood
IV. Solubility and diffusibility of oxygen

A. I and III
B. II and IV
C. I, III, and IV
D. I, II, and III

52. Large increases in intrathoracic pressure following initiation of positive pressure ventilation may typically result in:

I. Increased intracranial pressure
II. Decreases in central venous pressure
III. Reductions in venous return
IV. Decreases in intrapleural pressure

A. I and IV
B. II and IV
C. I and III
D. I, II, and III

53. Which of the following statements about the clinical usage of Apgar scoring is (are) true?

I. The 5-min score is generally lower than that at 1 min.
II. The last vital sign to deteriorate is the heart rate.
III. A score of 0–3 represents severe asphyxia.
IV. This system assesses the newborn's chances of having neurologic abnormalities.

A. II and III
B. I, II, and IV
C. II and IV
D. III only

54. An 18-year-old is seen in the emergency department following a near-drowning incident. The following data are charted at this time:

$Pa{O_2}$	38 mm Hg
$FI{O_2}$	10 L O_2 via simple oxygen mask
$Pa{CO_2}$	28 mm Hg
pH	7.34
HCO_3^-	12 mEq/L
BP	170/110
Pulse	130
Appearance	Profound cyanosis noted

Which of the following assessments are true regarding this patient's presentation?

I. Severe anemia is most likely responsible for the cyanosis.
II. PEEP or CPAP may be beneficial.
III. Refractory hypoxemia exists.
IV. Tachycardia and arterial hypotension exist.

A. IV only
B. II, III, and IV
C. I and IV
D. II and III

55. In reading a patient's chart, the respiratory therapy practitioner notes that the patient's pulmonary wedge pressures are consistently in the range of 3–4 mm Hg. These data are most consistent with:

A. Normal study
B. Left ventricular failure
C. Adult respiratory distress syndrome
D. Hypovolemia

56. The following pulmonary function data were obtained from a 61-year-old man as part of a routine preoperative screening program:

Test	Predicted	Observed
FVC	4.1 L	4.0 L
$\frac{FEV_1}{FVC}$ %	75%	70%
MEFR	8.1 L/sec	8.2 L/sec
FEF_{25-75}	3.4 L/sec	1.9 L/sec
Slow vital capacity	4.2 L	4.2 L

Which of the following is the most correct interpretation of the above data?

A. Moderate obstructive defect
B. Normal study
C. Small airways disease
D. Restrictive defect

57. Intensive therapy is in progress for a 7-year-old boy who was admitted in severe status asthmaticus. The patient is receiving intravenous aminophylline, methylprednisolone, and isoproterenol. In addition, metaproterenol is being administered every 3 hr via unpressurized nebulizer. Current blood gas results with the patient receiving 4 L oxygen via simple oxygen mask are as follows:

pH	7.20
Pa_{O_2}	67 mm Hg
Pa_{CO_2}	43 mm Hg
HCO_3^-	16.6 mEq/L
Base excess	–8.9 mEq/L

The physician does not want to begin mechanical ventilation and asks for a recommendation. At this time, the practitioner should suggest which of the following?

A. Increasing the dosage of metaproterenol
B. Discontinuing the intravenously administered aminophylline
C. Correcting base deficit to enhance bronchodilator effectiveness
D. Administering a continuous ultrasonic aerosol

58. In reading the chart of a patient who is being treated for a pulmonary embolus, the respiratory therapy practitioner would be *least* likely to note documentation of which of the following signs and symptoms?

A. Dyspnea
B. Chest pain
C. Increased pulmonary wedge pressure
D. Hemoptysis

59. A patient receiving continuous ventilatory support becomes distressed and exhibits diminished air entry over the left lung field. Other physical findings are nonspecific. Differential diagnosis can usually be accomplished rapidly by which of the following therapeutic modifications?

A. Advancing the endotracheal tube slightly
B. Stat chest roentgenogram
C. Inserting a 19-gauge needle into the chest wall
D. Retracting the endotracheal tube slightly

60. A 63-year-old woman is in the intensive care unit on a volume ventilator. Because of severe hypoxemia, it is decided to add PEEP in 5 cm H_2O increments. In so doing the following data were obtained:

	PEEP		
Parameter	5 cm H_2O	10 cm H_2O	15 cm H_2O
Temperature	38.1° C	38.1° C	38.1° C
Pa_{O_2}	51 mm Hg	73 mm Hg	82 mm Hg
$\dot{Q}_S/\dot{Q}_T$	24%	21%	18%
$\dot{Q}_T$	6.2 L/min	6.5 L/min	5.1 L/min
$C(a-\bar{v})O_2$	4.3 vol%	3.9 vol%	5.3 vol%
$S\bar{v}_{O_2}$	48%	53%	48%
Static effective compliance	20 cc/cm H_2O	25 cc/cm H_2O	20 cc/cm H_2O
FI_{O_2}	1.0	1.0	1.0
PWP (on ventilator)	8	9	12
Hb	12.3 g/dL	12.3 g/dL	12.3 g/dL

Which of the following assessments is (are) true regarding the above situation?

I. Some cardiovascular depression is noted at 15 cm H_2O PEEP.
II. The increase in PWP indicates the presence of adult respiratory distress syndrome.
III. The $S\bar{v}_{O_2}$ decreased at 15 cm H_2O PEEP because the Ca_{O_2} decreased.
IV. Tissue oxygenation is best at 10 cm H_2O PEEP.

A. II, III, and IV
B. I and IV
C. I, II, III, and IV
D. IV only

61. In reading the chart of a patient who was admitted with advanced chronic bronchitis, the respiratory therapy practitioner would expect to see documentation of all of the following *except:*

A. Cor pulmonale
B. Cough and sputum production
C. Cyanosis
D. Pulmonary hypotension

62. A 19-year-old patient with adult respiratory distress syndrome is receiving 8 cm H_2O PEEP with an FIO_2 of 0.7. Because of severe hypoxemia, the decision is made to increase the level of PEEP to 12 cm H_2O. The following data are collected at this time:

	8 cm H_2O PEEP	12 cm H_2O PEEP
$P(A–a)O_2$	400 mm Hg	400 mm Hg
SaO_2	75%	75%
$S\bar{v}O_2$	55%	47%
PWP (measured on ventilator)	7 mm Hg	8 mm Hg
Hb	15 g/dL	15 g/dL

The physician decides to leave the PEEP at 12 cm H_2O and asks the advanced respiratory care practitioner to recommend treatment for the decreased central venous oxygen content. The most appropriate response would be:

A. Increase cardiac output
B. Increase FIO_2
C. Decrease inspiratory flow rate
D. Induce hypothermia

63. A patient on a volume ventilator is noted to have both his peak and plateau pressures increase by 14 cm H_2O. Which of the following might have been responsible for this?

I. Atelectasis
II. Pneumothorax
III. Bronchospasm
IV. Acute gastric distention
V. Herniation of the endotracheal tube cuff

A. I, II, and III
B. I, III, and IV
C. III and V
D. I, II, and IV

64. The respiratory therapist is asked to collect appropriate weaning data on a comatose 20-year-old man who has a tracheostomy tube in place. The patient has been receiving continuous ventilatory support for the past 13 days following multisystem trauma sustained in a gang-related incident. He is currently on a volume-cycled ventilator in the assist/control mode with an FIO_2 of 0.4. The following information is presented to the physician by the therapist:

PaO_2	99 mm Hg
$PaCO_2$	33 mm Hg
pH	7.43
Vital capacity	Unable to obtain data
Negative inspiratory force	88 cm H_2O
Airway secretions	Minimal
Temperature	37.6° C
Resting minute volume	8.6 L/min
Pulse	80
BP	120/80

Based on the above information, which of the following is the most appropriate recommendation?

A. Place on SIMV.
B. Place on T tube with FIO_2 of 0.5.
C. Do not attempt weaning until patient has regained consciousness.
D. Lower FIO_2 to 0.35 and obtain an arterial sample.

65. Which of the following is (are) known to cause metabolic alkalosis?

I. Lasix administration
II. Diarrhea
III. Nasogastric suction
IV. Ileostomy loss

A. I and III
B. II and III
C. II and IV
D. I, III, and IV

66. A 25-year-old automobile accident victim is seen in the emergency department after sustaining extensive trauma. The following pertinent data were obtained from blood gas analysis:

PaO_2	64 mm Hg
FIO_2	0.40
$PaCO_2$	40 mm Hg
pH	7.33
HCO_3^-	19.6 mEq/L
V_D/V_T	0.78

Based on the above information, which of the following should the respiratory care practitioner recommend at this time?

A. Stat IPPB with 0.25 cc metaproterenol.
B. Increase FIO_2 to 0.7.
C. Initiate continuous ventilatory support.
D. Repeat blood gas studies.

67. The physician asks the respiratory therapy practitioner to modify all ventilator settings necessary to

help keep a 1000-g newborn's Pa_{CO_2} less than 60 mm Hg. Which of the following controls would the therapist be *least* likely to manipulate to help achieve this goal?

A. I:E ratio
B. PEEP/CPAP
C. Inspiratory time
D. Mandatory rate

68. When excessive levels of PEEP are administered, which of the following are commonly noted?

I. Decreases in $S\bar{v}O_2$
II. Decreases in effective static compliance
III. Narrowing of the $C(a-\bar{v})O_2$
IV. Decreases in PWP

A. I and IV
B. I and II
C. II and III
D. I and III

69. Which of the following describe liquid oxygen systems (LOX)?

I. They are unreliable at high flow rates.
II. They are portable.
III. No external power source is required.
IV. LOX is best for homebound patients.

A. I, II, and III
B. II and III
C. III and IV
D. I, III, and IV

70. Which of the following size (I.D.) endotracheal tubes should be selected for a newborn who weighs 1500 g?

A. 2.0 mm
B. 3.0 mm
C. 4.0 mm
D. 5.0 mm

71. Calibration of which of the following blood gas electrodes is usually achieved by using an analyzed gas with a concentration of 0% to establish the balance point?

A. pH electrode
B. Po_2 electrode
C. Pco_2 electrode
D. A and B

72. Which of the following would the respiratory therapy practitioner *not* recommend as a means of providing nutritional support to a 75-year-old patient with chronic obstructive pulmonary disease who is requiring prolonged, continuous ventilatory support?

A. 5% dextrose in water
B. 0.45% NaCl
C. Intravenous lipids
D. Nasogastric feeding

73. Which of the following is believed to be responsible for improvements in cardiovascular function reported after initiation of IMV and SIMV?

A. Normalization of Pa_{CO_2} levels
B. Decreased venous return
C. Improved distribution of ventilation
D. Decreased mean intrathoracic pressure

74. With a properly functioning, five-channel pulmonary artery catheter, it is possible to monitor which of the following parameters?

I. Cardiac output
II. Central venous pressure
III. Pulmonary artery systolic and diastolic pressures
IV. Mixed venous oxygen saturation
V. Left ventricular systolic pressure

A. I, III, and V
B. II, III, IV, and V
C. I, II, III, and IV
D. I, II, and III

75. Regarding the normal chest roentgenogram, which of the following statements is (are) true?

I. The width of the heart should be greater than one half the distance across the lungs at the level of the diaphragm.
II. The ribs should be an equal distance apart.
III. The left diaphragm is usually about one half a rib interspace higher than the right.
IV. The costophrenic angle should be considerably less than 90°.

A. II and IV
B. III and IV
C. II only
D. I, II, and IV

76. Clinical indications for pulmonary artery catheterization include:

I. Monitoring left ventricular function
II. Monitoring cardiac output
III. Monitoring mean peripheral venous pressure
IV. Accessing true mixed venous blood

A. I, III, and IV
B. I, II, and IV
C. III and IV
D. II and III

77. Pulmonary function tests performed on a patient with chronic bronchitis would most likely reveal:

I. Severely decreased D_LCO
II. Decreased FEV_1% FVC
III. Decreased expiratory flow rates
IV. Dramatic response to bronchodilator therapy

A. I and III
B. II and III
C. II and IV
D. III and IV

78. A 71-year-old, 80-kg woman with a history of chronic obstructive pulmonary disease is found semiconscious at home. After being brought to the emergency department, she is intubated and placed on a volume ventilator in the assist/control mode. Subsequently, the following data are collected:

FIO_2	0.4
PaO_2	54 mm Hg
$PaCO_2$	71 mm Hg
pH	7.47
Base excess	14 mEq/L
Pulse	120/min
ECG	Premature atrial contractions
BP	180/100
CVP	12 cm H_2O
HCO_3^-	40 mEq/L

Questioning the validity of the CVP measurement, the physician administers three successive 200-cc fluid challenges. The CVP, when measured following the third fluid challenge, is 13 cm H_2O. Based on the above information, the respiratory therapy practitioner should now recommend:

A. Another blood gas study
B. Pulmonary artery catheterization
C. Administration of an additional 200-cc fluid challenge
D. Switching the patient to SIMV

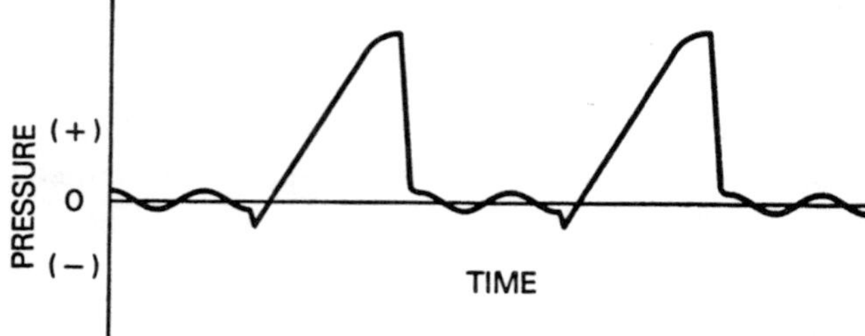

Figure 43.

79. The pressure waveform in Figure 43 is best described by which of the following terms?

A. SIMV
B. IMV
C. EPAP
D. CPAP

80. In reviewing a patient's chart, the respiratory therapy practitioner notes that the patient's urine output has been dropping steadily and is now approximately 15 cc/hr. This value is most consistent with:

A. Polyuria
B. Oliguria
C. Anuria
D. Normal urine output

81. When excessive levels of PEEP are used, which of the following are most likely to result?

I. Overdistention of pulmonary tissue
II. Increased physiologic shunting
III. Increases in airway resistance
IV. Increases in oxygen tissue transport

A. I and III
B. I and II
C. II and IV
D. I, II, and III

82. The respiratory therapy practitioner is monitoring a patient in the intensive care unit who is on a volume ventilator. The following parameters are noted at this time:

CVP	10 mm Hg
PWP	9 mm Hg
PA diastolic	31 mm Hg
PA systolic	48 mm Hg

These findings are most consistent with which of the following disorders?

I. Severe left ventricular failure
II. Pulmonary hypertension
III. Right ventricular failure
IV. Hypervolemia
V. Increased pulmonary vascular resistance

A. II and V
B. I, III, and V
C. I, II, and III
D. II, III, and IV

83. The respiratory therapy practitioner is assisting in a thoracotomy. On completion of the operation, chest tubes are connected to a three-bottle chest suction system. Subsequently, a large amount of bubbling is noted in the underwater seal chamber. What does this signify?

A. The chest tubes are leaking.
B. Too much suction has been applied to the unit.
C. Air is being evacuated from the pleural space.
D. The excess wall suction is being vented properly.

84. A 35-year-old patient received a vagotomy and partial pyloroplasty 8 days ago. Three days postoperatively he became septic and was taken back to the operating room to repair a perforated ileus. Since that time he has been on a volume ventilator with high levels of PEEP and FIO_2s of 0.7 or greater. Because of the danger of oxygen toxicity, the physician decides to raise this patient's PEEP to 28 cm H_2O and at the same time lower the FIO_2 to 0.5. Concurrent and pertinent information is noted below:

	20 cm H_2O PEEP	28 cm H_2O PEEP
$Pa{O_2}$	46 mm Hg	39 mm Hg
$P\bar{v}{O_2}$	32 mm Hg	24 mm Hg
$C(a-\bar{v})O_2$	3.5 vol%	5.8 vo1%
$\dot{Q}_S/\dot{Q}_T$	34%	28%
FIO_2	0.7	0.5
PWP (on ventilator)	7 mm Hg	9 mm Hg

Further orders are to leave the FIO_2 at the 0.5 level despite any cardiovascular depression noted at 28 cm H_2O PEEP. At this time, which of the following should the advanced respiratory care practitioner recommend to treat this patient's hypoxia?

A. Decrease venous return.
B. Administer diuretics.
C. Induce hypothermia to lower metabolic demands.
D. Optimize cardiac performance by whatever means possible.

85. A pulmonary function analyzing unit, when used to determine the functional residual capacity via the helium dilution method, must use which of the following in its circuit?

A. Nitrogen meter
B. Potentiometer
C. Carbon dioxide absorbing mechanism
D. Spectrophotometer

86. The respiratory therapist is monitoring a 48-year-old patient with bibasal viral pneumonia who is receiving continuous ventilatory support. The following data are obtained at this time with an FIO_2 of 0.5:

$Pa{O_2}$	78 mm Hg
$Pa{CO_2}$	31 mm Hg
pH	7.48
HCO_3^-	22 m Eq/L
PWP	26 mm Hg
Pulse	90
BP	150/100

Which of the following should the therapist recommend at this time?

A. Add 5 cm H_2O PEEP.
B. Decrease the FIO_2 to 0.4.
C. Administer a diuretic.
D. Administer $NaHCO_3$.

87. All five of the following patients are intubated and are receiving 100% oxygen via a volume ventilator. In addition, each one has a $Pa{O_2}$ of 50 mm Hg. The respiratory therapy practitioner would assess which one as having the largest intrapulmonary shunt fraction (assume an oxygen consumption of 250 mL/min for each patient)?

A. Patient A has a $C(a-\bar{v})O_2$ of 2.5 vol%.
B. Patient B has a $C(a-\bar{v})O_2$ of 3.5 vol%.
C. Patient C has a $C(a-\bar{v})O_2$ of 5.0 vol%.
D. Patient D has a $C(a-\bar{v})O_2$ of 6.0 vol%.

88. Which of the following chest radiologic findings would be noted in a patient with a massive right-sided atelectasis?

I. Mediastinal shift to the right side
II. Increased opacification on the right side
III. Elevation of the left hemidiaphragm
IV. Rib spreading over the affected area

A. I only
B. II and IV
C. I, II, and III
D. I and II

89. An 83-year-old patient is seen in the intensive care unit while receiving continuous ventilatory support with an FIO_2 of 0.7 and 8 cm H_2O PEEP. The following information is noted at this time:

$\dot{Q}_S/\dot{Q}_T$	18%
$C(a-\bar{v})O_2$	8.2 vol%
PWP	3 mm Hg
$P(A-a)O_2$	400 mm Hg
Oxygen consumption	250 mL/min

Which of the following should the respiratory therapist recommend to narrow the patient's $P(A-a)O_2$?

A. Increase PEEP.
B. Vigorously increase diuresis.
C. Increase FIO_2.
D. Administer fluids.

90. Which of the following pulmonary function tests is believed to give the best information about the patency of the smaller airways?

A. FEF_{25-75}
B. $FEF_{200-1200}$
C. FEV_1
D. FEV_2

91. The respiratory therapy practitioner is asked to calibrate a spirometer to ensure accuracy of measured flow rates. To do so properly, the practitioner should employ:

A. A potentiometer
B. An ultrasonic transducer
C. A rotometer device
D. A calibrated "super" syringe

92. For which of the following conditions would the respiratory therapy practitioner be *least* likely to recommend corticosteroid administration?

A. Postextubation laryngeal edema
B. Postoperative atelectasis
C. Idiopathic pulmonary fibrosis (Hamman-Rich syndrome)
D. Bronchial asthma

93. In which of the following types of hypoxemia will the sum of the $Pa{O_2}$ and the $Pa{CO_2}$ typically be greater than 110 mm Hg with the patient breathing room air?

A. Hypoventilation
B. Low V/Q
C. Shunting
D. Diffusion defect

94. In reviewing a patient's chart prior to therapy, the respiratory care practitioner notes that the patient has a history of respiratory insufficiency due to neuromuscular blockade. The above is most consistent with which of the following disorders?

A. Guillain-Barré syndrome
B. Pickwickian syndrome
C. Myasthenia gravis
D. Narcotic overdose

95. The physician wants the respiratory therapy practitioner to place a spontaneously breathing, 200-lb patient on a volume-cycled ventilator with an $FI{O_2}$ of 0.6. Which of the following are the most appropriate settings for this patient?

A. Tidal volume 1000 cc, backup rate 12, assist/control mode
B. SIMV mode, mandatory rate of 12, tidal volume 600 cc
C. Control mode with a rate of 20, tidal volume 1000 cc
D. A and B are correct.

96. Which of the following is (are) true regarding the presence of large right-to-left intrapulmonary shunts ($\dot{Q}_S/\dot{Q}_T$)?

I. Results when alveoli are ventilated but not perfused
II. Treatment includes application of PEEP therapy
III. Can be differentiated from low V/Q by administration of high concentrations of oxygen
IV. Treatment includes application of CPAP therapy
V. Generally leads to refractory hypoxemia

A. I and III
B. III and V
C. II, III, and V
D. II, III, IV, and V

97. A 58-year-old, 80-kg patient is seen in the intensive care unit while receiving continuous ventilatory support with an $FI{O_2}$ of 1.0 and 6 cm H_2O PEEP. The following information is charted at this time with the patient in the assist/control mode:

$C(a\text{-}\bar{v})O_2$	2.5 vol%
$\dot{Q}_S/\dot{Q}_T$	42%
Oxygen consumption	250 mL/min
PWP	15 mm Hg
$P(A\text{–}a)O_2$	600 mm Hg

Which of the following should the respiratory therapy practitioner recommend to treat this patient's arterial hypoxemia?

A. Increase PEEP.
B. Administer 500 cc lactated Ringer's solution.
C. Administer dobutamine (Dobutrex).
D. Switch to control mode.

98. In examining the chest roentgenogram of a critically ill patient, the respiratory therapy practitioner notes that the right costophrenic angle is considerably blunted. This finding is most consistent with which of the following disorders?

A. Noncardiogenic pulmonary edema
B. Idiopathic pulmonary fibrosis
C. Phrenic nerve paralysis
D. Pleural effusion

99. You have been asked to analyze a sample of fetal blood for carboxyhemoglobin level. If you use adult values for the extinction coefficient, how will your results be affected?

A. They will be accurate.
B. They will be in error from 4% to 7%.
C. They will be in error by as much as 20%.
D. You must multiply your result by 1.5.

100. A 54-year-old patient is admitted to the coronary care unit following a moderately severe left ventricular infarction. Important clinical data noted at this time with the patient receiving continuous ventilatory support are as follows:

Pa_{O_2}	48 mm Hg
FI_{O_2}	0.7
Pa_{CO_2}	31 mm Hg
Pulse	120
BP	180/130
PWP	30 mm Hg

Which of the following therapeutic modalities would be *least* beneficial for the respiratory therapy practitioner to recommend at this time?

A. Nitroprusside (Nipride)
B. Furosemide (Lasix)
C. Dobutamine (Dobutrex)
D. Phenylephrine HCl

Answer Key and NBRC Examination Matrix Categories

1. B, IIIC
2. D, IC
3. B, IA
4. D, IC
5. D, IIIC
6. C, IIIB
7. C, IIIC
8. C, IIID
9. C, IIB
10. D, IIIC
11. D, IIIB
12. C, IIIA
13. D, IIB
14. D, IIIC
15. C, IC
16. D, IIIA
17. A, IIIB
18. A, IIIE
19. B, IIIA
20. B, IB
21. D, IIA
22. D, IC
23. A, IIIA
24. A, IIIC
25. C, IA
26. A, IIIC
27. C, IIB
28. B, IA
29. A, IIIA
30. C, IIIC
31. D, IIA
32. A, IIIA
33. D, IA
34. D, IIIC
35. B, IIIB
36. B, IIIA
37. C, IA
38. A, IIIC
39. A, IIIB
40. B, IIIA
41. C, IC
42. B, IIIC
43. D, IIIB
44. D, IIIA
45. A, IC
46. A, IIA
47. D, IIB
48. C, IIIA
49. A, IIIB
50. D, IIB
51. C, IIB
52. C, IIIB
53. A, IIIA
54. D, IIIA
55. D, IA
56. C, IC
57. C, IIIC
58. C, IA
59. D, IIIC
60. B, IIIA
61. D, IA
62. A, IIIC
63. D, IIIA
64. B, IIIC
65. A, IC
66. C, IIIC
67. B, IIIB
68. B, IIIB
69. A, IIIB
70. B, IIIB
71. B, IIA
72. B, IIIC
73. D, IIIB
74. C, IIB
75. A, IB
76. B, IIIA
77. B, IC
78. B, IIIC
79. A, IIIB
80. B, IA
81. B, IIIB
82. A, IIIA
83. C, IIIE
84. D, IIIC
85. C, IIB
86. C, IIIC
87. A, IIIA
88. D, IB
89. D, IIIC
90. A, IC
91. C, IIA
92. B, IIIC
93. A, IIIA
94. C, IA
95. A, IIIC
96. D, IIIB
97. A, IIIC
98. D, IB
99. B, IB
100. D, IIIC